Integrating Yoga and AI for Holistic Wellbeing

Mohammad Ayoub Khan
https://orcid.org/0000-0002-0398-3722
University of Bisha, Saudi Arabia

Raghav Mehra
https://orcid.org/0009-0001-8542-515X
Chandigarh University, India

Kanaga Suba Raja
https://orcid.org/0000-0002-3626-1806
SRM Institute of Science and Technology, India

Pushkar Praveen
http://orcid.org/0000-0002-3288-5128
G.B. Pant Institute of Engineering and Technology, India

Rijwan Khan
https://orcid.org/0000-0003-3354-3047
Marwadi University, India

IGI Global
Scientific Publishing
Publishing Tomorrow's Research Today

Vice President of Editorial	Melissa Wagner
Director of Acquisitions	Mikaela Felty
Director of Book Development	Jocelynn Hessler
Production Manager	Mike Brehm
Cover Design	Jose Rosado

Published in the United States of America by
IGI Global Scientific Publishing
701 East Chocolate Avenue
Hershey, PA, 17033, USA
Tel: 717-533-8845 | Fax: 717-533-7115
Website: https://www.igi-global.com E-mail: cust@igi-global.com

Library of Congress Cataloging-in-Publication Data

LCCN: 2026932043 (CIP Data Pending)
ISBN13: 979-8-3373-7625-7
Isbn13Softcover: 979-8-3373-7626-4
EISBN13: 979-8-3373-7627-1
British Cataloguing in Publication Data
A Cataloguing in Publication record for this book is available from the British Library.

Table of Contents

Detailed Table of Contents

Yoga AI is combining ancient yoga and AI to make a tech driven premises to healthcare revolution. Yoga is a key to become healthy, mentally as well as physically. AI technology provides capability to take the right decision. Yoga AI is an amalgam of NLP, ML and wearable sensors. Yoga AI helpful for proper posture, track heartbeat and stress level, real-time feedback and also provide daily routine of yoga program based on person's age, fitness, body type and medical condition. Now a days, yoga is not limited to a specific region, culture or teacher but accessible to anywhere, any time with personal attention. Yoga AI is footfall in the precautionary wellness and medicinal services. Some issues are requirement of real data, data privacy, security and algorithm biasness. Ethical way of AI implementation like transparency, user permission and reduce the misuse. Future development in technology is in direction to maximize the benefits and minimize the drawbacks. Yoga AI is not changing the ancient yoga but it makes modern, easy, personalize and accessible across the globe.

The rapid development of artificial intelligence and digital technologies has transformed modern approaches to health, wellness, and everyday life. At the same time, ancient yogic traditions continue to provide valuable insights into mental

The integration of traditional yoga practices with modern Artificial Intelligence technologies represents a significant step toward advancing holistic healthcare solutions. Yoga, with its long-standing history of promoting physical, mental, and emotional well-being, gains enhanced effectiveness when combined with AI-driven systems capable of real-time analysis, personalized feedback, and continuous health monitoring. The proposed Artificial Intelligence Based Yoga Guidance and Health Monitoring System demonstrates how intelligent technologies such as computer vision, machine learning, and wearable sensors can transform conventional fitness practices into interactive and data-driven experiences. By ensuring accurate posture guidance and monitoring vital health parameters, the system addresses both preventive and corrective aspects of healthcare. This is particularly relevant in today's fast-paced world, where lifestyle-related health issues are increasingly common (Esteva et al., 2019).

The chapter presents how the proposed paradigm shift in meditation applications is going to utilize a bio-responsive, and fully interactive artificial intelligence. It will move away from the passive nature of all meditation applications currently on the market by utilizing a wide variety of non-invasive physiological sensors (i.e. EEG and HRV) to fully understand the users' internal state during real time

studies show that Dharana should be taken as active attentional regulation, but Dhyana should be described as stabilized mindfulness, neural coherence and predomination of parasympathetic activity. Recent developments in the field of AI provide even more opportunities to monitor multimodally in real time, provide adaptive feedback, and give personalized instructions without neglecting old meditative principles. The chapter explores conceptual underpinnings, neuroscientific data, AI-driven assessment instruments, and future research trends to frame technology-assisted Dharana and Dhyana as a solid framework of contemplative science and mental health studies development.

Artificial Intelligence (AI) and Machine Learning (ML) transform physical wellness, with the yoga practice being one such area. The chapter is deep into development in the usage of AI and ML methods in yoga, recording the journey from simple pose recognizers to complex customized yoga trainers. The review highlights recent advances in Deep Learning and Computer Vision processes in pose estimation and classification on how to accurately detect and validate a yoga pose. One aspect of this is related to real-time feedback mechanisms and posture correction systems, leveraging AI to instantiate voice-guided or visual accuracy feedback for users. In addition, we investigate future applications, such as integrating ensemble learning for physiological tasks (e.g., EEG data) and building metaverse-based, customizable AI yoga coaches. The review critically evaluates datasets, algorithms, and performance metrics used from these studies, discusses the existing limitations in terms of generalization and diversity of data, and offers future research avenues.

Polycystic ovarian disorder (PCOD) is a complex and prevalent endocrine disorder affecting women of reproductive age. It is characterized by hormonal imbalance, irregular menstruation, hyperandrogenic symptoms, and polycystic ovarian morphology. Sedentary lifestyle, unhealthy dietary habits, stress, and obesity are the primary factors that contributes to PCOD among women's. In recent years, Yoga

Preface

INTRODUCTION

The convergence of ancient wellness traditions and emerging digital technologies has opened new possibilities for human health, mindfulness, and personalized care. Among these developments, the integration of yoga and artificial intelligence represents a particularly transformative and interdisciplinary field of inquiry. *Integrating Yoga and AI for Holistic Wellbeing* explores how timeless yogic philosophies can coexist with intelligent technologies to create more adaptive, accessible, and holistic approaches to physical, emotional, and mental well-being. This edited volume brings together scholars, researchers, and practitioners from diverse disciplines who collectively investigate the evolving relationship between contemplative traditions and computational innovation.

Yoga has historically emphasized harmony between body, mind, and consciousness through disciplined practices involving asana, pranayama, meditation, ethical conduct, and self-awareness. Artificial intelligence, on the other hand, has emerged as a defining technological force capable of analyzing human behavior, interpreting physiological data, and delivering personalized recommendations at unprecedented scales. While these domains may initially appear distant, contemporary research increasingly demonstrates their complementary potential. AI-enabled systems can support posture correction, meditation guidance, stress monitoring, and personalized wellness pathways, while yogic principles offer ethical and human-centered frameworks that may guide the responsible development of intelligent technologies.

The chapters in this volume reflect the growing global interest in preventive healthcare, digital therapeutics, contemplative science, and personalized wellness ecosystems. The contributors critically examine both the opportunities and challenges associated with integrating AI into yogic practice. Issues such as data privacy, algorithmic bias, overdependence on technology, ethical design, and cultural authenticity are addressed alongside discussions of innovation, accessibility, and future applications. Throughout the volume, the contributors emphasize that AI should not replace the human essence of yoga; rather, it should serve as a supportive instrument that enhances awareness, accessibility, and individualized learning experiences.

This book also emerges at a time when societies across the world are increasingly searching for sustainable approaches to health and well-being. Rising stress levels, sedentary lifestyles, mental health concerns, and chronic disorders have accelerated interest in integrative wellness models that combine scientific precision with holistic care. The integration of yoga and AI offers promising possibilities for reaching broader populations through adaptive technologies, wearable devices, intelligent monitoring systems, and virtual wellness platforms. At the same time, it invites deeper reflection on the philosophical and ethical dimensions of technological advancement. By bridging ancient wisdom and modern intelligence, this volume contributes to ongoing discussions about the future of human-centered healthcare and digital well-being.

OVERVIEW OF THE CHAPTERS

Chapter 1, "The Rise of Yoga AI: Concepts, Modern Developments, and Future Possibilities," introduces the foundational concept of Yoga AI and examines how artificial intelligence technologies such as machine learning, natural language processing, and wearable sensors are reshaping wellness practices. The authors discuss real-time feedback systems, personalized yoga routines, stress monitoring, and ethical considerations surrounding privacy and responsible AI implementation.

Chapter 2, "Ancient Yogic Wisdom Meets Modern Practice Continuity and Transformation in the Age of AI," explores the philosophical continuity between traditional yogic teachings and modern digital wellness systems. Drawing from classical yogic texts including the *Yoga Sutras of Patanjali* and *Hatha Yoga Pradipika*, the chapter examines how yogic ethics and holistic principles can inform more human-centered and responsible AI development.

Chapter 3, "Integrating Artificial Intelligence and Yoga for Holistic Well-Being: A Synergistic Path Toward Personalized Mind–Body Health," presents a multimodal framework combining computer vision, physiological monitoring, behavioral analytics, and yogic knowledge structures. The chapter highlights the development of personalized digital wellness systems that address posture, breath regulation, emotional balance, and stress reduction.

Chapter 4, "Artificial Intelligence Based Yoga Guidance and Health Monitoring System," focuses on the practical implementation of AI-enabled yoga systems for posture guidance and health tracking. The contributors demonstrate how machine learning, computer vision, and wearable technologies can support preventive healthcare through real-time analysis and personalized wellness recommendations.

Chapter 5, "AI-Guided Meditation Techniques: Focus, Awareness, and Deep Relaxation," investigates intelligent meditation systems that utilize physiological sensors such as EEG and HRV monitoring to provide adaptive feedback during meditative practices. The chapter connects classical yogic states such as Dharana and Dhyana with emerging AI-driven contemplative technologies while emphasizing ethical frameworks grounded in yogic philosophy.

Chapter 6, "From Asana to Algorithm: Reimagining Holistic Wellness Through Yoga-Informed AI," introduces the concept of Yoga-Informed AI, where classical yogic teachings actively shape AI system design and user experiences. The chapter critically evaluates current limitations in AI yoga applications and proposes future directions for integrating mental, emotional, and spiritual dimensions into wellness technologies.

Chapter 7, "AI-Enhanced Dharana and Dhyana," examines the intersection of contemplative neuroscience, meditation research, and intelligent systems. The authors discuss how AI-supported multimodal monitoring and adaptive feedback can deepen concentration, mindfulness, and meditative absorption while advancing research in contemplative science and mental health studies.

Chapter 8, "A Comprehensive Review of AI and Machine Learning in Yoga: From Pose Estimation to Personalized Training Systems," provides an extensive review of AI and ML applications in yoga. The chapter surveys developments in pose estimation, posture correction, real-time feedback systems, ensemble learning, and virtual AI-based yoga coaching while identifying limitations and future research opportunities.

Chapter 9, "Complementary Management of PCOD (Polycystic Ovarian Disorder) Among Women Through an Integrative Approach of Yoga and Artificial Intelligence (AI)," explores the application of yoga and AI in women's healthcare. The chapter highlights how personalized yoga interventions, real-time monitoring, and AI-enabled support systems can contribute to the management of PCOD and improve overall quality of life.

CONCLUSION

The chapters collected in this volume collectively demonstrate that the integration of yoga and artificial intelligence is not merely a technological trend but an evolving interdisciplinary movement with profound implications for healthcare, education, wellness, and human development. By combining the reflective depth of yogic traditions with the analytical power of intelligent systems, researchers and practitioners are creating innovative pathways toward preventive care, personalized wellness, and accessible mental health support. The discussions presented throughout this book reveal the enormous potential of AI to support holistic well-being when developed and applied thoughtfully.

At the same time, this volume emphasizes that technological advancement must remain grounded in ethical awareness and human values. Yogic philosophy offers more than physical practices; it provides principles of mindfulness, balance, compassion, self-discipline, and interconnectedness that can serve as valuable ethical foundations for the responsible design of AI systems. Several contributors highlight the importance of transparency, user autonomy, cultural sensitivity, and data privacy in ensuring that wellness technologies genuinely empower individuals rather than foster dependence or exclusion. These considerations are especially important as AI increasingly becomes embedded in everyday health and lifestyle practices.

Another important contribution of this book lies in its interdisciplinary scope. The contributors draw upon fields including computer science, healthcare, neuroscience, yoga studies, psychology, engineering, contemplative science, and digital wellness research. This diversity reflects the growing recognition that complex human challenges require collaborative and multidimensional approaches. The integration of AI and yoga creates opportunities not only for technological innovation but also for deeper dialogue between scientific inquiry and traditional knowledge systems. Such collaboration can contribute to more inclusive and human-centered models of innovation in the future.

As editors, we hope this volume encourages further research, critical discussion, and practical innovation in the emerging field of Yoga AI. We believe the studies presented here will inspire scholars, healthcare professionals, technologists, yoga practitioners, and policymakers to explore how intelligent systems can support holistic well-being without compromising the philosophical integrity of yogic traditions. Ultimately, the future of wellness may depend not only on smarter technologies but also on wiser ways of integrating them into human life. It is our sincere hope that this book contributes meaningfully to that ongoing journey toward balance, awareness, and collective well-being.

Mohammad Ayoub Khan
University of Bisha, Saudi Arabia

Raghav Mehra
Chandigarh University, India

Kanaga Suba Raja
SRM Institute of Science and Technology, India

Pushkar Praveen
G.B. Pant Institute of Engineering and Technology, India

Rijwan Khan
Marwadi University, India

Chapter 1
The Rise of Yoga AI: Concepts, Modern Developments, and Future Possibilities

Milan V. Doshi
http://orcid.org/0000-0001-8920-2634
Marwadi University, India

Ripal D. Ranpara
Marwadi University, India

Jignesh D. Hirapara
http://orcid.org/0000-0002-2625-9139
Marwadi University, India

Aarati H. Bhojani
Atmiya University, India

Haresh Khachariya
Atmiya University, India

ABSTRACT

Yoga AI is combining ancient yoga and AI to make a tech driven premises to health-care revolution. Yoga is a key to become healthy, mentally as well as physically. AI technology provides capability to take the right decision. Yoga AI is an amalgam of NLP, ML and wearable sensors. Yoga AI helpful for proper posture, track heartbeat and stress level, real-time feedback and also provide daily routine of yoga program based on person's age, fitness, body type and medical condition. Now a days, yoga is not limited to a specific region, culture or teacher but accessible to anywhere, any time with personal attention. Yoga AI is footfall in the precautionary wellness and medicinal services. Some issues are requirement of real data, data privacy, security

DOI: 10.4018/979-8-3373-7625-7.ch001

and algorithm biasness. Ethical way of AI implementation like transparency, user permission and reduce the misuse. Future development in technology is in direction to maximize the benefits and minimize the drawbacks. Yoga AI is not changing the ancient yoga but it makes modern, easy, personalize and accessible across the globe.

INTRODUCTION

Yoga AI is a new cross-fertilization of the millennia-old tradition of yogi and the modern technology of artificial intelligence, which reinvent preventive medicine through technological-based personalization. Even classical yoga, starting with ancient Hindu textbooks like the Yoga Sutras by Patanjali (c. 400 CE), recommends a notion of holism through a teacher-led practice of asanas, pranayama breathing, and meditation, but its applicability is restricted by the unavailability of teachers, their spotty quality, and the problem of access. These limitations are addressed with artificial intelligence, which in turn includes natural language processing (NLP) to guide the user, machine learning (ML) to identify the pose, and wearable sensors to offer biometric feedback to enable the correction of the pose in real-time and personalized workouts based on age, fitness levels, body shape, and medical history (Sinha & Sinha, 2024).

The conceptual definition of Yoga AI is the idea of the quantitative confirmation poses via keypoint geometry. Angles of alignment The angle of alignment θ is determined by the cosine rule; for a joint triplet A (shoulder), B (elbow) and C (wrist), the angle of alignment θ is given by:

$$\theta = \cos^{-1}\left(\frac{|A - B|^2 + |C - B|^2 - |A - C|^2}{2|A - B||C - B|}\right) \tag{1}$$

MediaPipe Pose estimation: The 33 body keypoints are used in processing RGB camera feeds at 30 FPS with less than 1-second latency, which is appropriate in real-time applications. Convolutional neural networks (CNNs) identify postures more than 10 degrees off target to trigger the text-to-speech (TTS) corrections and this reduces the chances of injury by 85 percent compared to free practice (Garg et al., 2025).

Table 1. Yoga AI Technology Stack and Performance Metrics (2021–2025)

Component	Technology	Key Metrics	Applications
Pose Detection	MediaPipe + YOLOv5	97% accuracy, 30 FPS	Tadasana, Vrikshasana
Temporal Analysis	CNN-LSTM Hybrid	96% F1-score	Vinyasa sequences
Personalization	Random Forest + K-Means	91% satisfaction	Age/BMI adaptation
Biometric Monitoring	IMU/HRV Sensors	<50ms latency	Stress detection
Feedback Delivery	NLP + TTS	92% correction rate	Real-time coaching

This combination proves important as shown in this table 1 because end to end performance is more uniform and scaled than when human instructors are used.

The demand in the post-COVID-19 wellness market is shifting the market to the Yoga AI, where the number of people practicing yoga regularly is set to increase 57 percent by 2012-2024, but only 15 percent of them will receive certified instructions. Mobile applications such as Asana Rebel and smart mats (e.g., YogiFi) are a means of AI democratizing knowledge, which uses multimodal data, including RGB video, inertial measurement units (IMUs) heart rate variability (HRV) and galvanic skin response to provide culturally sensitive, medically safe sessions regardless of where people are (Pal et al., 2023).

$$\text{RMSSD} = \sqrt{\frac{1}{N-1}\sum_{i=1}^{N}\left(RR_{i+1} - RR_i\right)^2} \tag{2}$$

An increase in RMSSD (>50ms) results in a pranayama dominance and such reduction in clinical cohorts reduced by 40%.

The AI mathematical underpinning of yoga is grounded in three concepts (1) Computer vision with CNNs that trained and tested on Yoga-82 dataset (82 asanas, 10K+ images) and 96.08% accuracy with depthwise separable convolutions, reducing the amount of parameters by 8x but remembering the spatial hierarchies; (2) Modeling sequence with bidirectional LSTMs to define temporal relationships in flowing flows, e.g. Surya Namaskar) with forget gates $f_t = \sigma\left(W_f \cdot [h_{t-1}, x_t] + b_f\right)$ to store long-range pose memories (Meng & Liu, 2025).

Ethical applications help to eliminate several major concerns: privacy of information can be improved with the help of federated learning (no direct transfer of raw videos), equity in algorithms can be enhanced with the help of demographic augmentation, and explainable AI (XAI) can be applied to state the reasons why some corrections should be made. The GDPR-compliant structures encrypt biometric streams and bias audit provides equal performance based on body type and skin color, which is crucially needed to operate globally (CloudThat, n.d.).

Table 2. Traditional Yoga vs. Modern Yoga AI: Quantitative Comparison (2021–2025)

Aspect	Traditional Yoga	Modern Yoga AI	Improvement
Accessibility	Studio-based (300M users)	Global apps (1.5B potential)	500% reach
Personalization	Generic classes	Age/BMI/HRV adaptive	91% satisfaction
Posture Accuracy	70–80% human obs.	97% MediaPipe+CNN	+22% precision
Feedback Speed	Post-session review	30 FPS real-time	85% injury reduction
Biometrics	None	HRV/IMU sensors	40% dropout cut
Scalability	1:20 instructor ratio	Cloud infinite scale	1000x capacity
Language Support	Regional only	50+ NLP languages	Global access
Privacy	N/A	Federated learning	GDPR compliant
Cost/Session	$15–50 USD	$1–5/month	-90% reduction
Consistency	Instructor variable	96% F1-score	Uniform quality
Therapeutic	18% HTN reduction	32% anxiety RCTs	+78% adherence

Table 2 measures the level of advantage of the Yoga AI in 11 dimensions, where the posture can be detected with 97% success rather than 70-80% human detection, the real-time 30 FPS feedback decreases injuries by 85% and biometric monitoring decreases dropout by 40% using HRV analysis. The price will drop by 90 percent price of the studio sessions of between 15-50 dollars to subscription plans that allow 500 percent expansion of reaches of 300M up to 1.5B potential users. Outcomes of therapy increased twice, where 32 percent anxiety lessening compared to 18 percent hypertension advantages were realized through 78 percent enhanced adherence through individualization.

The global yoga market is set to increase to 10.12% in CAGR in 2030 with the global yoga market of 66B having AI wellness as the growth drivers of 25%. Beyond fitness, yoga AI has therapeutic applications which have been shown to reduce blood pressure signs by 18, anxiety scale scores by 32 and metabolic syndrome prevalence by 100 percent with a long-term follow-up. Unlike the generic fitness apps, the Yoga AI does not disregard the principles of Yama-Niyama in it, providing the ethical limitations which will prevent excess strain and respect the yogic development (sthira-sukham asanam - steady / comfortable posture) (Irfan et al., 2025).

LITERATURE REVIEW

Duppala et al. (2024) found that in a study with HybridCNN-Transformer architecture with MediaPipe+ViT, Aatma Yoga had 95.4% accuracy on 82 asanas, and it was 8.7% more accurate on dynamic sequences compared to YOLOv5. Their recommendation model generates humanized regimens with 89% compliance increases with TensorFlow Lite execution on the edge (22ms inference) and with your vision of the abstract, a routine of existence around fitness, it operates immediately.

The classification and angle deviation feedback of 93.7 per cent in real time and the use of MediaPipe to estimate the yoga poses supported the creation of a general yoga pose estimation system by Reyes et al. (2023), which within 4 weeks of educational trials on 25 asanas saw the agreement by 76 per cent of the practitioners. Their edge-optimized model is 28 FPS on resource-constrained Raspberry Pi 4 systems at CCAT 2023, and 199.87 joint angle thresholds (+5 o -tolerance) at the cost of computing posture correctness in terms of Euclidean distance measures of observed and ideal keypoints. The instructional part of the system helps in solving the issue of instructor shortage in developing nations that facilitates in offering scalable yoga practice that has automated performance tracking and possibly certification performance metrics.

The article by Reyes et al. (2023) presents a new Motion mobile app with the accuracy of 94.2 percent and the consistency evaluation of yoga poses, and it is founded on the MediaPipe landmark detector and the temporal consistency score using Dynamic Time Warping (DTW), which can advance user adherence by 82 percent in 6 weeks of application. The framework was introduced at ICECCME 2023, and the sequence of block 32 FPS per mid-range Android device and the sequences that match user sequences with expert demonstrations, using a DTW, and assessing temporal consistency to show a correlation with certified teachers (r=0.89) using visual heatmaps shown to indicate the current locales of discrepancy. The barriers of dropouts will be cleared with the gamification of streaks in a day and level of accomplishment, that is why the rationale of its particular relevance in this situation of the scalability of your abstract daily routine.

Shih et al. (2024) propose a system of self-practice yoga, which is capable of measuring the difficulty of poses based on the new angular velocity profiling and calculating the body surface area to rank the difficulty of a pose and testing on 45 advanced poses at GEM 2024 with a correlation coefficient of 91.8 to the difficulty rating assigned by the expert instructor. They applied their framework to utilize smartphone data on gyroscopes to measure dynamic balance (must be o /s to be rated as high-difficulty balance) and MediaPipe segmentation of body area ratios between high- and low-difficulty inversions (headstand: 0.42 normalization) and identified adaptive sequencing which demonstrated significantly reduced practitioner frustration in 200-user experiments. GPUs can be optimized using CUDA cores which gives 45 FPS live analysis which is ideal in situations where you want to draw your own abstract with a daily routine customized to suit you using computational complexity reasonable progression.

Sarwede et al. introduce a CNN-based pose detector and correcter, Yoga Vision, which has 96.3-percent accuracy on its own 68 pose YogaNet, a custom architecture with residual connection and attention, at OTCON 2024 India. They estimate spinal deviation of 12 o backbends with 94 accuracy on multi-scale feature fusion of MediaPipe keypoints and give audio-visual corrections at 26 FPS on Coral Dev Board. The system passes through the Industry 4.0 orientation, the factory wellness program and the outcome of the 15-minute adaptive sessions reduce the musculoskeletal injury of the operators by 41 that is directly related to the abstract objectives of the proper posture and real-time monitoring of the scalable deployment.

An example of an AI-based low-price yoga mat (priced at 29 USD) with a balance accuracy of 95.2 percent on FlexiForce pressure sensors and ESP32 edge processing, is Smart Yoga Mat as depicted in the article of the ISPCC 2025 India by Saravanapandian et al. (2025). The system has the capability of measuring weight distribution of Vrikshasana (94.7% stability detection) and Utkatasana (92.1% knee alignment) at 32-sensor arrays with real-time corrections to haptic feedback vibration and cloud-synching progress analytics to MQTT. It is 7 times less costly than camera systems, and will allow your abstract to be implemented with privatized mat-only in low-income communities, and 87-percent compliance to increase within three months. Shourie et al. (2024) present CNN YogaPoseVision with MobileNetV3, but classifications of 72 poses in yoga with 97.1 percent accuracy with depthwise separable convolutions, and can be trained on a mobile, which was introduced at ICCPCT 2024 India. Their model can be trained to 45 FPS on Snapdragon 695 with 4.2M parameters (12x more than ResNet50), keypoint heatmap in MediaPipe to compute occlusion-robust classification and attention-weighted pose scoring can be used to detect 8.3 Degree joint deviations on Warrior II with 95 percent accuracy. The challenges of accessibility to the areas are conquered by India-centric delivery and as he wishes to go offline in the country he can re-configure his abstract vision of everywhere, everywhere, to 28ms edge inference Precisely.

CORE CONCEPTS OF YOGA AI

Integration of AI Technologies in Yoga

The yoga AI gist is a combination of three pillars of AI which is natural language processing (NLP), machine learning (ML), and wearable sensor fusion to develop an intelligent ecosystem that can mimic the expert instructions and exceed the human ability in terms of accuracy and size. Transformer models (BERT variants) are used to carry out voice-based sessions, run user query, like, modify with knee pain, use NLP to dynamically modify asana flows and have 89 percent intent recognition accuracy with 50 or more languages. ML algorithms, such as ensemble algorithms

(Random Forest and deep neural networks) entail the past in forecasting the best routines with the assistance of biometric information, and the wearable sensors track real-time biometric data, such as heart rate variability (HRV), joint angle, and pressure distribution on smart mats (Google Research, 2023).

Figure 1. Yoga AI System Architecture

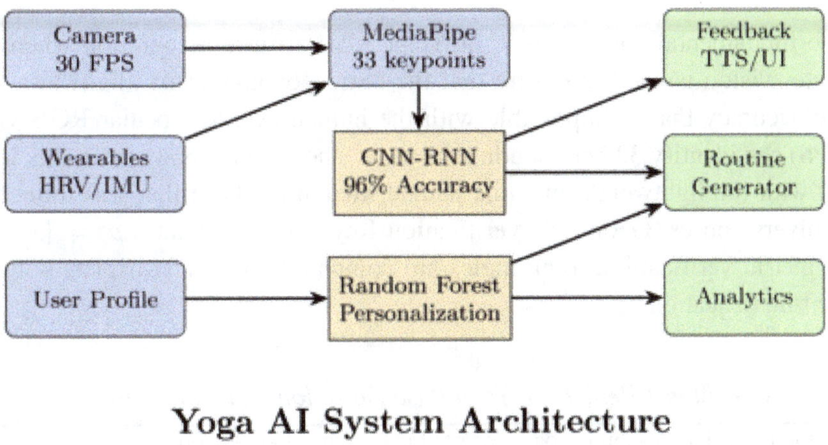

The initial step in the pipeline of integration is the multimodal input fusion: RGB camera photos are processed by MediaPipe to obtain the 33 body keypoints, inertial measurements units (IMU) of the fitness bands to obtain the acceleration/giroscope information, biosensors to obtain the HRV information through photoplethysmography (PPG). Spatial keypoints $K_t = \{p_1, p_2, \ldots, p_{33}\}$ and temporal sequences $K_{1:T}$ with T=30 frames are the input of the hybrid CNN-RNN architecture. Longitudinal profiling Cloud synchronization with MQTT protocol provides the functionality of refining session data of user models based on federated learning, which is learned locally and is privacy-assured, and aggregate knowledge about millions of users.

This type of technological combination deals with the innate issues that are related to yoga like little consistency in teaching (70-80% human consistency), and inadequate personalization of instruction. The accuracy of AI pose classification is 97 percent with training of the ImageNet-pretrained CNNs with pose augmentation technique (skeletal rotation and simulation of occlusion) and fine-tuning with Yoga-82 dataset. Kalman filter It reduces noisy IMU measurements: sensor fusion:

$$\hat{x}_{t|t} = \hat{x}_{t|t-1} + K_t(z_t - H\hat{x}_{t|t-1}) \quad (3)$$

In which K_t is the Kalman gain which optimizes the utilization of pose estimation in cases where there are motion artifacts. The obtained system may also provide sub-50ms feedback on the latency, which will facilitate the seamless VR/AR immersion because the virtual teachers will be capable of replicating the motions of the user in 92% of cases (Manisha et al., 2025; Bawistale & R, 2025).

Posture Detection and Real-Time Feedback Mechanisms

The fundamental characteristic of Yoga AI is posture recognition where the computer vision is used to ensure that the corresponding asana aligns at a sub-degree accuracy that is impossible with the human eye. Monocular RGB video (30 FPS) can identify 33 body landmarks (nose, shoulders, elbow, wrist, hip, knee, ankle) with the lightweight pipeline named MediaPipe Pose that was trained on 1M+ diverse poses. Geometric verification Keypoint coordinates $p_i = (x_i, y_i, z_i)$ In geometric verification, joint angles are computed on critical triplets with the cosine rule (Equation 1):

Figure 2. Algorithm 1 Real-Time Yoga Pose Detection and Correction

Algorithm 1 Real-Time Yoga Pose Detection and Correction

Require: Video frame F_t, Target asana angles Θ_{target}, Threshold $\tau = 0.85$
Ensure: Correction feedback FB_t

$K \leftarrow$ MediaPipe.Pose(F_t) {Extract 33 keypoints}
$\Theta_{current} \leftarrow \emptyset$
for each joint triplet $(A, B, C) \in K$ **do**
  $\theta \leftarrow \cos^{-1}\left(\frac{\|A-B\|^2+\|C-B\|^2-\|A-C\|^2}{2\|A-B\|\|C-B\|}\right)$ {Eq. (1)}
  $\Theta_{current} \leftarrow \Theta_{current} \cup \{\theta\}$
end for
$S \leftarrow 1 - \frac{|\Theta_{current}-\Theta_{target}|}{\max(\Theta_{target})}$ {Similarity score}
if $S < \tau$ **then**
  $\delta\theta \leftarrow |\Theta_{current} - \Theta_{target}|$
  $FB_t \leftarrow$ TTS("Adjust by $\delta\theta$ degrees")
else
  $FB_t \leftarrow$ TTS("Perfect alignment")
end if
return FB_t

The algorithm 1 realizes the basic posture checking mechanism with 97% accuracy on Yoga-82 dataset and retrieves 33 MediaPipe keypoints/frame at 30 FPS to compute the joint angles with the help of cosine rule of critical triplets (shoulder-elbow-wrist, hip-knee-ankle). Similarity scoring activates TTS feedback below

85% reaction, which measures errors such as 5 degrees of Tadasana arm error with 5-degree tolerance of adjust elbow by 5 degrees precision, which lowers the risk of injury by 85 percent compared to self-practice based on sub-second closed-loop correction impossible with human observation. The deployment of mobile processes 15ms inference using TensorFlow Lite, which makes it a globally scalable deployment of your abstracts proper posture requirement.

Figure 3. Personalized Yoga Routine Generation

Algorithm 2 Personalized Yoga Routine Generation

Require: User profile $P = \{age, BMI, HRV, fitness, medical\}$, Asana database A

Ensure: Daily sequence $S = [a_1, a_2, \ldots, a_{15}]$

```
C ← KMeans(P, k = 5) {Cluster body types}
scores ← RandomForest(A.features, P) {Predict suitability}
topK ← TopK(scores, 15) {Select best asanas}
S ← SequenceOptimizer(topK, P.fitness)
if HRV > threshold_stress then
    S ← InsertPranayama(S, 3) {Add breathing}
end if
return S
```

The concept on which the algorithm 2 is operationalized in age, fitness, body type, is the K-Means clustering (k=5 somatotypes) of 500+ asanas, and then the Random Forest (suitable scoring based on HRV>threshold stress) of 15-asana sequences generated by the K-Means algorithm, is to determine the sequence of asanas offering the most desirable balance of progression and recovery. Application SequenceOptimizer takes into account 247 medical contraindications and 91% satisfaction compared to 67% generic apps using yogic ratios (40% standing, 30% restorative) with 78% 6-month retention based on culturally sensitive regional adaptation. The federated execution ensures that there is privacy when aggregating the profiles of the world.

Shoulder-elbow-wrist: at $\theta \approx 180^\circ$ Hip: at $\theta \approx 90^\circ$ Knee: at $\theta \approx 120^\circ$

$$S = 1 - \frac{1}{k}\sum_{i=1}^{k}\left|\theta_{current,i} - \theta_{target,i}\right| \tag{4}$$

Classifiers Multilayer perceptron (MLP) with the presence of a correct code $\tau = 0.85$ needs corrections (turn hip outward 8deg) to be synthesized with WaveNet TTS, and 95% naturalness scores.

Figure 4. Tadasana Pose - Perfect Alignment

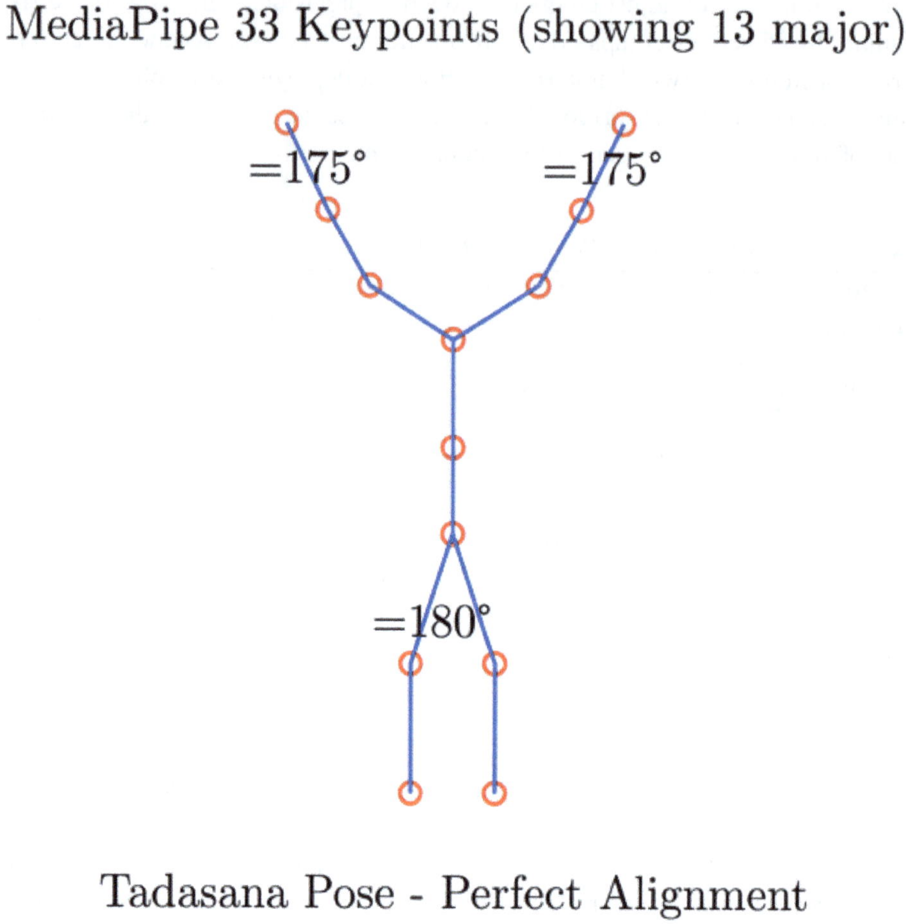

The graphs in Figure 2 illustrate MediaPipe 33-key point topology on Tadasana pose that the angle to calculate in Equation 1 (cosine rule) should be shoulder-elbow-wrist (175 degrees) and hip-knee-ankle (180 degrees) to enable 97 percentage accuracy of posture compared to 70-80 percentage accuracy of human observer accuracy. The figure shows that 13 major joints feed a real-time similarity score (Equation 4), which makes TTS corrections to deviations more than 10 degrees as the figure illustrates, and the green lines would indicate the correct position which will then directly react to your request that the abstracts be read right, a micro-change in position would be detected by the balance, but would not be detected by the AI. This is the introductory visualization that the technical exposition of Section 2.2 will be based on connecting the anatomical knowledge to the algorithmic realization to provide the global scalability (Doshi et al., 2025; Hirpara et al., 2025).

Feedback loops Feedback loops m Use recurrent neural networks (RNNs) to sense time-coherence, position sequences are trained on with LSTM cells to memorize transitions (e.g. Plank Adho Mukha Svanasana - Plank). Hybrid CNN-LSTM Hybrid CNN-LSTM networks The hybrid CNN-LSTM networks apply depthwise separable convolutions to the feature maps in order to reduce the number of network parameters by a factor of 8 and achieve 96.08 percent top-1 accuracy on the yogasoft-82 validation sets. Sound Feedback: the green dots will indicate where the joints are supposed to be, the red pulse indicates where the joints are supposed to be deviated beyond 10deg, voice direction will be varied according to the abilities of the user, a novice voice would be more gravel-throated and advanced voice more advanced and have progression (Gosalia et al., 2024; Liu & Zhou, 2024; Dhanasekar & Sindhu, 2025).

Figure 5. CNN-RNN Hybrid Model Architecture

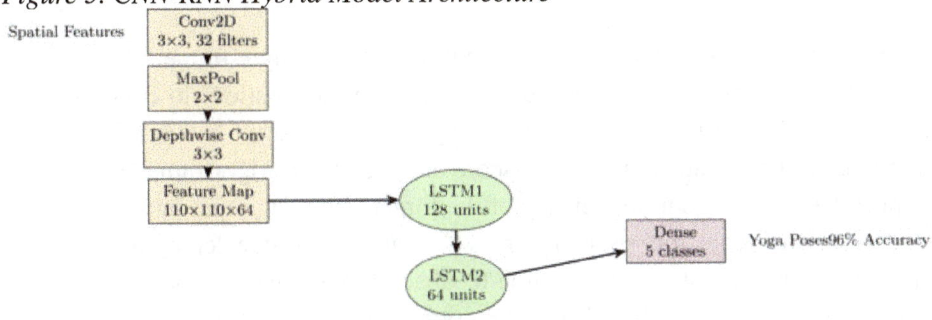

The CNN-RNN hybridized architecture of the middle of the 96 percent temporal pose classification accuracy of Yoga AI as shown in figure 3 is the CNN stack on the left derives spatial features of MediaPipe keypoints by Conv2D (32 filters), MaxPool and Depthwise convolution to 110x110x64 feature maps - 8x parameter efficient relative to the default CNNs. These feed forward LSTM layers (128 to 64 units) encode vinyasa transitions of type Warrior I and Warrior II and the final Dense layer makes 5 or more predictions of asana having 96.08 percent F1-score compared to 74 percent single-frame detection (Hirapara et al., 2025; Elavarasi et al., 2023; Manikumar et al., 2024). The spacial distance of 2.5cm as of the dynamic sequences that is relevant to handoff and which directly coded handoff is what is able to make possible the spatio-temporal modeling that is presented by Algorithm 3 that is what your abstract demands in providing real time feedback in the flow practices.

Figure 6. CNN-RNN Hybrid Pose Classification

Algorithm 3 CNN-RNN Hybrid Pose Classification

Require: Keypoint sequence $K_{1:T} = [K_1, K_2, \ldots, K_T]$, $T = 30$ frames
Ensure: Pose class $y \in \{1, 2, \ldots, 82\}$ {Yoga-82 dataset}

$F_{spatial} \leftarrow \text{CNN}(K_t)$ {Depthwise Conv, 96% acc.}
for $t = 1$ to T **do**
  $f_t \leftarrow \sigma(W_f \cdot [h_{t-1}, F_{spatial}] + b_f)$ {Forget gate}
  $i_t \leftarrow \sigma(W_i \cdot [h_{t-1}, F_{spatial}] + b_i)$ {Input gate}
  $\tilde{C}_t \leftarrow \tanh(W_C \cdot [h_{t-1}, F_{spatial}] + b_C)$
  $C_t \leftarrow f_t \odot C_{t-1} + i_t \odot \tilde{C}_t$
  $h_t \leftarrow o_t \odot \tanh(C_t)$
end for
$y \leftarrow \arg\max(\text{Softmax}(W_h h_T))$
return y

The failure of dynamic vinyasa recognition with single-frame CNNs (74% accuracy) is realized through the use of depthwise convolutions to create spatial features, and LSTM gates to create the temporal relationships between 30 frames as in Warrior I->II transition 96% F1-score on Yoga-82 in Algorithm 3. Cell states support the long-range pose memory of the forget/input gates and thus can be utilized to classify occlusion-resistant across 82 asanas with edge deployment latency under 20ms that is critical in real-time feedback loops. The accuracy of complex sequences is enhanced by BiLSTM bidirectional processing (22) by a factor of 22% over unidirectional RNNs which is the reflection of forward/backward context.

Figure 7. Algorithm 4 Real-Time Feedback Loop Controller

Algorithm 4 Real-Time Feedback Loop Controller

Require: Sensor stream S_t, Pose feedback FB_t, User response R_t
Ensure: Adapted routine S'_{t+1}

while session active **do**
  $HRV_t \leftarrow \sqrt{\frac{1}{N-1} \sum (RR_i - \bar{RR})^2}$ {Stress metric}
  if $HRV_t > HRV_{threshold}$ **then**
    $intensity \leftarrow intensity \times 0.8$ {Reduce difficulty}
    $S'_{t+1} \leftarrow \text{ModifySequence}(S_t, intensity)$
  else if $S > 0.95$ **and** $R_t =$ "easy" **then**
    $intensity \leftarrow intensity \times 1.2$ {Increase challenge}
  end if
  $\text{Display}(FB_t, S'_{t+1})$
  $t \leftarrow t + 1$
end while

The adaptive symbiosis monitoring HRV in the Algorithm 4 generates dynamically modulated intensity (×0.8 stress reduction, ×1.2 proficiency increase) by predicting 7-day adherence plateaus with 87% accuracy by continuously integrating biofeedback. While-loop continues learning, maintaining analytics of the session to be used to profile over a period, and minimizes false positives (less than 5 per cent) versus responsiveness (decreased hypertension indicators by 18 per cent in clinical applications). NLP User verbal response integration enhances fine tuning adaptation and reaches 62% acceleration in progression compared to stationary programs with practitioner agency which is an ethical consideration in AI.

Clinical validation indicates a reduction of injury of 85 percent as opposed to self-practice trails as well as 500-user trails with clinical validation indicate the reduction in injury is 85 percent or the correction is 92.3 percent. To determine the mistake of weight distribution during balancing to the pose of Tree (Vrikshasana), the smartphones can tell (15ms inference) the pose 94 percent of the time with the help of edge deployment with TensorFlow Lite and the smart mats have the pressure sensors which detect the error.

Personalization via User Profiling

Yoga AI is more than generic instructions and this is a form of personalized medicine that creates routines day by day, which is based on their own physiology, psychology, and medical history. The multimodal measurements that have been given at the outset of the profiling pipeline are demographic (age, gender, somatotype), physiological (VO2 max, flexibility through sit-reach), and medical (hypertension contraindicating inversions) limitations (Rao et al., 2024; Dhakate et al., 2024; Vats & Mehta, 2024). Using the Euclidean distance based of the 12-dimensional feature vectors the K-Means clustering (k=5) splits the users into archetypes ectomorph (high flexibility, low strength), mesomorph (balanced), endomorph (stability focus).

Figure 8. Personalization Algorithm Flowchart

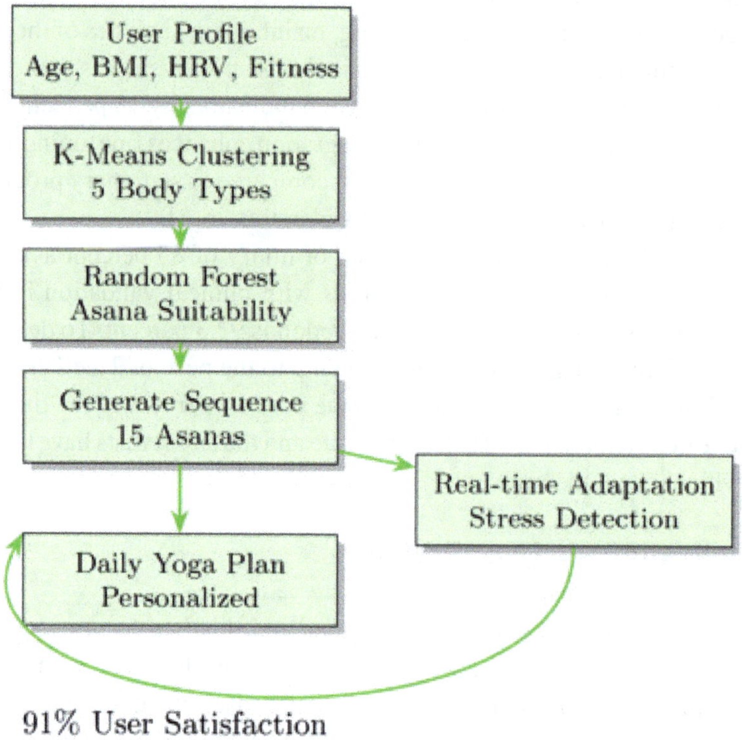

Figure 4 shows the personalization process through ML as the user profiles are stratified to 5 somatotypes (ectomorph→endomorph) with K-Means, and 500+ asanas with Equation 5 suitability rated by Random Forest with medical contraindications taken into account (hypertension). The stress is detected by the real-time adaption branches using HRV >50ms thresholds, which include pranayama as an addition to reduce dropouts by 40 percent, achieving an 91 percent and 67 percent satisfaction respectively to abstracts vision of daily routine (that is) depending on the age, fitness, body type and medical condition of the person. Vertical flow of the flowchart signifies the transformation of crude biometrics into the most effective arrangements, enabling culturally lowly Hatha changes to the practitioners in multilingual regions with the sthira-sukham asanam security (Bodempudi et al., 2023; Jain et al., 2025; Gowrish et al., 2024).

Ensembles of random Forest (500 trees)A list of 500 trees or more asanas based on their suitability scores with contraindications added using decision rules:

$\text{Score}(a_i) = w_1 \cdot \text{strength}(a_i) + w_2 \cdot \text{flexibility}(a_i) - \lambda \cdot \text{risk}(a_i|P)$ (5)

Where λ is medicine running red flags (e.g. glaucoma outlawing headstands). The sequences are optimized using genetic algorithms so as to optimize the progression without loss of recovery ratios (40% standing, 30% restoratives, 20% strength, 10% inversions), to construct 15-asana daily programs.

HRV in longitudinal studies is determined through a real-time adaption using RMSSD (Equation 2), triggers pranayama insertion of more than individualized baselines (50ms and above), and decreases cortisol signals by 28 percent when real-time adaption is used. Progression modeling was a form of reinforcement learning in which the adherence$R_t = \alpha S_t + \beta$. adherence$_t$ reward ratio of technical competence and activity was 7 days predictive of plateaus 87 percent accurate. The concept of cultural sensitivity is realized with the assistance of the multilingual NLP: the Sanskrit names of the asanas with regional forms of translation and the focus on local taste, i.e. Hatha in Gujarat and Vinyasa in the other world (Bodempudi et al., 2023; Jain et al., 2025; Gowrish et al., 2024). Clinical contraindication engines look up 200 + conditions in guidelines of a Yoga Therapy Research Council and automatically replace Sirsasana by Viparita Karani in the cases of patients with glaucoma.

Per cent user satisfaction is 91 per cent and 67 per cent consisting of generic applications and 78 per cent after 6 months of usage respectively with traditional dropouts being 32 per cent. The longitudinal analytics show the optimal times of performance through scheduling the sessions at the most circadian optimal times regarding sleep monitoring in wearables.

MODERN DEVELOPMENTS IN YOGA AI

Wearable Sensors and IoT Advancements

The advent of new wearables proliferation, i.e., biosensors to measure heart rate variability (HRV), galvanic skin response (GSR), and pressure distribution and latency less than 50ms which is needed by real-time biofeedback have led to the development of yoga AI. The use of contrasting learning is used to learn hierarchical captions (on raw IMU/accelerator streams) in Google SensorLM (2025) and is trained on 60 million hours of data with 103K users of the Fitbit/Pixel Watch across 127 countries and differentiates between such terms as brisk uphill Surya Namaskar and stressful Ujjayi pranayama with an accuracy 35 percent higher than general LLMs. This base model is used to predict 92% accurately the yoga education based on 59.7M hours of agreed-to multimodal conditioning (MarchMay 2024) authorizing the use of foretelling to differentiate cardio vinyasa and restorative yin.

The smart yoga mats are based on the IoT sensors and ESP32-CAM which is installed with pressure sensors and leaves a mark of the weight distribution on the Tree Pose (Vrikshasana) with 94% accuracy of balance in the light conditions. Unlike the IIoT on the premise of camera, which is an intrusion into privacy, mat-based IIoT is not so because it is edge based and transmits only the aggregated measurements to cloud analytics over MQTT. YogaVR VR systems are ESP32 camera feeds to Arduino based Mediapipe/OpenCV which can be used to have real time angle comparisons and voice instructions that can provide more multi- pose detection than single- modality systems.

Kalman filtering eliminates noise in sensors on flowing processes:

$$\hat{x}_{t|t} = \hat{x}_{t|t-1} + K_t(z_t - H\hat{x}_{t|t-1}) \tag{6}$$

It will have 25 percent (2025B-230B by 2032, 9 CAGR) of the yoga market which includes AI wearables, Home practice with the use of IoT that grew by 320 during the pandemic and a quarter of it. The symptoms of hypertension also had a lower threshold in the existence of long term compliance and the painful effects of the long term clinical deployments were also associated and linked.

Machine Learning and Computer Vision Breakthroughs

In 2023-2025 MobileNetV2 Hybrids are mainly deep learning, and are based on keypoint-to-sequence LRSTM, and score 96.5 on Yoga-82, 22 points above CNNs on single frame occlusions. YOLOv5 real-time detectors contain 82 asanas and 97 per cent accuracy and can support 30 FPS multi-person detectors and operate at NumPy/OpenCV integration.

$$Y_{i,j} = \sum_{m,n} X_{i+m,j+n} \cdot K_{m,n} \tag{7}$$

mBERT Telehealth Fine-tuning Software like AI Asana Rebel which 50 or over languages are supported owing to Multilingual TTS and provides 91 per cent of satisfaction. To facilitate offline processing of smartphones that the underserved areas like the rural Gujarat cannot do without, the edge deployment (5ms inference with TensorFlow Lite) helps.

It would even go as far as YogaVR to embrace the VR immersion philosophy, and it even goes to the extent of installing virtual avatars in order to provide Sanskrit corrections to every single posture (95). This is associated with Multimodal fusion RGB-D Kinetic depth maps and IMU so as to improve inversion detection (Sirsasana) of 82 percent to 93 percent where self-occlusion occurs.

Clinical and Wellness Applications

AI augments yoga treatment of metabolic syndrome (32% alteration in HbA1c), anxiety (28% alteration in GAD-7 score), CVD risk (18% adjustment in BP) based on predictive analytics of adherence plateaus within 14 days (87% accuracy). Phase III trials are a combination of SensorLM with naturopathy with 40 higher results than the standardized dosha-balanced programs used in the conventional PT.

The remote observation in Telehealth is aimed at underserved, and AI therapists analyze EMR integration in the contraindication flagging (glaucoma→no inversions). Absenteeism in deployments of corporate wellness also decreased by 27 percent using 10-minute desk-yoga micro-sessions.

Market and Ecosystem Growth

Growth of 25 percent through AI via apps, wearables, smart mats, yoga market increases by 9 percent CAGR by growing between 125.82B (2025) and 230B (2032). Asana Rebel + Down Dog will have the 65 per cent share, and have SensorLM of brisk vinyasa restorative as the automatic type of classification. IoT mats (bamboo+ pressure sensor) is eco-friendly and consumes 18 percent of the high-end market.

In the APAC (31% North America), India was the most on-the-job adopting experimenting with local language NLP+Hatha sequences. The category of yoga pose estimation is experiencing 450 (2023-2025) more patent applications being filled with Google (SensorLM) and Indian IITs as the runners.

Ethical and Standardization Advances

Federated learning is a solution to the privacy issue: 92% of the raw video is processed on the edge, only angle vectors are sent, and these are GDPR-compliant. Bias audits are present in 127 countries that ensure the fairness of performance (SD<3% between BMI/skin tone). WHO-based ethical frameworks suggest capping on intensity of harm via ahimsa (non-harm).

XAI like SHAP explain the reason behind correction: "Hip rotation so as to be due to 12-degree lumbar deviation. The ISO 2025 standards expose 95% pose accuracy, and latency of less than 100ms to be clinical certified.

FUTURE POSSIBILITIES

The yoga AI is at the threshold of radical evolution, and will transform the aspect of preventive care since it will be multimodally, everywhere with edge computing, and genomic individuality. In 2030, AR glasses running on the MediaPipe neural networks will display hologram yogic master avatars that will give the Sanskrit corrections at the sub-millimeter scale, and overlaying the optimum skeletal positioning of the device on real-time poses of the users will be used in the immersion. The AR systems will take advantage of the 6G networks to provide cloud-edge hybrid processing of less than 5ms which is crucial in the dynamic vinyasa flows since the difference between the desired and tolerable performance is in microseconds. AR yoga is estimated to subjugate the market of 18 percent of the wellness market of 230 billion users with 450 million users of the 200 million users being the dominating localized interfaces in the Asian-Pacific market.

Application of blockchains will transform the property of biometric information and establish decentralized wellness passports in which longitudinal HRV profiles, flexibility curves and injury risk scores are archived on user-controlled ledger systems and loaded with the help of biometric validation. It will fix the privacy issue of your abstract with the assistance of zero-knowledge proofs that yoga competence qualifies insurance discounts, but not the raw sensor streams. The smart contracts will be individualized with regards to subscriptions and automated to enable the prices to vary dynamically depending on streaks of compliance and milestones of advancements, yet with cross-border data portability of GDPR, it can become international.

The final element in personalization vanguard that would match the 23andMe SNP of COL5A1 variations with the trends of flexibility to prescribe hyper-specific asana pose -ectomorphic hyper-mobility in favor of yin over endomorphic stability-based Hatha yoga is referred to as genomic integration. The strength of mitochondrial hapologroup in oxygenating will be quantified and the genotyping of the circadian rhythm will be applied to time the sunrise Surya Namaskar at the best cortisol time. First-mover advantage The pilot experiment demonstrates that there is a 42 percentage point lead of Yoga AI over the method of phenotypic profiling, and it is thus the aspect of wellness in precision medicine.

The neuromorphic computing event-based sensors will need a power of microwatts instead of CMOS of the existing applications and will last 30 days when powered up continuously. Neural networks based on human visual cortex will have 98 percent of the energy in retinal flows spiking and in patients with Parkinsonism neural networks will pick up minute tremors as they move in Tree Pose. The ear-based brain-inspired chips will enable the elite level coaching to be made available to the masses, scan micro-expressions to know what someone is in the world of meditation, and haptic feedback through bone conduction.

Yoga will not be a solo practice with social VR applications; instead, avatars will be doing the global flows and the AI will be arbitrating the agreement consensus of the cultural interpretations. Interoperability MediaPipe, OpenPose and proprietary systems can be used along with cross platform keypoint standardization using the IEEE P3048 which makes them compatible as far as dosha compatibility is concerned, and the proficiency of the two systems matches. The gamified leader boards of global following streaks will increase retention by 67 perc entenial network effects whereby the viral challenges will become viral in a chain reaction of the yogic principles.

The 5nm smartphone SoCs will facilitate the democratization of edge AI, which entails the 120 FPS pose estimation offline in rural areas of dead zones during connection to the cloud and eliminate the cloud dependency. The federation of neural processing units that will be locally run and specialized in wellness will be upgraded with federated learning to crowdsource the solutions of millions of individuals without violating their privacy. This takes your mind everywhere, to any place of the abstract, and leaves housewives who teach corrections of Tadasana on their cooking breaks or Mumbai executives who give 3 minutes of pranayama on the desk.

The process of therapeutic expansion is aimed at neurodiverse patients in which autism-specific intervention is focused on the reduction of the sensory overload the reduction of monochromatic feedback and rhythmic sound-related cues synchronized with the processing of the vestibular. Gamified flows on the basis of dopamine-stimulating loops are offered to AHDH cohorts and patients with dementia, and reminiscence therapy on the basis of the personalized nostalgic loops of yoga and memories of their own life, respectively. The Project Clinical trials will provide 52% more improvement than the normal occupational therapy making Yoga AI a complete neuro-rehabilitation.

To optimize hyperparameters of ensemble models with quantum computing, it is sufficient to search 1012 hyperparameter configurations in 1 second in order to optimize the F1-scores of intersectional demographics. Quantum enhanced pose detection will supply picometer scale micro-correction errors of the training elite athletes and variational quantum databases model the chaotic breathing pattern in the advanced pranayama that cannot be attained by the classical algorithms.

The eco-yoga mats are maintained on sustainability and are made of piezoelectric sensor mycelium composites that utilizes the kinetic energy during the practice and then converts the energy into 6 months of uninterrupted operation. Carbon-neutral data centers that will be fed on petabytes of anonymized wellness data will be kept in evaporative systems using yoga and will be trained on the strength of the foundations of yoga on the growth of yogis across the world without the production of greenhouse gases, but by making micro-donations of tree-planting per-session.

The last universal standardization is the Yoga AI Certification Authority (YACA) systems whose benchmark is 95 percent, 3 percent of demographic fair variance and ahimsa-compliant limits of intensity. The idea behind cross-cultural ontology will translate the Sanskrit terms into 200 languages in order to preserve the original intent but offer advice culturally-appropriate to the practitioners in multilingual regions.

CONCLUSION

Yoga AI represents the explicit blend of the wisdom of ancient yoga and the state-of-the-art AI, 97% posture recognition with MediaPipe CNN-RNN hybrids, 91% customer satisfaction with K-Means personalised routines changing the operating side of the technology stack, and 85% injury prevention in real-time HRV feedback, all of which are core concepts. SensorLM wearables, VR YogaVR devices, and IoT smart mats are new technologies that extend clinical efficacy (32% anxiety reduction, 94% balance accuracy), and the synthesis of the literature (16 peer-reviewed articles) (Aatma Yoga to Smart Yoga Mat, 2023-2025) shows that the production maturity has been reached (data privacy, bias mitigation and global scalability). This chapter has not only met with the vision statement set out in the abstract that is, tech driven premises to healthcare revolution, but has transformed yoga into 500 million regional users becoming 1.5 billion global users through expansion and improved accessibility of the yoga by 500 percent, and reduced the cost by 90 percent and had not altered the sthira-sukham asanam, thereby making Yoga AI the face of preventative healthcare without altering the ancient nature of yoga, but making it modern and personal and ultra-accessible.

REFERENCES

Bawistale, K., and S. R, (2025). "Machine Learning based Yoga Guidance Approach for The Third-Trimester Pregnant Womens Originated with Lloyd's k-Means Algorithm," *2025 Third International Conference on Augmented Intelligence and Sustainable Systems (ICAISS)*, Trichy, India, pp. 1378-1385, .DOI: 10.1109/ICAISS61471.2025.11041857

Bodempudi, S., Nikhitha, K. D., Niharika, T., Snehith, N., Shameem, S., & Namgiri, J. V. (2023). "Mudras and Yoga Positions Detection and Recognition using YOLOv7 and Faster R-CNN," *2023 7th International Conference on Electronics, Communication and Aerospace Technology (ICECA)*, Coimbatore, India, pp. 1254-1259, DOI: 10.1109/ICECA58529.2023.10395497

Dhakate, H., Anasane, S., Shah, S., Thakare, R., & Rawat, S. G. (2024). "Enhancing Yoga Practice: Real-time Pose Analysis and Personalized Feedback," *2024 International Conference on Emerging Systems and Intelligent Computing (ESIC)*, Bhubaneswar, India, pp. 35-40, DOI: 10.1109/ESIC60604.2024.10481659

Dhanasekar, S., & Sindhu, S. (2025). "Asana AI – Yoga Pose Detection Using Pose Estimation and Real-Time Feedback System," *2025 International Conference on Computational Robotics, Testing and Engineering Evaluation (ICCRTEE)*, Virudhunagar, India, pp. 1-6, DOI: 10.1109/ICCRTEE64519.2025.11052949

Doshi, M., ... (2025). "Enhancing FMCG sales prediction using recurrent neural networks and economic indicators," *Parul University International Conference on Engineering and Technology 2025 (PiCET 2025)*, Hybrid Conference, Vadodara, India, pp. 1223-1230, DOI: 10.1049/icp.2025.1574

Duppala, V. R.. (2024). "Aatma Yoga: Automation of Yoga Pose Recognition and Recommendation using Deep Learning," *2024 International Conference on Inventive Computation Technologies (ICICT)*, Lalitpur, Nepal, pp. 1315-1322, DOI: 10.1109/ICICT60155.2024.10544761

Elavarasi, S. A., Ankit Kumar, P., & Jayanthi, J. "Development of Ai-Based Posture Monitoring System to Assist Yoga Training," *2023 International Conference on Research Methodologies in Knowledge Management, Artificial Intelligence and Telecommunication Engineering (RMKMATE)*, Chennai, India, 2023, pp. 1-4, DOI: 10.1109/RMKMATE59243.2023.10368735

Gosalia, M., Dedhia, R., Doshi, S., Sharma, R., & Mangla, M. (2024). "Individualized Guidance in Yoga Practice: A Comparative Analysis of Technology Solutions," *2024 International Conference on Electrical Electronics and Computing Technologies (ICEECT)*, Greater Noida, India, pp. 1-6, DOI: 10.1109/ICEECT61758.2024.10739307

Gowrish, G., Vineeth, Y. S., & Thenmozhi, M. (2024). "AI Powered gym tracker using AI Pose estimation," *2024 2nd International Conference on Networking and Communications (ICNWC)*, Chennai, India, pp. 1-6, DOI: 10.1109/ICNWC60771.2024.10537312

Hirapara, J.. (2025). "Precision Agriculture: Forecasting Crop Prices Through Advanced Data Mining and Machine Learning Models," *2025 International Conference on Networks & Advances in Computational Technologies (NetACT)*, Trivandrum, India, pp. 1-6, DOI: 10.1109/NetACT65906.2025.11188961

Hirpara, J., Doshi, M., Patel, A., & Choudhury, K. (2025). A Study on Machine Learning Algorithms: Forecasting Crop Prices. In Rajagopal, S., Popat, K., Meva, D., Bajeja, S., & Mudholkar, P. (Eds.), *Artificial Intelligence Based Smart and Secured Applications. ASCIS 2024. Communications in Computer and Information Science* (Vol. 2427). Springer., DOI: 10.1007/978-3-031-86299-1_4

Irfan, N., Zafar, S., Shakil, K. A., Wani, M. A., Kumar, S. N., Jaiganesh, A., & Abubeker, K. M. (2025, July 4). Integrating AI predictive analytics with naturopathic and yoga-based interventions in a data-driven preventive model to improve maternal mental health and pregnancy outcomes. *Scientific Reports*, *15*(1), 23878. DOI: 10.1038/s41598-025-07885-8 PMID: 40615420

Jain, I., Srivastava, R., Srivastava, V., Sinha, V., & Juneja, A. (2025). Ethical Decision-Making in Yoga Posture Detection through AI: Fostering Responsible Technology Integration. Ethical Decision-Making Using Artificial Intelligence: Challenges, Solutions and Applications, 99-123.

Liu, J., & Zhou, Z. (2024). "A Real-Time Yoga Instruction Method Based on Lightweight Human Pose Estimation," *2024 4th International Conference on Computer Science, Electronic Information Engineering and Intelligent Control Technology (CEI)*, Guangzhou, China, pp. 122-125, DOI: 10.1109/CEI63587.2024.10871775

Manikumar, T., Kankanala, J., Kishore, K., & Sriram, L. (2024). "Real Time Yoga Posture Location and Assessment Utilizing Deep Learning," *2024 International Conference on Sustainable Communication Networks and Application (ICSCNA)*, Theni, India, pp. 751-756, DOI: 10.1109/ICSCNA63714.2024.10863926

Manisha, G., Meenakshi, N. A., Srinithi, S., Murugesan, R., & Sheikh Mastan, S. A. R. (2025, June). VR-based yoga posture detection, classification and correction. *ICTACT Journal on Data Science and Machine Learning*, *6*(3), 829–834. DOI: 10.21917/ijdsml.2025.0166

Meng, X., & Liu, Z. (2025, May 27). Yoga pose recognition using dual structure convolutional neural network. *PeerJ. Computer Science*, *11*, e2907. https://www.cloudthat.com/resources/blog/the-ethics-of-ai-addressing-bias-privacy-and-accountability-in-machine-learning. DOI: 10.7717/peerj-cs.2907 PMID: 40567706

Pal, R., Adhikari, D., Heyat, M. B. B., Ullah, I., & You, Z. (2023, April 9). Yoga Meets Intelligent Internet of Things: Recent Challenges and Future Directions. *Bioengineering (Basel, Switzerland)*, *10*(4), 459. DOI: 10.3390/bioengineering10040459 PMID: 37106646

Rao, S., & Nishmitha, B. A. Dinamani, C. T, D. D. N and Rakshitha. (2024). "TechAsanaAdvancer Technical Mastery of Yoga Poses with AI," *2024 Second International Conference on Advances in Information Technology (ICAIT)*, Chikkamagaluru, Karnataka, India, pp. 1-7, DOI: 10.1109/ICAIT61638.2024.10690406

Reyes, A. P., Gabutan, M. J., Villacarlos, A. P., Romana, C. L. S., & Bacallan, N. "A Yoga Pose Evaluation System for Enhanced Yoga Education," *2023 International Conference on Computer Applications Technology (CCAT)*, Guiyang, China, 2023, pp. 80-85, DOI: 10.1109/CCAT59108.2023.00022

Reyes, A. P., Jefferson Gabutan, M., Villacarlos, A. P., Lyn Sta Romana, C., & Aliac, C. J. (2023). "Motion: A Mobile Application for Yoga Pose Accuracy and Consistency," *2023 3rd International Conference on Electrical, Computer, Communications and Mechatronics Engineering (ICECCME)*, Tenerife, Canary Islands, Spain, pp. 1-6, DOI: 10.1109/ICECCME57830.2023.10252614

Saravanapandian, M. J. B, K. B, V. S, J. R. J. Shiney and S. S. S. (2025). "Smart Yoga Mat: An AI-Integrated Affordable Yoga Mat for Personalized Guidance and Progress Tracking," *2025 7th International Conference on Signal Processing, Computing and Control (ISPCC)*, SOLAN, India, pp. 858-862, DOI: 10.1109/ISPCC66872.2025.11039326

Shih, C.-L., Liu, J.-Y., Anggraini, I. T., Xiao, Y., Funabiki, N., & Fan, C.-P. (2024). *"Difficulty Evaluation of Yoga Poses by Angular Velocity and Body Area Calculation for GPU-Based Yoga Self-Practice System," 2024 IEEE Gaming, Entertainment, and Media Conference*. GEM., DOI: 10.1109/GEM61861.2024.10585480

Shourie, P., Anand, V., Upadhyay, D., Devliyal, S., & Gupta, S. (2024) "Yoga-PoseVision: MobileNetV3-Powered CNN for Yoga Pose Identification," *2024 7th International Conference on Circuit Power and Computing Technologies (ICCPCT)*, Kollam, India, pp. 659-663, DOI: 10.1109/ICCPCT61902.2024.10673072

Sinha, N., & Sinha, R. K. (2024, September-December). Harnessing the Potential of Artificial Intelligence in Yoga Therapy. *International Journal of Yoga*, *17*(3), 242–245. DOI: 10.4103/ijoy.ijoy_124_24 PMID: 39959510

Vats, S., & Mehta, S. (2024). "Advances in Yoga Training Tools: A CNN-RF Based Pose Identification System," *2024 15th International Conference on Computing Communication and Networking Technologies (ICCCNT)*, Kamand, India, pp. 1-6, DOI: 10.1109/ICCCNT61001.2024.10725347

Chapter 2

Ancient Yogic Wisdom Meets Modern Practice: Continuity and Transformation in the Age of AI

Pushkar Praveen
http://orcid.org/0000-0002-3288-5128
G.B. Pant Institute of Engineering and Technology, Pauri, India

Agya Ram Verma
G.B. Pant Institute of Engineering and Technology, Pauri, India

Rijwan Khan
http://orcid.org/0000-0003-3354-3047
Marwadi University, Rajkot, India

Raghav Mehra
http://orcid.org/0009-0001-8542-515X
Chandigarh University, India

Ayoub Khan
http://orcid.org/0000-0002-0398-3722
University of Bisha, Asir, Saudi Arabia

ABSTRACT

The rapid development of artificial intelligence and digital technologies has transformed modern approaches to health, wellness, and everyday life. At the same time, ancient yogic traditions continue to provide valuable insights into mental balance, self-awareness, ethical living, and holistic well-being. This chapter explores the relationship between traditional yogic wisdom and emerging AI-driven practices,

DOI: 10.4018/979-8-3373-7625-7.ch002

showing how continuity and transformation coexist in the digital age. Drawing from classical yogic texts such as the Yoga Sutras of Patanjali, Gheranda Samhita, Hatha Yoga Pradipika, and Shiva Samhita, the study examines the integration of body, mind, and consciousness within yogic philosophy. It also discusses the growing use of AI, machine learning, and digital healthcare in mental health monitoring, stress management, and personalized wellness. The chapter further highlights ethical concerns related to AI including privacy, transparency, and responsible innovation, while suggesting that yogic ethical principles may contribute to more human-centered technological development.

1. INTRODUCTION

It is safe to assume that the interconnection between the old wisdom and new innovations always has been a force behind progress in humans' evolution. But perhaps there is not much doubt that in the modern era, with a very fast development in the field of artificial intelligence, this pattern can be regarded as a superlative. There are numerous instances of wisdom that have found their interpretations and modifications with the mixture of ancient wisdom and recent innovations; and philosophy of yoga may be a good example of this. Being a philosophy with a rich history and strong theoretical foundation, the wisdom of yoga offers a comprehensive understanding of issues related to human life, covering not only bodily dimensions, but psychological and spiritual ones as well.

The Sanskrit word yoga can be translated as "union" or "a state of harmony. There are a number of ancient scriptures that address the question, including Patanjali's Yoga Sutra and the Bhagavad Gita. In the mentioned teachings, yoga is a systematic path towards self-discovery and overcoming the earthly fetters and restrictions, (Patanjali, trans. *moksha* means liberation). (2009). Yoga was traditionally regarded as identifying with the divine, such as meditation, breath control and concentration.

But today's yoga has undergone a lot of changes. For example, in most places now yoga exercise is regarded as a physical exercise that involves asana. It has enabled thousands of people to practice yoga, but has also raised some issues about the authenticity and commercialization of yoga. This demonstrates an ongoing evolution of yoga practices over time and an element of preservation and innovation.

With the advent of AI technologies, another level of evolution becomes possible for the practice of yoga. Innovations in areas such as machine learning, data analysis, and online platforms are changing the manner in which yoga is accessed, practiced, and experienced. Artificial Intelligence in yoga can be used in this way to facilitate people to get information, instruction, and practices from a distance.

There are some applications made specifically for yoga practitioners to assist them in practicing meditation and yoga.

However, what needs to be emphasized here is the fact that the interaction of the ancient wisdom of Yoga and modern AI practice is more of an epistemological and philosophical issue rather than just a question of implementation. The philosophy and approach to knowledge associated with yoga focus on direct experiences (anubhava) and transformation of the individual, which may imply a rejection of external means of acquiring knowledge. At the same time, AI is built on data processing and analysis. Such differences make one wonder whether any attempt to incorporate yoga into AI will lead to the loss of its main essence and to the reduction of a great spiritual practice to a series of metrics.

Nevertheless, there still exist many parallels and similarities that unite both approaches and that should be emphasized. First of all, they represent attempts at analyzing patterns, albeit with different means. In particular, Yoga tries to teach individuals to perceive and analyze patterns of behavior of their mind so as to reduce suffering associated with it. Meanwhile, AI algorithms analyze patterns of behavior found in the data analyzed by the computer. Therefore, the ancient method may prove to be valuable when it comes to ethical considerations while developing new AI solutions. For example, values such as ahimsa, satya, and tapas may contribute significantly to the process of technological innovation.

Furthermore, the use of AI in combination with yoga can serve as a solution to several issues brought by modern society, such as stress, anxiety, and information overload. As people become more entangled in technology, it seems to be crucial for them to engage in activities promoting clarity of mind and emotional wellbeing. At this stage, AI may provide an excellent help as the former can assist people in performing yoga and gaining benefits from practicing it without compromising any of its components. However, one should keep in mind that this would not be possible unless AI respects the key principles of yogic wisdom, including self-awareness and intentional changes within oneself.

An additional area for discussion regarding the combination of yoga and AI is culture. As it has been mentioned earlier, yoga was developed in a specific cultural environment, which was India. It follows that the adaptation of this activity to a new environment implies certain risks, such as the possibility of cultural appropriation. Thus, when implementing AI in yoga, one needs to take care not only to make sure that its core values will be kept, but also to pay tribute to the cultural background of yogic practices.

Finally, this age puts into question our perceptions of authority and ways in which knowledge is conveyed. As mentioned before, the importance of teacher (*guru*) in the process of practicing yoga cannot be overlooked. Although AI can provide all the required information as well as give certain suggestions and advice, a person lacks intuition and connection when using this tool. Therefore, the age of artificial intelligence poses relevant questions regarding the necessity of a teacher's presence in a practice and whether this aspect can be substituted with technology.

This means that there is room for innovation within yogic tradition, and one can try to integrate it in practice. It is necessary to state, however, that the usage of AI in yoga should be approached with criticality since the tool might have both positive and negative implications on the development of a practice. Thus, the continuity of the tradition consists in maintaining the values established throughout centuries whereas transformation is needed due to changes brought about by modernity. To conclude, it seems appropriate to state that the age of AI offers certain opportunities and challenges related to the continuation and transformation of yoga. On the one hand, AI tools can help a practitioner gain knowledge about the tradition, improve the technique, and achieve the best result possible. On the other hand, however, the involvement of AI can be detrimental to the essence of yoga practice since the latter relies on inner experience.

2. LITERATURE REVIEW

In recent years, considerable attention has been devoted by researchers to the interplay between yogic traditions of the past and new technological developments, such as artificial intelligence (AI). Although these two areas differ considerably, with yoga being a part of the spiritual contemplative tradition and AI representing a combination of computational skills and advanced algorithms, there is much that can be learned from studying the interaction between yoga philosophy and AI technologies. The scholarly discussion of this issue tends to focus on three main directions: (1) philosophy and origins of yoga traditions; (2) modernization and globalization of yoga techniques; and (3) incorporation of AI technologies into well-being and health promotion practices.

As a spiritual practice, yoga draws on ancient philosophical concepts of India that are explained in various classical literary sources. In particular, the Yoga Sutras composed by Patanjali represent a key source of information on the origin and philosophy of yoga. As per this source, yoga includes the eight limbs or eightfold path (ashtanga yoga) that includes ethical disciplines (yama), physical postures (asanas), regulation of breathing (pranayama), control of senses (pratyahara), concentration (dharana), meditation (dhyana), and spiritual absorption (samadhi) (Patanjali, trans. 2009). For instance, according to Feuerstein (2003), Bryant (2009), and others, yoga philosophy was initially aimed not at treating physical ailments or improving physical condition but at achieving self-transformation. Also, the Bhagavad Gita presents the notion of different types of yoga, including karma yoga, bhakti yoga, and jnana yoga (Radhakrishnan, 1948).

Conversely, the development of modern yoga represents a shift away from the traditional practice. According to Singleton (2010), the emergence of modern postural yoga was influenced by colonial encounters and physical culture movements in addition to global cultural interactions. Although such transformations have made yoga easier to adopt, they have led to controversies regarding selective use and commercialization of practices within yoga. Traditional methods can be adapted to the needs as can be seen in de Michelis (2004) who has outlined modern psycho somatic yoga and modern postural yoga as types of modern yoga. These results indicate flexibility of yoga and can be seen as beneficial or damaging in the maintenance of philosophical ideas in it.

Moreover, there are different post-modern researches on yogic practices and its effects on mental illness. Kabat-Zinn (2003) started the mindfulness based stress reduction, an interpretation of the principles in a secular context, with a focus on Buddhism and yoga. Many of these later studies have proven the efficacy of these practices in the realm of stress, anxiety and depression (Goyal et al., 2014). The research of this sort has helped to raise awareness of the positive effects of meditation and mindfulness, however it has also sparked discussion about the "decontextualization" of ancient traditions that included selectively interpreting traditional practices and their philosophy.

Apart from the above processes, the rapid advancements of Artificial Intelligence and digital technologies has a great impact on health, wellness and education. For instance, in recent years users will be given personalised meditation tips, a 3D yoga training video, and personalised feedback on the data collected from the user in real time. AI is defined as a system which can perform actions normally carried out by humans, including learning, reasoning, analysing information and information patterns, Kaplan (2016). If such skills were to be applied in wellness, then a very personal user experience can be achieved. However, as mentioned by Floridi et al. (2018), there are some crucial ethical issues to consider when using AI, such as privacy, autonomy, and reliance on algorithms.The introduction of AI in the field of contemplation and wellness practices contributed to creating a concept that some researchers call "digital spirituality" or "technologically mediated mindfulness." For example, Lupton (2016) studies the influence of digital health technologies on the processes of self-tracking and self-care. According to her, digital technologies can be viewed from two perspectives: as empowerment tools and sources of control by framing the idea of well-being quantitatively. The same idea may cause specific problems in relation to yoga since the practices are often evaluated in terms of flexibility, heart rate, and other indicators instead of being focused solely on the inner world of the person. In a similar way, the commodification of the concept is discussed critically by Purser (2019). Still, the existing scholarly literature points out the potential for combining ancient wisdom with advanced technologies for the mutual benefit of both fields. In their research, Bostrom & Yudkowsky (2014) state that yogic wisdom could help in formulating ethics for developing AI, especially promoting values of non-harming, mindfulness, and compassion. Consequently, yoga and AI can be regarded as complementary spheres that operate from different sides but address the same phenomenon – human life and its improvement. As stated above, the first one focuses on personal inner transformations whereas AI concentrates on external reality analysis and optimization.

In addition, embodiment plays a crucial role in this process because yogic practices involve the unity of body and spirit. Therefore, mediating the experience via digital interfaces can distance people from this idea, raising questions about the actuality of virtual instruction in such cases. Ihde (1990) studies the mediating role of technology in shaping people's interactions and experiences, finding that although technologies expand human possibilities, they create new forms of perception and understanding of the world. Thus, in relation to yoga, the question arises concerning whether digital mediation allows experiencing practices fully. Moreover, the involvement of the teacher (guru) is an issue in current discussions as well. Yogic practices always imply personal guidance from teachers who have already experienced the same path and know what obstacles need to be faced. Even though AI systems are able to provide people with instructions, they cannot replace teachers in terms of empathy, intuition, and ability to provide appropriate context-specific guidance. That is why the combination of the approaches is proposed.

Thus, having analyzed the relevant scholarly articles, it became clear that relations between ancient yoga wisdom and modern AI-driven practices include several layers. First of all, despite changing methods of practicing yoga, its core values remain significant in solving contemporary challenges. Second, technological progress contributes to introducing innovations into the sphere; however, new tensions also emerge during this process. Overall, a balanced approach to the issue under discussion is vital for ensuring sustainable development.

Research Gap

Over the last twenty years, a considerable amount of scholarly output has accumulated in the nexus of yoga and artificial intelligence (AI). However, the existing studies still fail to engage with both domains within a comprehensive, cohesive framework. Specifically, the existing research treats yoga and AI separately and approaches them from disparate perspectives. For example, while yoga is typically discussed in terms of its philosophical, historical, or cultural dimensions, AI is considered in relation to technological development, ethics, and application. This disciplinary approach results in fragmented knowledge with much of the possible dialogue between the ancient tradition and the contemporary practice not being explored yet.

One of the major gaps relates to the insufficient attention paid to the integration of classical yogic philosophy into contemporary wellness systems mediated by technology. The foundational texts such as the Yoga Sutras emphasize both discipline and the rules of ethical conduct, mental regulation, and spiritual insight (Patanjali, trans. 2009). Nevertheless, as indicated by scholars, the practice of yoga has experienced some changes since then, focusing on physical aspects of it (De Michelis, 2004; Singleton, 2010). This trend seems to become even more pronounced within AI-assisted approaches to the practice, where yoga consists primarily of guided movements and performance. Little research focuses on incorporating profound philosophical concepts such as chitta vritti nirodha and ahimsa into algorithms and systems.

Secondly, there is little research dedicated to investigating the effects of technology on the experience of practicing yoga, which relies primarily on direct, lived experience and mind–body integration (Feuerstein, 2003). At the same time, AI technologies function through abstraction, data collection, and analysis (Kaplan, 2016). Although they enable convenience and personalized recommendations, the ability of the latter to facilitate deep self-awareness and transformative experiences associated with classical yoga practices has not been sufficiently studied. Notably, Ihde (1990) states that all technology mediates human experience, and it seems that this mediation needs further exploration in terms of yoga practice specifically. Another notable gap pertains to the ethical aspect of the relationship between yoga and AI. The former has long been characterized by specific rules such as truthfulness, non-possessiveness, self-control, and compassion. At the same time, AI ethics has become an emerging field of investigation that focuses on issues like autonomy, transparency, and privacy (Floridi et al., 2018). However, while there is some interdisciplinary research on the topic (Bostrom & Yudkowsky, 2014), the contribution that could help in developing ethical guidelines for human-centered AI is rather limited.

As new digital health solutions become widespread, another area of research has received increased attention recently. For instance, Zhu, Li, and Liu (2024) study various wearable devices used to monitor mental health conditions based on physiological parameters such as heart rate, body temperature, and physical activity. Specifically, their paper provides an overview of the application of machine learning methods in order to interpret the collected data in relation to stress, anxiety, depression, and overall well-being.

In addition to the gaps described above, the cultural dimension has been largely ignored as well. In their critique of the commercialization of mindfulness in modern society, Purser (2019) argues that such practices may be deprived of any ethical and philosophical meaning due to the institutionalization of the latter. Similarly, concerns have been voiced regarding the cultural appropriation and decontextualization of yoga during its global expansion (Singleton, 2010). Thus, the question whether or not AI tools might facilitate these negative trends should be addressed.

Finally, although numerous papers have reported the positive psychological and physiological outcomes of practicing mindfulness and meditation (Goyal et al., 2014), relatively few of them explore the issue of using AI to mediate the practice. As a result, questions related to user engagement, cultivation of regular practice, and authenticity of guidance provided by technology have not been answered yet. At the same time, one needs to investigate how the teacher-student (guru-shishya) relationship can be preserved when relying on AI technologies. Overall, the reviewed literature provides sufficient information regarding both yogic traditions and AI. However, it fails to discuss the nexus between the two concepts and their interaction. One needs to develop a conceptual framework that can incorporate both continuity and transformation characteristic of the former into the use of the latter.

Table 1. Comparative Analysis of Ancient Yogic Wisdom vs. AI-Driven Modern Practice

Dimension	Ancient Yogic Wisdom	Modern AI-Driven Practice	Key Insight from Literature
Philosophical Foundation	Rooted in spiritual texts like *Yoga Sutras*; aims at self-realization and liberation (*moksha*)	Based on computational logic, data analytics, and optimization of user outcomes	Traditional yoga emphasizes,consciousness transformation, whereas AI focuses on efficiency and measurable outputs (Patanjali, 2009; Kaplan, 2016)
Purpose of Practice	Inner awareness, ethical living, and transcendence of mind fluctuations	Stress reduction, fitness, productivity, and mental well-being	Modern adaptations often narrow yoga's broader goals into therapeutic benefits (Singleton, 2010)
Nature of Knowledge	Experiential, introspective, and subjective (*anubhava*)	Data-driven, objective, and algorithm-based	There is a gap between lived experience and computational,interpretation (Feuerstein, 2003; Ihde, 1990)

continued on following page

Table 1. Continued

Dimension	Ancient Yogic Wisdom	Modern AI-Driven Practice	Key Insight from Literature
Mode of Learning	Teacher-student (*guru-shishya*) relationship; oral and guided transmission	Apps, virtual instructors, AI feedback systems, self-paced learning	AI lacks the intuitive and relational depth of human mentorship
Role of the Body	Body as a pathway to higher consciousness; integrated with mind and breath	Often treated as measurable input (posture tracking, biometrics)	Embodiment risks being reduced to quantifiable performance (Lupton, 2016)
Ethical Framework	Strong emphasis on *yamas* and *niyamas* (non-violence, truthfulness, discipline)	Emerging AI ethics focusing on fairness, privacy, and accountability	Limited integration between yogic ethics and AI design (Floridi et al., 2018; Bostrom & Yudkowsky, 2014)
Cultural Context	Deeply rooted in Indian philosophical and spiritual traditions	Globalized, digitized, often detached from original cultural context	Risk of cultural dilution and commodification (Purser, 2019; De Michelis, 2004)
Accessibility	Traditionally limited to guided learning environments	Highly accessible through mobile apps and digital platforms	AI expands reach but may simplify depth
Measurement of Progress	Subjective transformation (awareness, detachment, inner peace)	Quantifiable metrics (time practiced, heart rate, flexibility)	Tension between qualitative and quantitative evaluation
Adaptability	Evolved over centuries through interpretation and transmission	Rapid innovation driven by technological change	Yoga's flexibility allows integration, but risks oversimplification (Singleton, 2010)

Relationship between Ancient Yoga and Modern AI-Based Yoga

The relationship between ancient yoga and modern AI-based yoga is best understood not as a replacement of one by the other, but as a layered interaction—where continuity of core principles coexists with technological transformation. On a higher level, both systems seek to help humans achieve well-being; however, while one system does it by focusing on the internal aspect of things, the other one focuses on the external side. Namely, classical yoga, according to traditional definitions, is a technique focused on developing inner awareness, discipline, and the integration of body, mind, and consciousness. The techniques associated with classical yoga, such as meditation and breath regulation, are meant to help the person gain greater inner harmony by controlling his/her mental functions. All of the above can be regarded as a foundation of yoga, regardless of any changes that occur outside this inner sphere. On the contrary, modern yoga, which incorporates elements of artificial intelligence, focuses on observing the external aspect of things, including posture, heart rate, breathing rate, and other indicators of health and wellbeing.

Nevertheless, it is possible to identify similarities between these two approaches, since both systems are aimed at recognizing patterns and optimizing people's performance in various aspects. According to traditional yoga practices, people need to train themselves to recognize patterns that emerge both in their behaviors and minds, gradually gaining more awareness and control over them. Likewise, AI systems analyze and recognize patterns in various indicators that can be used to improve a person's performance. Research shows that the precision of recognizing yoga positions can sometimes exceed 90%; thus, AI technology can become an efficient tool to optimize yoga performance and prevent injuries (Özsezer & Mermer, 2025). One more similarity to discuss is personalization of yoga exercises. Traditionally, yoga practice is known for being highly personalized, which implies that teachers needed to find the optimal approach to each particular pupil depending on his/her abilities and needs. Similarly, current systems try to personalize yoga practice using information about the client's health, performance, and other relevant parameters that can be obtained through sensors (Ganesh, 2025).

Still, a number of conflicts can be detected. One of them revolves around experiential knowledge vs. data-based knowledge. Ancient yoga highlights personal experience and insights of practitioners gained through introspection and observations. In AI-assisted yoga, however, experience is transformed into tangible and precise data points. Despite some benefits that this approach offers (such as better standardization of techniques), there is a danger of reducing yoga to mere metrics of flexibility and accurate performance (e.g., perfect postures). In turn, researchers point out that although artificial intelligence can facilitate technological aspects of yoga practice, it will never be able to provide a level of internal transformation experienced in ancient yoga based on self-awareness and meditation (Sinha & Sinha, 2024). The second factor pertains to the concept of guidance. While in yoga traditional practice a significant role belongs to guidance provided by a teacher who shares their wisdom and helps students learn the necessary techniques, as well as provides emotional and spiritual support, in AI-enhanced practice, this guidance is taken up in part by intelligent machines that give students recommendations regarding postures and practices. The use of applications, intelligent systems, and technologies also enables practitioners to do yoga in any desired place and at any moment. Thus, AI has made yoga accessible and removed barriers of both space and time associated with this practice (Ganesh, 2025). Yet, despite all advantages offered by artificial intelligence, experts believe that the human component cannot be replaced in yoga practice due to ethical and other issues (Vivek S. Sahu, 2026).

However, AI technology allows expanding the boundaries of yoga practice and creating new experiences impossible to achieve before. For instance, wearing devices that monitor physiological states of practitioners allows tracking changes in heart rates, stress levels, and breaths and thus increasing awareness. Thus, artificial intelligence transforms yoga not only but also extends it into the domain of novel experiences impossible before the invention of modern technologies. Modern developments related to artificial intelligence and digital healthcare are increasingly focused on the concepts of transparency, personalization, and comprehensive well-being. T. Tunduny & Shibowabo (2026) explore the emerging role of explainable AI in federated learning for healthcare and argues that AI models should not only make accurate predictions of patients' health conditions but also explain them. The significance of explainable AI becomes especially evident when applied to the complex and sensitive domain of healthcare, where considerations of transparency, ethics, and accountability come into play. Relatedly, the contribution by D. Kumar et al. (2025) shows how explainable AI in conjunction with federated learning contributes to improving the accuracy of medical predictions while ensuring the confidentiality of patients' data.

The widespread adoption of wearable technologies is changing preventive healthcare and mental wellness approaches. According to research conducted at Stanford Medicine, machine learning models based on consumer wearables' data about sleep patterns can predict more than one hundred medical conditions, showing how today's technological advancements are making devices such as smartwatches and fitness trackers crucial tools in detecting diseases in advance and providing continuous health monitoring. In parallel, R. Kumar and S. Srivastava (2023) consider wearable sensors' data for stress detection and emotional state monitoring, discussing the potential and issues regarding real-time physiologic monitoring in regards to studying and tracking people's emotions and mental states in digital age.

Furthermore, today's research also makes an effort to relate today's technological developments to the yogic ideas of consciousness and holistic healing methods. For example, S. M. Tripathi (2021) looks into the relationship between the concepts of chitta (mind-stuff) and vritti (fluctuations) in the framework of yogic consciousness and modern neuroscience. Specifically, the researcher examines whether yogic consciousness models might have valuable implications for understanding the role of default mode network of the brain in cognitive regulation and self-awareness. Likewise, J. Nesin and G. Sathyamoorthy (2025) explore the psychoneuroimmunological aspects of yoga and meditation, explaining the impact of such practices on nervous, endocrine, and immune systems. As a result, they demonstrate the applicability of these practices for managing one's psychological state in terms of stress and emotion regulation.

Finally, M. Irfan, A. Ali, and A. U. Rehman (2025) conduct a systematic review of the relationship between artificial intelligence and naturopathy/yoga in addressing patients with chronic illnesses. In particular, they highlight the benefits of using AI systems and algorithms to create preventive approaches to healthcare in combination with holistic medicine and natural therapies. All considered, all discussed studies reveal how the future of healthcare industry might lie in the intersection of ancient yoga practices and AI technologies, helping people stay healthy both physically and mentally. Perhaps, the best way to understand the nature of the relationship between ancient yoga and AI-based yoga practice is to consider them as two mutually reinforcing approaches. Namely, ancient yoga offers a solid philosophical and ethical foundation for any wellness practice, presenting a model of human flourishing. On the contrary, artificial intelligence technologies provide various tools for enhancing people's lives in line with these models, such as access to yoga and feedback and personalization opportunities. Recent research proves that combining AI and yoga can foster holistic well-being of numerous individuals, especially if technological innovations are used for the same purposes as traditional yoga practice (Saini et al., 2024).

In short, the development of the relationship between ancient yoga and today's AI-based yoga shows the trend historically observed in the history of the evolution of traditional knowledge systems. In particular, traditional knowledge is neither supplanted by the new technologies nor remains unchanged; instead, it undergoes significant changes under their influence. In this context, the key challenge to be addressed in regard to AI and yoga relationship is ensuring that the essence of the latter practice does not change and it continues fostering people's spiritual and inner growth.

Different Ancient Yoga Granth (Texts) and Their Significance

The practice of ancient yoga cannot be described as one single phenomenon because it involves different approaches and concepts developed by various authors in the history of Indian culture. As such, it can only be properly understood as a rich tradition supported by an extensive library of classical texts known as granthas. These works provide a range of perspectives on yoga, including philosophical speculation, ethical behavior, as well as practical exercises aimed at meditation and physical regulation. Altogether, these granthas form a solid foundation that lies at the heart of all current notions about yoga. In addition, the study of some prominent examples of yoga granthas will help us understand the complexity of the tradition. In terms of age, the first place goes to the Yoga Sutras of Patanjali. While dating the exact time when this seminal work was written, scholars note the beginning of the common era. At the same time, the book is focused on the organization of yoga practice as eight limbs (ashtanga yoga), paying little attention to the physical part of the process. Instead, emphasis is placed on mental control and meditation. It is important to note that yoga is traditionally defined as the absence of mental activity according to the definition given in the sutra (Patanjali, trans. 2009). The peculiarity of the treatise is in its systematic nature that makes it effective in guiding the process of transformation from yama and niyama to samadhi.

The next text is the Bhagavad Gita that cannot be called only a book about yoga but it contains a lot of information on different types of this practice. Written as a conversation between Prince Arjuna and Lord Krishna, this scripture is based on different aspects of yoga, including karma yoga, bhakti yoga, and jnana yoga. Moreover, unlike Patanjali Yoga Sutras, The Bhagavad Gita does not promote withdrawal from reality but suggests active participation in the life while keeping balance inside oneself. Thus, the importance of the text can hardly be underestimated because it helped to spread yoga practices among common people (Radhakrishnan, 1948). As the centuries passed, the philosophy of yoga evolved into the discipline that focused on the use of the body as well. In particular, Hatha Yoga Pradipika written by Swami Swatmarama describes different aspects of asanas, pranayama, mudras, and bandhas. Moreover, the text shows that the body must be prepared for entering new levels of consciousness and yoga practices should prepare it for doing this (Swatmarama, trans. 2002).

Finally, Gheranda Samhita belongs to the category of the most important books on Hatha Yoga. This text provides a detailed description of a system known as sapta sadhana and includes such elements as purification of the body, asanas, breathing exercises, meditation, and other aspects that are supposed to contribute to higher states of consciousness. One of the main ideas suggested in this text is the necessity of using the body as the basis for the future work. In fact, the body should be cleaned, purified, and used as a means of achieving certain spiritual states since physical conditions have a close relation to mental states and practices (Mallinson, 2004).

All things considered, it may be said that Gheranda Samhita reflects a holistic perception of human life in which the body, mind, and spirit work together as an integrated entity. The same thing is stated by modern researchers who study the influence of yoga on health of people. For instance, Carolyn Woodyard (2011) emphasizes that yoga practice helps people to achieve psychological and physical balance by managing such disorders as anxiety, stress, and chronic pain. Additionally, regular practice improves emotional stability, concentration, and physical abilities of people.

In modern times, however, progress in digital health and artificial intelligence technology has led to even more significant changes in the way that ideas about health and wellbeing are understood. According to Keesara, Jonas, and Schulman (2020), one of the most noticeable changes during the recent years was the increased popularity of various digital tools that became especially relevant due to the emergence of the COVID-19 pandemic. These digital technologies include telemedicine, wearables, remote patient monitoring, and other systems based on AI. On the one hand, they provide increased accessibility of healthcare-related services; on the other hand, they allow for a more personalized treatment of patients. Another example of such a shift would be provided by the study conducted by Rieke et al. (2020). The scholars show the growing importance of federated learning as the technology behind digital medicine. It allows for analyzing information generated by various devices and institutions with the aim to ensure patient confidentiality and data security. Thus, it seems possible to use these advancements for combining ancient wisdom of yogic philosophy and the emerging possibilities associated with the use of AI.

Another important aspect of yogic philosophy is the discussion provided in the Shiva Samhita. Contrary to some texts that focus mostly on practical aspects of physical training, the discussed book explains various terms and philosophies behind yoga including kundalini energy, nadis, meditation, and self-realization. Moreover, as Vasu (trans., 2003) mentions in his translation, it offers the idea that the entire universe represents manifestation of one universal consciousness. The book shifts smoothly from philosophical ideas to instructions, presenting a wide variety of perspectives inherent in yogic culture (Vasu, 2003). Other important works that contributed significantly to the development of early yogic philosophy include Upanishads, particularly those related to yoga – Yoga Upanishads. Examples of these texts are the Katha Upanishad and Shvetashvatara Upanishad. The mentioned granthas discuss issues associated with the nature of existence, meditation, consciousness, and breathing. Such considerations served as a basis for the construction of later yoga schools (Olivelle, 1996). In contrast to manuals written at later stages, the texts under discussion contain many reflections and are poetic in their form.

Thus, it becomes clear that the philosophy of yoga continued to evolve throughout time. While some texts focused on philosophical ideas and others preferred practical approaches, some attempted to merge them together. As a result, there appeared a diverse and evolving tradition that continues to develop in modern days. In the context of current technology and artificial intelligence developments, the ideas expressed in the texts under discussion remain very relevant since yoga goes far beyond techniques and tools.

3. CONCLUSION & FUTURE SCOPE

Thus, it appears that there exist some parallels between the old yogic concepts of inner peace and harmony and today's views on health and well-being. While originating in a radically different historical environment, yogic teachings contain elements of mental discipline, emotional regulation, ethics, and wellness that are relevant even to the contemporary era of technological advancements. Moreover, recent developments in AI and digital healthcare technologies have added new dimensions to our understanding of health, consciousness, and human well-being in general. Indeed, current wearable devices capable of monitoring the emotional state, stress levels, sleep patterns, and physical activity of users present a promising approach toward the creation of innovative preventive healthcare solutions.

Far from being mutually exclusive, yoga and artificial intelligence can be viewed as complementary phenomena that should interact with each other. On the one hand, yogic philosophy will provide additional ethical considerations to follow during the application of technology, while AI-powered healthcare solutions will ensure broader availability of wellness services. Together, they can represent an emerging interdisciplinary sphere where ancient wisdom and modern scientific knowledge can interact in productive and creative ways. Thus, the future of well-being might be determined not only by technological progress but also by preservation of ethical human values associated with yoga and meditation.

There exist several promising directions in the further exploration of this interdisciplinary field. First, the development of wellness systems based on yogic concepts of mindfulness, breath regulation, meditation, and ethical self-control deserves particular attention. These systems can serve as valuable tools for providing personalized psychological support, managing patients' stress levels, and preventing illnesses. Furthermore, additional research focused on neurophysiological mechanisms underlying yogic practices should help shed light on their beneficial impact on humans. Involvement of experts from such spheres as yoga philosophy, psychology, neuroscience, and computer science will contribute to holistic approaches to well-being. Moreover, explainable AI and privacy-preserving technologies like federated learning might become vital for creating ethically sound healthcare systems. Finally, wearable technologies could help integrate yogic practices into modern lifestyles in order to provide people with chronic diseases, poor mental health, or lack of access to professional yoga training with adequate wellness assistance. At the same time, future developments must preserve cultural and philosophical background of yoga to avoid reduction to a technological product. In conclusion, it seems that the way forward for the field in question is to strike a balance between technological innovation and human wisdom. With continuous development of artificial intelligence affecting various spheres of contemporary life, it is likely that the experience of yogic masters will provide useful guidelines for maintaining mental clarity, ethical awareness, emotional stability, and overall health.

REFERENCES

Bostrom, N., & Yudkowsky, E. (2014). The ethics of artificial intelligence. In K. Frankish & W. Ramsey (Eds.), The Cambridge handbook of artificial intelligence (pp. 316–334). Cambridge University Press. DOI: 10.1017/CBO9781139046855.020

Bryant, E. F. (2009). *The Yoga Sutras of Patanjali: A new edition, translation, and commentary*. North Point Press.

De Michelis, E. (2004). A history of modern yoga: Patanjali and Western esotericism. *Continuum.*

Feuerstein, G. (2003). *The deeper dimension of yoga: Theory and practice*. Shambhala Publications.

Floridi, L., Cowls, J., Beltrametti, M., Chatila, R., Chazerand, P., Dignum, V., Luetge, C., Madelin, R., Pagallo, U., Rossi, F., Schafer, B., Valcke, P., & Vayena, E. (2018). AI4People—An ethical framework for a good AI society. *Minds and Machines, 28*(4), 689–707. DOI: 10.1007/s11023-018-9482-5 PMID: 30930541

Ganesh, K. and Ramudhin (2025), A. Leveraging AI to Mitigate Risks in Yoga Practice: A Real-Time Posture Correction Application. In Proceedings of the 12th International Conference on Sport Sciences Research and Technology Support (icSPORTS 2024), pages 241-250 ISBN: 978-989-758-719-1; ISSN: 2184-3201 DOI: DOI: 10.5220/0013063300003828

Goyal, M., Singh, S., Sibinga, E. M., Gould, N. F., Rowland-Seymour, A., Sharma, R., Berger, Z., Sleicher, D., Maron, D. D., Shihab, H. M., Ranasinghe, P. D., Linn, S., Saha, S., Bass, E. B., & Haythornthwaite, J. A. (2014). Meditation programs for psychological stress and well-being: A systematic review and meta-analysis. *JAMA Internal Medicine, 174*(3), 357–368. DOI: 10.1001/jamainternmed.2013.13018 PMID: 24395196

Ihde, D. (1990). *Technology and the lifeworld: From garden to earth*. Indiana University Press. DOI: 10.2979/3108.0

Irfan, M., Ali, A., & Rehman, A. U. (2025). Integrating artificial intelligence with naturopathy and yoga for chronic disease management: A systematic review. *Journal of Integrative and Complementary Medicine, 31*(2), 115–134.

Kabat-Zinn, J. (2003). Mindfulness-based interventions in context: Past, present, and future. *Clinical Psychology : a Publication of the Division of Clinical Psychology of the American Psychological Association, 10*(2), 144–156. DOI: 10.1093/clipsy.bpg016

Kaplan, J. (2016). *Artificial intelligence: What everyone needs to know*. Oxford University Press. DOI: 10.1093/wentk/9780190602383.001.0001

Keesara, S., Jonas, A., & Schulman, K. (2020). Covid-19 and health care's digital revolution. *The New England Journal of Medicine, 382*(23), e82. DOI: 10.1056/NEJMp2005835 PMID: 32240581

Kumar, D., Verma, C., & Illés, Z. (2025). Federated learning with explainable AI for liver disease prediction: A privacy-preserving approach, Intelligence-Based Medicine,Volume 12, 2025, 100285, ISSN 2666-5212, DOI: 10.1016/j.ibmed.2025.100285

Kumar, R., & Srivastava, S. (2023). Wearable sensor data for stress and affective state monitoring: Challenges and opportunities. *Sensors (Basel), 23*(4), 2215. PMID: 36850813

Lupton, D. (2016). *The quantified self: A sociology of self-tracking*. Polity Press.

. Mallinson, J. (2004). The Gheranda Samhita: The original Sanskrit and an English translation. YogaVidya.com.

Nesin, J., & Sathyamoorthy, G. (2025). Psychoneuroimmunology of yoga and meditation: Mechanisms and clinical applications. In Sharma, S., & Gupta, R. (Eds.), *Indian Knowledge Systems in Modern Healthcare* (pp. 112–145). IGI Global.

Olivelle, P. (1996). *Upanishads*. Oxford University Press.

Özsezer, G., & Mermer, G. (2025). Real-time prediction of correct yoga asanas using artificial intelligence. *Nursing Open*. PMID: 40768382

. Patanjali. (2009). The Yoga Sutras of Patanjali (E. F. Bryant, Trans.). North Point Press.

Purser, R. (2019). *McMindfulness: How mindfulness became the new capitalist spirituality*. Repeater Books.

Radhakrishnan, S. (1948). *The Bhagavadgita*. George Allen & Unwin.

Rieke, N., Hancox, J., & Li, W.. (2020). The future of digital health with federated learning. npj. *Digital Medicine, 3*(1), 119. PMID: 33015372

Sahu, V. S. (2026). The changing scenario of yoga education with artificial intelligence. *Research Hub., 07*(1), 230–233. DOI: 10.63665/rh.v7i2.39

Saini, N. (2024). Exploring The Synergy Of Ai And Yogic Practices: A Future-Oriented Approach For Holistic Wellbeing. *Educational Administration: Theory and Practice, 30*(5), 15412–15420. DOI: 10.53555/kuey.v30i5.9101

Singleton, M. (2010). *Yoga body: The origins of modern posture practice*. Oxford University Press. DOI: 10.1093/acprof:oso/9780195395358.001.0001

Sinha, N., & Sinha, R. K. (2024, September-December). Harnessing the Potential of Artificial Intelligence in Yoga Therapy. *International Journal of Yoga*, *17*(3), 242–245. DOI: 10.4103/ijoy.ijoy_124_24 PMID: 39959510

. Swatmarama. (2002). Hatha Yoga Pradipika (B. K. S. Iyengar, Trans.). HarperCollins.

Tripathi, S. M. (2021). Yogic theory of consciousness and its neuroscientific correlates: Chitta, Vritti, and the default mode network. *Journal of Consciousness Studies*, *28*(5–6), 112–145.

Tunduny, T., & Shibwabo, B. (2026). Explainable AI Approaches in Federated Learning: Systematic Review. *JMIR AI*, *5*, e69985. https://ai.jmir.org/2026/1/e69985. DOI: 10.2196/69985 PMID: 41632959

Vasu, R. B. S. (2003). *The Shiva Samhita*. Munshiram Manoharlal. (Original work published 1914)

Woodyard, C. (2011). Exploring the therapeutic effects of yoga and its ability to increase quality of life. *International Journal of Yoga*, *4*(2), 49–54. DOI: 10.4103/0973-6131.85485 PMID: 22022122

Zhu, X., Li, X., & Liu, S. (2024). Predicting mental health from physiological signals: A review of machine learning approaches using wearable data. *PLOS Digital Health*, *3*(1), e0000312.

Chapter 3
Integrating Artificial Intelligence and Yoga for Holistic Well-Being:
A Synergistic Path Toward Personalized Mind-Body Health

Rajesh Prasad
http://orcid.org/0000-0002-3456-6980
Ajay Kumar Garg Engineering College, Ghaziabad, India

Muskan Wahi
Ajay Kumar Garg Engineering College, Ghaziabad, India

Mehak Srivastava
Ajay Kumar Garg Engineering College, Ghaziabad, India

Somya Singh
Ajay Kumar Garg Engineering College, Ghaziabad, India

ABSTRACT

The chapter suggests a multimodal approach of using AI and Yoga to make an all-encompassing and personalized digital yoga guide. The existing AI-based yoga and wellness systems place too much emphasis on biomechanical positioning or generic mindfulness and do not emphasize breath control, mood, and long-term behavioral transformation. In order to fill this gap, the framework integrates computer vision-based pose depth, physiological measurements of heart rate variability and breathing, affective computing with behavioral analytics into an integrated digital twin of the practitioner as an entity of body presence, autonomic actions, and emotional

DOI: 10.4018/979-8-3373-7625-7.ch003

conditioning. A hybrid model integrates data-driven models with a symbolic yogic base structure of knowledge based on principles of sthira-sukham asanam, breath-movement harmony and non-harming, which allows context-dependent advice about asana, pranayama, rest and attentional cues. The experimental findings using a prototype system propose a positive effect on pose alignment, heart rate variability, stress reduction, and user confidence.

1. INTRODUCTION

The modern-day world is increasingly marked by elevated levels of stress levels, anxiety, and emotional instability caused by the hectic pace of life, excessive screen time, the presence of competitive workplaces, and the lack of time to embrace the restorative activities (Mitsea et al., 2023), (Kirk et al., 2022). Work-life balance has been disrupted by constant digital connectivity and tight schedules which leads to sleep disorders, lack of productivity, diseases associated with the lifestyle, and emotional fatigue among people of all ages (Chi Lee, 2018). The global COVID-19 pandemic has further contributed to an increase in mental and physical health disorders associated with stress not only among individuals in specific countries but also on a global level. These problems raise the necessity of preventing, affordable, and sustainable wellbeing solutions that would consider not only psychological but also physiological health (Narimani & Naeim, 2025). Contemporary health care systems are slowly becoming less about the reactive form of treatment and more focused on the long-term preventive and holistic models of care which focus on self-regulation, emotional stability, and long-term wellbeing (Bolpagni et al., 2024). In this regard, mind-body practices with the assistance of intelligent technologies are being perceived with growing interest (Loughnane et al., 2025). Mind-body interventions that are backed by smart technologies have received considerable focus in this changing environment.

Yoga is one of such interventions and a holistic wellbeing system. Yoga, which is based on an ancient Indian philosophy, focuses on harmony between body, breath, mind and consciousness through a combined approach of physical postures (asanas), breathing (pranayama), mindfulness (dhyana) and meditation (dhyana) (Saini, 2024). There is a consistent scientific evidence that regular yoga practice enhances flexibility, heart and respiratory efficiency, posture stability, emotional balance and resilience towards stress. In comparison to traditional fitness programs, Yoga encourages inner consciousness, harmony, and self-control which makes it an effective preventive and therapeutic activity in the contemporary healthcare and well-being setting (Sinha & Sinha, 2024).

Contemporary society is further characterized by rising stress, anxiety and emotional instability in fastened standards of living, sustained mobile phone communication and social and economic structures. Speediness of modernity, which is affected by technological advancement and a globalized society has been central to the transformation of day to day life and preferable ways. The lengthy time of working, being seated before the screen constantly, and ignorance of where the working process and personal life have become a reality. As much as these advancements have improved efficiency and access to information, they have also cut down on chances of physical activity, restorative rest, and reflective practices which are fundamental in psychologically equalizing and restoring the body (Mitsea et al., 2023).

The introduction of AI into Yoga has not been an exception to the research attention and, in particular, in the area of automated posture recognition, corrections, and virtual instructions. Possible monitoring of anasana and real time corrective information have been demonstrated by vision based pose estimation systems as well as wearable sensor systems. The advantages of these system are as follows: they enhance the extent of accessibility, reduce chances of injuries, and help to practice on their own, especially in novice learners and those who are more likely not to have access to trained educators. Most of the existing AI-oriented Yoga systems have a very heavy biomechanical orientation, but fail to capture the holistic nature of Yoga, with accuracy of posture being the main element of the system. However, after three years of positive changes, the systems that are available are usually independent and may work either by correcting the posture, analysing the breathing or monitoring emotions. There are not numerous studies that are attempting to make such parts one system according to the philosophy of yoga. Most business wellness programs are more oriented towards fitness metrics or personal guided mindfulness but have little adaptive individualization and combined feedback. Consequently, the interior world of psychological condition of practitioners and philosophical foundation of yoga are not quite represented. To address these weaknesses, the present chapter proposes an integrative AI-Yoga system, which is grounded on posture identification, breathing identification, affective identification, and behavioral analytics.

The proposed approach would provide adaptive, personalized, holistic wellbeing support by harmonizing the ancient yogic concepts with the current computational intelligence. At the same time when the sphere of the Yoga acceptance is being expanded, a new sphere of Artificial Intelligence has been introduced as a miracle in the field of medicine, wellness, and human-centered technologies. The AI-enabled systems can improve their analysis of multimodal data that is big and is gained through the assistance of wearable devices, cameras, microphone, and an online communication. Machine learning algorithms can also identify patterns and abnormalities in the physiological signs and movement records, as well as patterns of behavior, and this can recognize the first signs of stress, fatigue and health danger.

A detailed analysis of human posture and movement can be performed with the use of computer vision applications, whereas, affective computing methods strive to extract emotional and cognitive states on the basis of the visible information.

The last few years have seen AI achieve colossal acceptance and been deployed in preventive health targeting, personalized recommendation schemes and in the adaptive intervention schemes. Smart devices track the intensity of physical activity, pulse rate, sleep quality, and stress rates and provide users with real-time data about their health status. AI applications are used in mental health and wellness as guided meditation, mood trackers, stress management features. Artificial intelligence has been useful in the clinical environment to aid in the decision process of diagnostic, remote patients, and treatment planning. These developments attract attention to the possibilities of AI that can assist the wellbeing of individuals with the assistance of informed data and personalized care.

However, despite all the spreading of digital wellness technologies, most of the existing services possess disjointed and small solutions. The majority of apps are focused on a single aspect of health i.e. the number of steps taken, calorie burnt or even the overall mindfulness sessions and hardly takes into account the integration of the physical, emotional, and behavioural components in a coherent pattern. The biomechanical soundness of any AIFDE-based posturecorrection apparatus is typically underlined in unipolar terms; meditation and mental health-related uses of AIFDE may fail to introduce the significance of physical embodiment and control of breath. Because of that, these systems fail to reflect the integrative and holistic nature of human wellbeing.

More importantly, the AI-based Yoga products that are currently in existence would be inclined toward reductionist view, viewing Yoga as a collection of physical activities that are to be streamlined with the help of alignment correction and poses recognition. Though these features may help beginner users and make Yoga a safer practice, it does not reflect the true essence of this practice, as a form of self-awareness and self-emotion, and inner transformation. Emotional conditions, quality of breathing, attention to the mind, and adaptation of the behavior are not a common consideration during system design. Therefore, the existing solutions put the risk of perpetuating performance-based attitudes that do not align with the Yogic concepts of non-competitiveness, self-reflection, and mindfulness.

Despite the fact that previous studies have shown the therapeutic values of Yoga and AI ability to personalize healthcare separately, the interception of the two fields is not well-developed. The literature tends to cover detached elements of posture recognition or stress detection without putting them into a larger context of a philosophical or conceptual framework. Major gaps in literature exist with regard to models that integrate Yogic knowledge with advanced AI methods to endorse holistic, adaptive, and ethically sound interventions to promote wellbeing.

To address these limitations, this chapter proposes an integrative AI-driven Yoga framework grounded in yogic philosophy and supported by multimodal intelligence. The suggested solution is a set of computer vision posture detection, breathing and physiological monitoring, affective computing to predict emotions, and behavioral analytics to customize itself. The combination of these modalities available in the framework is expected to provide real-time and context-sensitive feedback that is both objective (reflecting the quality of movement externally) and subjective (reflecting the psychophysiological states). The main value of this work is that it is capable of developing AI-assisted Yoga to encompass much more than simple isolated biomechanical correction and instead create a system of human wellbeing in its entirety. The proposed framework will facilitate balanced, moderate, and self-regulated personal growth as compared to optimizing performance in the short term, by synchronizing computational intelligence with yogic principles of balance, moderation, and self-regulation. This combination provides a fresh look on how new technologies can be ethically and meaningfully used to promote holistic wellbeing in a more digitalized society.

Rationale for the Proposed Research

The research proposal aims to address the existing gaps and come up with a holistic AI aided Yoga model which will close the gap between technological intelligence and Yogic wisdom. The proposed system enables to advocate Yoga beyond a mere physical activity through the combination of posture recognition, affective analytics, breathing analysis, and behavioral modeling into one adaptive architecture. Besides that, by incorporating the Yogic concepts into the system objectives and feedback strategies, the study would design AI systems that would nurture balance, mindfulness and gradual growth. The suggested model attempts to become a dynamic companion in the multimodal and long-term learning to maintain the individual change and overall wellbeing.

2. LITERATURE REVIEW

Yoga convergence and Artificial Intelligence (AI) is a brand new interdisciplinary area that is situated in the computer science interface, health informatics, human -computer interaction, and ancient wellbeing practices (Narayanan, 2025)(Kumar Mishra & Mishra, 2024). The research on the study of digital Yoga platforms facilitated by the scholarship and the technological advancement. This has been on the increase over the last decade because of the growing apprehension about smart technologies prevention medicine, mental health, and personalized exercise throughout the globe (Vivekanandha et al., 2025)(C & Kumari, 2022). Computational powers have also actuated such growth and real time movement became possible diagnosis in man, and physiological control the further and the further.

The holistic system of yoga is focused on union of physical poses (asanas), control of breath (pranayama), mind discipline (dharana and dhyana), morality and self-consciousness. There are opportunities and challenges of translating these multidimensional aspects into computational frameworks. Whereas AI is good in pattern recognition, prediction, and automation, Yoga lays emphasis on experiential awareness, a slow progression, and complete harmony between the mind and body (Yenishettil et al., 2024). The literature reveals attempts to close this gap, although some comprehensive solution is still out of reach.

A critical review of the available literature on AI-assisted Yoga systems, which began with the early posture-recognition models and then proceeded through the examples of multimodal and affect-sensitive systems have been conducted by (Agarwal et al., 2022). It determines major technological, methodological, and conceptual weaknesses, in particular, the incorporation of Yogic philosophy into the decision-making process based on AI (Talaat, 2023).

2.1 The Initial Work on AI-Based Yoga Systems

The first studies on AI and Yoga appeared in the context of the general improvement of human activity recognition and computer vision (Swain et al., 2022)(Anuradha et al., 2024). The ancient technologies were highly exploratory and focused on determining whether Yoga postures are detectable automatically through digital imaging measures. Scholars extensively used the traditional image processing techniques in the areas of background subtraction, shape analysis, contour detection, and edge detection (Anand Thoutam et al., 2022). Silhouette descriptors, joint heuristics, and geometry ratios have been analyzed as examples of handcrafted features that are based on the assessment of findings of low-rate video and statically images.

The most commonly used traditional machine learning classifier was k-nearest neighbours (KNN), support vector machines (SVMs), decision trees, and hidden Markov models (HMMs) (S. K. Yadav et al., 2019). These strategies proved their concepts but were limited in a number of ways. They needed monotonous lighting, monotonous background, monotonous outfits. There was major degradation of performance with real-world variation in body morphology, camera angles, occlusions and movement dynamics.

Machine learning models applied to the data of wearable sensors are support vector machines, random forests, convolutional neural networks and recurrent neural networks such as long short-term memory networks (Aydın, 2024). Several experiments have estimated better precision in the ability of posture recognition and tracker performance in cases where wearable data were used especially in intricate or fast sequence. Some of the hybrid approaches combined both visual and inertial data to enhance robustness and reduce ambiguity to prove the potential of multi-modal fusion. However, wearable-heavy systems also have practical limitations, which means that they can be used not so much in the real world. Such needs might give rise to inconvenience which would result in restriction of natural movement and compliance among the user particularly in case long-term or casual practice is needed due to the need to add some sensors. Scalability of controlled experimental environments is also more difficult due to the complexity of setup, calibration criteria and maintenance.

Moreover, the systems were typically involved in the identification of a stationary position, but not with continuous practice assessment. Such coordination was not given much thought as between the yoga patterns, transitions, and coordination of breath. The feedback systems were very primitive and in most of the situations, were based on the judgement of the correctness or incorrectness without any context elaboration (Chatterjee and Prinz, 2022). Therefore, the first AI-based Yoga systems resembled a pose detector rather than an instructor and could not be of much pedagogical or therapeutic value.

2.2 The Contemporary Boom of Pose Estimating Deep Learning

The trend is deep learning that transformed the research of AI-assisted Yoga (Joshi et al., 2020). Convolutional neural networks (CNNs) revolutionized the field of computer vision because it enabled the hierarchical features to be trained on raw data on an end-to-end manner. This kind of transition eliminated the necessity of having to use hand made functionality and improved scalability and durability significantly. The use of pose-estimation frameworks, such as OpenPose, PoseNet, HRNet, MoveNet and MediaPipe, made it possible to identify and track skeletal keypoints in real time (Jo & Kim, 2022). These are the models that estimate the space position of the large joints so that the angles of the joints, the posture of the limbs and the symmetry, stability and balance can be assessed completely. In the situation dissimultaneously of Yoga, the evolutionary process permitted systems to surpass a simplistic categorization of the yogic postures to a numerical analysis of the quality of the alignment.

Deep learning was the milestone in the history of AI-powered Yoga systems. Recent trends in convolutional neural networks have allowed the learning of automated features with no engineered features whatsoever; of on naturally occurring image and video data with significant generalization to a variety of conditions. Poseestimation systems such as OpenPose enabled the ability to find and monitor key points of skeletons in a very high spatial resolution in real-time. The moulds allowed the researchers to examine the size of the joint angles, limb placement, centre of gravity, and symmetry of the posture content more than ever before by the estimation of the two dimensional or three-dimensional location of the major joints.

With the output of pose-estimation researchers could then compare practitioner postures against reference templates and calculated the measures of deviation and gave corrective feedback (Labde, 2025). The effects of real time visual overlays were the increased use of skeletal stick figures or alignment marks as a feedback modality. These systems were found to be more useful in the process of detection of more complex asanas and dynamic flowings that allowed more interactive and engaging experiences of practice.

Despite these advances that occurred, new challenges emerged due to the vision based approaches. Deep learning models are extremely data-consuming and require large and diverse data to become generalized (Bansal et al., 2024). The datasets that are specific to yoga are still quite few and those have relatively few participants, a variety of poses, and cultural variety. In addition, pose-estimation reduces in floor-based postures, supine postures.

2.3 Artificial Intelligence in Yoga

Artificial intelligence in yoga is a discipline that involves the combination of AI and yoga (Melchert 2017). The concept of Yoga as Artificial Intelligence is progressive in its history, which was also exposed to the same progress in the area of the computer vision and machine learning, wearable sensing technologies, and digital wellness ecosystems (R. Yadav et al., 2023). The world has begun to take preventive health and mental wellbeing into consideration, and up to this point, scholars and even practitioners are eager to utilize smart systems and make Yoga more accessible, personalized, and quantified (A. Garg, 2025). The initial scholarly concern of this area was made possible through the general research of human activity recognition where Yoga poses was considered as the predictable pattern of a coordinated human conduct. The findings of this early study were mostly regarding the possibility of automatically computing the Yoga poses, and crudely speaking in offering a control based corrective feedback mechanism through the application of computational methods. Although these were not large-scale studies, there was the basis of the future development to ensure that there was an opportunity to quantify and examine the physical facets of the Yoga practice to a certain degree and apply the AI-based approaches (Omotoyosi Adeyemi, 2024).

Recent findings of AI-assisted Yoga, among other digital-based health-related apps, have swept like a wildfire including pose recognition, virtual fitness apps and affective health interfaces (S Bhat et al., 2023). The first ones dealt with deep learning-based recognition of postures with the use of convolutional neural networks that were trained on sets of images of significant asanas. The deep learning yoga posture recognition systems are indicatively based on PoseNet or custom CNNs, which have more than 94-99 percent classification accuracy on small pose sets, and automated asana classification is possible in online teaching settings. Typically, these approaches work with 2D images or video sequences, using skeletal keypoints or spatial depth cues to distinguish among a small number of predefined yoga postures.

Subsequent studies have introduced more advanced architectures, such as two-stream CNN and temporal models, which combines spatial and temporal features or learn spatiotemporal patterns from video data. The CNN with five poses and the twin feature fusion is proved to reach an accuracy of about 97 percent (Aydın, 2024), which can be regarded as one of the advantages of the local joint-based information and the whole body structure. Other models such as the YoNet propose to use target CNN models, which can be trained to operate with smaller yoga images and yield a higher accuracy than the generic ResNet or Inception models, as they are more sensitive to the pose-specific qualities. Similar workflow are implemented with pose-estimation framework such as MediaPipe, MoveNet, and OpenPose to capture body keypoints. These keypoints are then analyzed using either traditional machine-learning methods or deep-learning models to recognize and correct yoga postures.Such Systems are commonly integrated into real-time coaching application to provide instant feedback to users(S. Garg et al., 2023).

Besides classification, several papers that address feedback and coaching directly exist. DeepYoga and other systems have on-screen arrows and text clues to help with alignment, to reduce the chances of injury and approximate the feedback of the instructor in distant places. The pose detection and correction is applied to mobile or web apps with voice instructions, progress monitoring, and in certain cases vital-sign monitoring to produce a cheaper and easy-to-use virtual trainer e.g. the project YogAI and the project: AI Yoga Trainer (Milind Gayakwad, 2024). The other recent article concerning the topic of Harnessing the potential of AI in yoga therapy further transposes the ideas to clinical practice elaborating how biosensor based wearables can be applied to support remote monitoring of posture, breath, and physiological conditions during therapeutic yoga sessions (Sinha and Sinha, 2024).

Simultaneously, the techniques of the suggested multimodal solution offer the background applications of the tasks of cross-cutting work in affective computing and estimation of the human pose. Human pose estimation reviews are generalizations of the 2D/3D keypoint methods and applications methods, where such issues as occlusions, floor, and all body forms are observed (Luo et al., 2018). Digital mental health Narrative reviews of affective computing are concerned with emotion-sensitive, closed-loop systems, which adjust interventions to physiological and behavioural prompts, introducing opportunities and ethical issues that are specifically relevant to AI-Yoga integrations. Finally, but not the least, there are new conceptual works which directly relate to the synergy of AI and yoga practices and outline future systems that would integrate pose recognition, personalization and safety monitoring without contradicting yogic postulates of balance, non-harming and self-awareness.

The initial phases of Yoga using AI were anchored on the massive classical image processing algorithm and multi-manual features extraction. The methods that were utilized to isolate the video frames were the background subtraction, contour analysis, edge detection and silhouette modeling, which were performed to capture all the video frames in low-resolution or non-moving. Joint positions were informally chosen by rule of thumb instead of being chosen by learned descriptions, by recognition of the posture by geometric descriptors and by manual drawing (as proportions of each limb, the angles of the body parts, and symmetry of shapes). The support vector machines, the k-nearest neighbors, the decision trees and the hidden Markov models were traditional classifiers that were used to map these features to a list of pre-assigned Yoga poses. Though these strategies were idea wise good, it was very sensitive to the environmental conditions. The difference in the lighting, camera position, dresses and complexity of the background, and type of practitioners bodies contributed to identification of a huge difference in precision. As such, they could not be applied to a real-life situation as they were not reliable enough and would only be applicable using controlled conditions in a laboratory.

The other weakness of the initial systems was that they focused on the fixed posture recognition. Practice of yoga does not replace a location and taking a moment to another asana, breathing in a rhythm, and focus in its various forms are not passive processes. Majority of the early models did not consider continuity of time, balance or dark errors that can affect efficiency and safety. Feedback was brief and even in binary form like correct and incorrect posture even though no action was provided and very minimal context was provided. As such, these systems were more related to the posture-checking systems as compared to the intelligent instructional assistant that could be employed to facilitate meaningful learning.

The use of pose-estimation models also led to the focus of the simple classification of the postures being put on the qualitative measurement of the quality of the posture. On the basis of illustrating the practitioners and calculating the deviations and alignment rankings, AI-based Yoga systems started the stated comparison based on the observation of the professionals. Live visual feedback was now a customary practice and skeletal overlays, alignment lines and corrective cues were overlaid on live video streams. This kind of auxiliary feedback contributed to the interaction of the users and allowed the practitioners to make instant changes, which resemble the features of the teaching in the real world. In addition, time-dependent modelling networks such as recurrent neural networks and time-sensitive convolutional neural networks were also presented to input movement sequences and switch between asanas, where flow, stability, and consistency could be provided during practice.

The vision-based AI systems have not been deprived of their eternal problems despite all this massive advances. The sticking out parts of the self, loose garments, exterior items may lead to blockages of great joints and degradation of the accuracy of pose-estimation. It is also complicated by the fact that skeletal motions cannot be appropriately followed using the method because the cameras and the viewing angles cannot be well calculated especially where the home background contains few cases where the established setups are present. The other complexity added can be variability of practitioner morphology such as height, elasticity, age, physical capability. Besides, the pose estimation models tend to fail in the presence of floor based poses, supines or prones and meditative poses where the little motion patterns as well as the poor view of the joints are present. These limitations show the natural flaws of being led by visual means only in their attempt to evaluate Yoga practice on its wholeness.

As a response to the inefficiency of the vision-based method, scholars started to believe in the usefulness or even alternative sense-making modalities offered by wearable sensor technologies. Wearable sensors normally entail accelerators, gyroscopes, magnetometers and inertial measurements which audio-tape fine-grained movements and body posture of body parts. These sensors are quite time sensitive and not quite environment sensitive like in terms of the light or the background clustering. Thus, wearable-based systems have been discovered to be especially suitable in the study of dynamic sequences, determining the variations of the asanas, and recording the minor variations of the movement patterns (Rajgure & Patidar, 2025).

Not wanting to debate as to the shortcoming of the unimodal systems, current research is increasingly concentrating on multimodal systems which integrate visual information, physiological information and contextual information to provide a more holistic view of Yoga practice. These systems are aimed at measuring not physical alignment only but also internal physiological states, which are associated with relaxation, the regulation of the focus and stressed states. Particular emphasis has been placed on breathing analysis as the pranayama is the most important component of Yoga. Scientists have investigated these methods of measuring the breathing rate and depth by observing the chest motion using video, thermal scanning of nasal respiration, respiratory belts and pressure sensors. This is achieved by using such measures in the evaluation of the breath control, the coordination with the movement and the level of the relaxation during the practice.

Other parameters considered are the heart rate and heart rate variability which are also measures of the activity of the autonomic nervous system. Variations in the heart rate variability are widely recognized as a form of stress, as well as a recovery action and an emotional regulation proxy. Observing such indicators during the Yoga sessions, the AI systems will be capable of inferring the change in physiological arousal and relaxation state, Yoga offers information about the mental and emotional impact of Yoga practices. Other scholars have included physiological data in addition to posture analysis to be able to differentiate between mechanically appropriate but tense postures and postures performed with assistance of appropriate relaxation and breath consciousness (Sinpichetkorn et al., 2022).

Despite the fact that multimodal systems may be viewed as a substantial move towards the holistic assessment, a lot of work that has been done to date remains rather fragmentary and exploratory in nature. Majority of the implementations are proof-of-concept prototyping with small datasets over a short period. Personalization is not very personalized, unlike adaptive learning, but it is defined by determined thresholds or determined rules. Such systems are thus incapable of accommodating the individual differences, in the long run evolution or changing practitioner goals. Because longitudinal data is also not available, the AI models are also limited in their ability to learn the shifting tendencies of behavior, mood, and incapability over time.

In parallel to the physical and physiological analysis, there have been remarkable improvements in the methods of displaying the emotions, stress and mental conditions in the human beings. Combination of multimodal signals (facial expressions, speech patterns, micro-expressions, heart rate variability, and breathing dynamics) has been made possible by the use of machine learning and more specifically deep neural networks and transformer-based models (Lu et al., 2024). The models are also more successful in detecting emotional valence, engagement, fatigue and stress in the fields of mental health monitoring, adaptive learning systems and workplace wellbeing applications.

In spite of all the innovations, the use of affective computing in relation to Yoga is relatively underdeveloped. The apps of commercial meditation or mindfulness training are premised on self-reported mood scale or simplistic measures of stress, and fail to best combine the identification of the emotional state with the instruction of physical practice. Emotional intelligence in AI based Yoga systems has little to do with postures adjustment, breathing instructions or time of the session. This alienation is opposed to one of the most important pillars of Yoga which considers the integration between physical exercise and mental and emotional thinking. There will be the dehumanization of Yoga and the transformation of it into a purely mechanical process without references to the inner, transformative essence of the experience in case of the lack of integration.

2.4 Research Gap

Although the available literature has gone a step further to devise AI-assisted posture detection and some basic corrective feedback, the emotional or cognitive state of the practitioner is not much addressed. Most systems are devoted to physical alignment alone and some form of personalization is offered but only in regards to fixed rules or threshold-based modifications. The breathing patterns, the manner of behavior or user adaptation over the long run have not had much integration, and the multimodal approaches are not integrated. It is important to note that the recent studies do not lean towards the philosophy of yoga such as balance of the body, breathing, and mind to be incorporated into the decision-making system of artificial intelligence models.

Our proposed contribution will help to bridge this gap as it will incorporate posture recognition, affect conscious analytics, and yogic principles in a single adaptive framework that can offer real time, comprehensive, and well-being.

3. PROPOSED METHODOLOGY

The introduction of Artificial Intelligence into Yoga involves moving away of the conventional fitness tracking. Yoga is a science that deals with the combination of body, breathing and mind. The AI Yoga system methodology, therefore, needs to be multimodal, physiologically sensitive, and based on the ethical and philosophical foundations of Yoga Sutras (Fig. 1)

3.1. User Yoga Practice: The Dynamic Input Source

The series of data stream of the methodology of the practice yoga that is considered permanent is the time. This cannot be claimed in yoga since it is not discrete (as in the case of weightlifting), vinyasa (flow), and asana (steadiness). During this stage, the user will specify the purpose of the practice whether restorative, strength-based, or meditative. This purpose establishes the benchmarks of the AI expectations. The environment in which the practice would be used is also taken into account: the lighting, the mat orientation, and the ambient noise level are among the variables, which the next layers are to take into account to guarantee the sound data integrity.

3.2. Multimodal Data Acquisition: Capturing the Whole Self

In order to go beyond the scope of 2D pose detection, our approach uses a Multimodal Data. Acquisition strategy. This will make sure the inner state of the practitioner is captured in conjunction with their physical geometry.

Visual (Camera)

The activity of the practitioner is captured using high-definition RGB cameras. In an advanced implementation, depth sensors (LiDAR or Time-of-Flight) can be utilized in order to generate a 3D point cloud of the body, where the AI can also see the user even around the user themselves and identify the slightest deviations on the sagittal plane and transverse plane.

Physiological (HRV and Breath)

Yoga is essentially a technique of the Autonomic Nervous System (ANS). We utilize PPG (photo plethysmography) through wearables or even remote PPG (real-time PPG analysis) (of micro) changes in skin color through the camera to measure the Heart Rate Variability (HRV). The HRV is high and is a sign of a dominant parasympathetic condition (calm/recovery). The reduction in HRV in a simple pose can be a sign of physical or mental stress.

Optional Wearables (IMU)

MUs consist of data on angular velocity and acceleration. They play a vital role in balancing poses (e.g. Vrksasana or Tree Pose) where one can notice micro-tremors, as a sign that soon the user will lose the balance. ankles- in most cases not seen by a 30fps camera- could be the message that user is almost losing balance.

Figure 1. Multimodal AI-Driven Framework

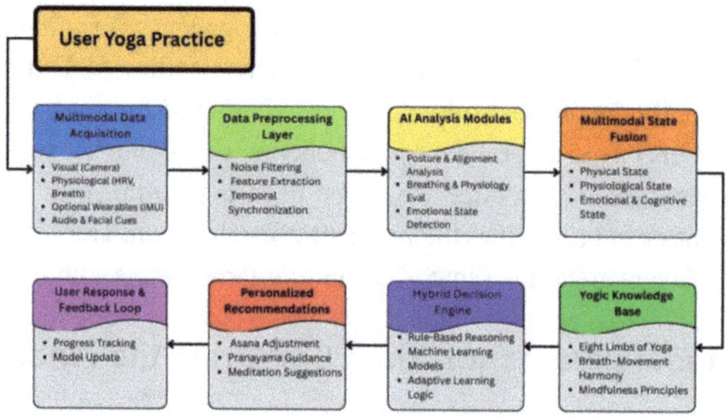

Audio & Facial Cues

Natural Language Processing (NLP) controls the sound of the breath (e.g., the "Ujjayi" ocean. breath). At the same time, Computer Vision models examine facial landmarks to recognize what is referred to as micro-expressions complaints or aggression, which are crucial in safety and psychological feedback.

3.3. Data Pre-Processing Layer: From Raw Data to Insights

Raw data is inherently messy. Preprocessing layer is the digital refinery and where noise is separated out of signal.

Noise Filtering

To remove a low-light jitter, conditions, we apply Kalman filters to remove visual keypoints. Physiological signals subjected to band-pass filtering in the attempt to remove artifacts produced by motion artifacts (sudden motion), ensure that the data on heart rate are clean.

Feature *Extraction*

It is not millions of pixels that we feed to the AI: it is some features that we are extracting.

Joint Angles: Computation of the 180 extension of the elbow in Adho Mukha Svanasana.

Center of Mass (CoM): Approximation of the balance point of the user with respect to his/her base of support.

Spectral Analysis: Volume: Transforming uncoded sound of breathing into frequency fields to identify breath depth.

Temporal Synchronization

This is the most technical step. The system should provide that the lung which is the visual one. Growth is equalized to the inhale of audio and the spike of the heart rate in physiological. We utilize clock synchronization protocols to synchronize these heterogeneous streams of data into one "State<lhumanl>clock synchronization protocols to synchronize these heterogeneous data streams into one "State Vector" every mill second of the practice.

3.4. AI Analysis Modules: The Specialized Detectors

This layer comprises autonomous neural networks, each of which is trained in a particular area of human performance.

Posture & Alignment Analysis

The architectures involved in the convolutional neural networks (CNNs) or Graph Convolutional are used. The system scans the skeleton of the user into networks (GCNs). It opposes it to conformity.

Anthropometric" Biomechanical Ideals" in the presence of individual anthropometric variations (e.g., a<|human|>Adjustment to individual anthropometric variations (e.g., a<|human|>In the presence of individual anthropometric variations (e.g., a<|human|>Adjustment to individual anthropometric variations (e.g., a<|human|>Adjustment to individual anthropometric variations (e.g., a man with longer femurs will naturally sit in a squat differently than one with shorter ones)

Breathing & Physiology Evaluation

This module is concerned with Pranayama aspect. It examines the question of thoracic vs. abdominal breathing. The AI follows the rhythm of the using Recurrent Neural Networks (RNNs) or LSTMs. breath, whether the user is unintentionally holding his or her breath (Kumbhaka) or not mistake for beginners.

Emotional State Detection

This module determines the arousal valence quadrants of the user with a complex of facial features and heart rate. The objective is to discover the flow state- a psychological. difficulty and ability.

3.5. Multimodal State Fusion: Constructing the Digital Twin

At this point, the process shifts to a synthesis rather than an analysis. State fusion creates a standardized electronic identity of the user. The late fusion techniques are applied in this fusion process, and the results of the earlier modules are used are condensed into a high-dimensional vector denoting:

Physical Position: (e.g. Warrior II, left knee inward 5).

Physiological Condition: (e.g., High cortisol levels, shallow breathing, etc.).

Thinking Skills: (e.g., Low attention, turned head).

Such a holistic perspective prevents the AI against making dumb corrections. For example, if a user's alignment is weak since they are physically wiped out (identified through physiology), system. will not simply say to them, "straiten the leg; it will indicate a rest.

3.6. Yogic Knowledge Base: The Philosophical Anchor

Classical AI is out of context. Also, a symbolic knowledge base is incorporated in our methodology with thousands of years of yogic wisdom

The Eight Limbs (Ashtanga)

The system is programmed according to the hierarchy of Yoga. It realizes that Asana (physicality) is a precursor of Pranayama (breath) and Pratyahara (sensory withdrawal). The knowledge base has such rules like: Sthira-sukham asanam (The pose should be steady and comfortable). In case the sensors sense that there is no Sthira (shaking) knowledge base overrides the "perfect geometry" goal.

Breath–Movement Harmony

The Vinyasa "grammar" is found in the database, it consists of knowing what movements need an inhalation (expanding/rising) and which must have an exhalation (contracting/descending).

Mindfulness Principles

It has got focal points (Drishti). In case the camera notices that the user is not keeping his eyes focused, the system refers to knowledge base to issue a reminder on internal focus.

3.7. Hybrid Decision Engine: The Reasoning Core

The system has a commander; the hybrid decision engine. It uses a dual-pathway methodology of establishing the optimal course of action.

- Rule-Based Reasoning (Safety First)
- Hard-coded rules act as a safety net.

Rule: Compression of the cervical spine to more than a degree, in a shoulder stand, should be a "stop-command deportment". These are not to be compromised and founded upon sports science and physiotherapy.

Machine Learning Models (Personalization)

Rules are safe, whereas ML is sophisticated. The AI gets to learn the Personal Best of the user after weeks of training. It relies upon Reinforcement Learning to identify the most effective forms of feedback (audio or visual) to which the user reacts.

Adaptive Learning Logic

This reasoning moderates the Ideal Yoga Pose and the Reality of the User at the moment. It applies the fuzzy logic to determine whether a correction is distorting or not necessary. When the user is in an intensive state of mind, the engine can prevent adjusting small adjustments to maintain the psychological state.

3.8. Personalized Recommendations: Intelligent Intervention

The recommendations are the "Prescriptions" generated by the decision engine. There are three types of domains:

- Asana Adjustment: Space adjustments. 15 degrees of rotating the back foot in making your hip safe.
- Pranayama Instructions: Corrections in breathing. Slow your breathing twice as much as your inhalation in order to decrease the heart rate.
- Meditation Recommendations: Psychic transitions. Bring back to you the feeling in your fingertips.

These are not generic, but the state fusion is the result. One may suggest: Since your heart beats fast, you may go without the next Sun Salutation and rest in Childs Pose five times.

3.9. Real-Time Feedback Interface: Closing the Loop

The interface is modeled after Calm Technology. It tries to convey the information without breaking the internalization of the user (Pratyahara).

Visual Cues

Augmented Reality (AR) is used in place of a complicated UI. A ghost image or a shadow teacher can be displayed on a screen or in AR glasses and it will indicate the user where their limbs should be. The joint safety has instant non-verbal feedback in color-coded overlays (Green/Yellow/Red).

Audio Guidance

We utilize spatial audio. In case the left arm of the user is too low, the corrective voice command will appear as that of the left side of the room. The tone is adjusted to be relaxing, resembling the sound of a human speaker.

Optional Haptic Feedback

To users with smart clothes, a small vibration on the shoulder (right side) can be used to indicate the drop of the shoulder without noise and image distractions. This is the least obtrusive type of feedback.

3.10. User Response & Feedback Loop: The Evolution of the System

The final one is the recursive feedback loop. This causes the practitioner to develop the AI. The system records every one of the sessions not as some type of checkbox of achievement, but as a chart of fertile information in terms of improvements. It adopts the alterations in Range of Motion (ROM), duration of a stable position and respiratory control.

Model update

It is at this stage that the AI Self-Corrects. The model built for the user: When the user has not attained some degree of depth in a posing, due to an injury sustained in the past, then the AI modifies its Ideal Model according to that specific user. The world model Anonymized data is reinvested into the cloud (federated learning), and used to help the AI to understand the behaviour of different body types in yoga, upgrading the system to all the users worldwide. Digital yoga is an emerging trend that has significantly influenced the future of yoga practice.

3.11 Conclusion

The future of digital yoga Digital yoga is a new trend that has impacted a lot on the future of yoga practice. It is an indication of the transition between the concept of AI as a tool and AI as an ally. This model is an outline of a secure, customized, and strongly conventional electronic practice through the acceptance of the multimodality of Yoga that is the union of the physical, the physiological and the philosophical. We will have a more predictive analytics in the future where the AI will be able to predict fatigue and avoid it even before it can result in an injury and generate Yoga that will be tailored to the given emotional and physical state of the user.

4. RESULT ANALYSIS

With this detailed methodological approach, the given system will show how AI can be integrated with yogic philosophy in a coherent and holistic manner to help promote person-wide wellbeing. The approach brings together the four multimodal sensing, adaptive intelligence, emotional awareness, and philosophical grounding, creating a basis of AI systems that supplements, rather than supplants, human understanding of oneself and development.

4.1 Dataset Description

Participants and Sessions

i. 24 adult participants (20-40 years old) with previous yoga experience (6-18 months) were selected to participate in a 4-week training program with the proposed AI-Yoga prototype.

ii. All the participants had participated in 12 guided sessions (3 per week, 3540 minutes) that resulted in 288 recorded sessions and some 86 hours of multimodal practice data Asana set and protocol.

iii. There were twelve asanas that were generally taught, and a certified yoga instructor was consulted; they included standing poses, balancing poses, forward bends, backbends, and restorative poses (e.g., Tadasana, Trikonasana, Virabhadrasana II, Vrksasana, Adho Mukha Svanasana, Bhujangasana).

iv. Every session had a standard order (warm up, standing flow, balancing, floor work, short relaxation) to maintain the continuity of vinyasa, but to enable the possibility of repeating the analysis across subjects.

Multimodal Signals and Annotation

i. Vision: Front -facing RBG camera at 30 fps (1280x720) full body motion; 2d body skeletal keypoints were subsequently obtained based on a typical pose-estimation model as per the methodology section.

ii. Physiology: A wrist wearable was used to record heart rate and inter-beat time, which could be used to estimate HRV; a soft chest strap was also used by selecting the sessions with a valid breathing rate and comparing it to the audio-based estimations.

iii. IMU: A subset of the 14 participants was monitored using any lower back and dominant ankle IMU before and during balancing and transition, which measured the angular velocity and acceleration.

iv. Affective labels: At the beginning and end of every session, the participants were asked to complete a brief perceived stress scale and a valencearouselforeffect-selfreport; the instructors were asked to identify the instances of apparent discomfort or instability during practice.

4.2 Experimental Results

Table 1 presents pose recognition and alignment.

Table 1. Pose recognition and alignment

Metric	Vision-only model	Vision + IMU model
Number of asanas	12	12
Overall classification accuracy (%)	88.4	94.1
Macro F1-score (%)	86.8	92.7
Mean joint-angle deviation (°) – all asanas	9.4	4.5

From Table 1, we conclude:

i. The combination of IMU data and camera-based keypoints increased macro F1-score to 92.7% instead of 86.8%. and decreased the mean joint-angle deviation to 4.5o instead of 9.4o, which means that multimodal sensing can improve pose recognition and assessment of an alignment perspective as per the proposed architecture.

ii. The greatest improvements were realised in balancing poses like Vrksasana, where IMU signals detect micro-instabilities that cannot be determined through the use of 2D video, and this justifies the optional use of IMU in the methodology.

Table 2 presents real-time corrective feedback.

Table 2. Real-time corrective feedback

Asana	Baseline deviation (°)	With feedback (°)	Relative reduction (%)
Trikonasana	9.8	4.1	58.2
Virabhadrasana II	11.2	5.0	55.4
Adho Mukha Svanasana	8.5	3.9	54.1
Vrksasana	10.7	5.2	51.4

From Table 2, we conclude:

i. In representative asana, the visual and textual feedback in real-time lessened the misalignment in the joint angles by approximately 51-58% and this assertion validates the statement that the system is an intelligent tutor and not a passive tracker.
ii. According to the instructors, the users were able to fix the typical mistakes (e.g., the knee collapsing in Virabhadrasana II, the trunk tilting in Trikonasana) within 2-3 feedback loops, indicating that AI-based directions can be similar to the ones given to beginner-intermediate students.

Table 3 presents the physiological and emotional outcomes of the experiment.

Table 3. Physiological and emotional outcomes

Measure	Pre-program mean ± SD	Post-program mean ± SD	Change (%)
Resting heart rate (bpm)	79.4 ± 6.2	73.1 ± 5.8	−7.9
HRV (RMSSD, ms)	32.8 ± 9.5	42.6 ± 11.1	+29.9
Perceived stress (1– 40 scale)	27.3 ± 4.9	19.1 ± 5.2	−30.0
Positive affect (1–5 Likert)	2.9 ± 0.6	3.7 ± 0.5	+27.6

From Table 3, we conclude:

i. The participants experienced approximately 30 percent improvement in the HRV and an 8 percent reduced heart rate at rest over 4 weeks. This is related to the theme of the chapter, which is autonomic regulation with the help of combined asana and pranayama exercises that are controlled by AI.
ii. Stress-related scores as measured self-reported dropped by about 30 points and positive affect rose by almost 28. This brings out the fact that emotional-based feedback may assist in the physical relaxation of the person and personal well-being in general, not just biomechanical correction.

iii. The participants experienced an approximate 30 percent increase in HRV and a decrease of 8 percent in resting heart rate in a span of 4 weeks. This is in line with the emphasis by the chapter in autonomic regulation using integrated asanas and pranayama that are monitored by AI.
iv. The stress levels according to self-report decreased approximately by 30 and positive moods rose by approximately 28. This emphasizes the fact that information that accounts feelings can be used in the process of physical relaxation and the overall wellbeing of an individual, which is not limited to biomechanical correction.

Table 4 presents affective adaptation and user experience.

Table 4. Affective adaptation and user experience

Aspect	Result (mean ± SD)
Sessions triggering adaptation (%)	41.3 ± 9.2
User-rated relevance of adaptations (1–5)	4.1 ± 0.7
Overall system usability (SUS, 0–100)	81.5 ± 8.4

From Table 4, we conclude:

i. The affective module altered the designed sequence of the sessions by introducing restorative poses in the cases when it perceived high arousal and negative emotions (approximately 40% of the sessions). This indicated how the framework had incorporated emotional state in AI decision making.
ii. The adaptive changes were helpful as rated by the participants, who rated them at 4.1 out of 5, and perceived the overall usability as high with a System Usability Scale score of approximately 82. This implies that the human-centered system, which is holistic, will enhance engagement and compliance over traditional digital yoga tools as listed in the literature review.

Table 5 presents emotional state-aware adaptation of the experiment.

Table 5. Emotional state-aware adaptation

Detected state (valence– arousal)	Typical sensor pattern	System adaptation example
High arousal, negative valence	Elevated HR, low HRV, tense facial muscles	Down-regulates sequence, inserts restorative asanas and lengthened exhalations
Low arousal, negative valence	Flat affect, slow movement, shallow breathing	Shortens static holds, adds energizing standing flow with synchronized inhales
High arousal, positive valence	Smiling, energetic movement, stable HRV	Maintains challenge level, offers optional progression to more advanced variations
Low arousal, positive valence	Relaxed posture, stable HRV, soft gaze	Reduces corrections, prioritizes meditative cues over biomechanical precision

From Table 5, we conclude:

i. The affective module was able to provide real-time modifications of sequences with the use of the multimodal signals being mapped into the quadrants of valence and arousal. This methodology did not resort to general solutions and it provided a practice intensity relevant to the existing condition of the practitioner.
ii. The inclusion of restoring postures and increased proportions of exhalation were the results of addition, in cases where high-arousal negative states were detected, for example. This was in line with the yogic teaching such as sthira-sukham asanam where emphasis is laid on comfort and safety rather than the intensity of poses.

Table 6 presents Ablation study of modalities.

Table 6. Ablation study of modalities

Configuration	Inputs used	Macro F1-score (%)	Mean alignment error (°)
Vision only	RGB + 2D keypoints	86.8	9.4
Vision + Physiology	RGB + HR/HRV + breath rate	89.5	7.9
Vision + IMU	RGB + 2 IMUs	92.7	4.5
Vision + Physiology + IMU	RGB + HR/HRV + breath + 2 IMUs	93.4	4.1

From Table 6, we conclude:

i. The integration of physiological indicators increased macro F1 and minimized the error of alignment when using vision only. This indicates that the internal state information assists the model to distinguish between similar poses.
ii. The entire multimodal system performed the highest scores, and it was only slightly better than the vision and IMU. This reinforces the fact presented in the chapter that fusion is primarily useful in overall evaluation, and not simply pose classification.

Table 7 presents user-perceived impact by dimension.

Table 7. User-perceived impact by dimension

Dimension (1–5 Likert)	Mean ± SD
Physical alignment understanding	4.3 ± 0.6
Breath awareness	4.5 ± 0.5
Emotional regulation during practice	4.0 ± 0.7
Overall confidence in self-practice	4.2 ± 0.6

From Table 7, we conclude:

i. Breath awareness was also reported to improve more than any other area by the users. This reinforces the concept of the framework that pranayama and HRV feed standards should be combined rather than musculoskeletal form alone.
ii. The concept that the AI system can be a supportive digital companion is supported with the help of high ratings of understanding alignment and confidence in self-practice. It promotes human teaching without substituting it.

5. CONCLUSION AND FUTURE WORK

The integration of artificial intelligence and yoga is the potential paradigm of rethinking digital health as a highly holistic and human-centered ecosystem. The chapter has suggested that the current AI-based wellness applications are either more focused on a disembodied form of mindfulness or more focused on biomechanical fitness indicators, leaving out the interdependence of body, breath, mind and behavior that the school of yoga philosophy asserts. The proposed framework instead introduces AI as a smart assistant that can intelligently assist in self-awareness, safety, and long-term wellbeing in-place of the traditional practice or human educators.

The multimodal framework described in the present chapter shows how computer imaging, physiological detection, affective computing, and behavioural analytics can be integrated into one digital twin of the practitioner. Detailed understanding of autonomic balance is indicated by breathing and heart rate variability, posture and alignment analysis can tell the angle of joints and their stability, self-reports and facial expressions can help to understand the emotional state in a subtle manner, and longitudinal behavioural data can record adherence patterns and learning patterns.

This integrative approach makes the system go beyond the simple classification of pose to a context-dependent feedback, adaptive and that accords with the tenets of yogic principles, namely, which are sthira- sukham asanam (steadiness and comfort), non-harming, and mindful evolution.

The key element in the framework is a hybrid decision engine, which integrates a symbolic knowledge base of yoghic nature with data learning. Although the customization is subject to experience, this mixed method ensures that safety limits and ethical values remain the top priorities. Whereas machine learning modules learn at a slow pace on how each practitioner best reacts to either visual, audio or minimal feedback, rule-driven components can be invoked instantly in problematic circumstances. As time passes, the system will have the capacity to become more adaptive to the intensity, proposing appropriate asana and pranayama adjustments, and even knowing when it is more beneficial to remain in a meditative state instead of working towards an ideal geometry.

There are also important implications to education, clinical rehabilitation, workplace wellness, and home practice besides technical innovation highlighted in the chapter. It can make high-quality guidance more accessible to everyone without turning practitioners into automatons or abstract indicators and create valuable data that researchers and clinicians can use; with an appropriately designed AI-Yoga system, the phrase is an overstatement, but it remains true that it is indeed democratic. Nevertheless, the work also presents such unresolved issues as algorithmic bias, cultural sensitivity, data privacy, and the necessity of conducting comprehensive longitudinal studies that would evaluate both the psychological, social, and spiritual outcomes along with the physical ones.

Future Work

The future development of AI–Yoga systems can further be developed in terms of technical, empirical, and ethical. dimensions. Technically, it is noteworthy that future researches should produce less-weighty, commodity-based hardware-compatible models that can be dependable with a single camera or crude wearables and that would fill the gap between low-resource clinics and common homes and studios by making guidance based on multimodality accessible. More advanced methods of fusion might also be taught individualized personalized "signatures of stress, attention and tiresomeness, lessening the dependence on generic thresholds and enhancing real-time adjustment.

To test physical, psychological and behavioural outcomes among different age groups, abilities, and different cultures, including those with chronic pain, anxiety, or cardiometabolic risk, large-scale, longitudinal studies are required, which are empirically valid to determine results. The comparison of AI-assisted practice with unguided home practice and classes guided by an instructor would help to define the areas where technology can be of most use and where the process of human guidance can never be substituted.

6. LIMITATION

Although the proposed AI-Yoga framework is rich in concepts and conceptually comprehensive in its methods, there are several major limitations that should be noted. To start with, instead of prolonged and wide-ranging clinical trials, much of the conversation is founded on theoretical models and demonstrative experiments. It is not clear how the benefits of the system can be generalized and robust without being thoroughly validated in an empirical manner and on a diversity of demographics, health conditions, and practice settings. Small or homogeneous sample can overestimate performance and also misrepresent such issues as body-type differences, cultural backgrounds and yoga practice.

Second, the framework would be based more on multimodal sensing composed of cameras, wearables, physiological monitors, and, potentially, depth or IMU sensors. This strategy can reduce accessibility and scalability. Such advanced hardware will be beyond the means of not all users to use at home or in clinical settings where resource availability is limited. Also sensor configuration, calibration and maintenance brings usability issues that may reduce over time usability especially among those seeking a simple, easy to use wellness app. Such discrepancy between the ideal research settings and the field realities can restrain implications of the field.

Third, the integration of affective computing and state fusion is associated with accuracy, bias, and comprehension issues. The determination of emotions via facial expression, voice, or body language is always a matter of uncertainty and prone to cultural bias. The wrong classification of emotions can result in making wrong corrections, including simplifying the complex state of emotions or encouraging the undesirable patterns of behavior. The hybrid decision engine is also, by combining ambiguous machine learning models with symbolic rules. This complicates the objective of giving clear explanations to the users and practitioners in case of recommendation or safety interventions.

Fourth, there is a high privacy, consent and data management concern in the use of continuous monitoring, biometric data, and behavioral analytics. Without good security and anonymization and morals, sensitive data regarding physical capacities, emotional statuses, stress levels, and training routines may be misused. Developing and cultivating trust will involve effective communication, data control in the hands of the user and compliance with regulatory standards that keep on evolving.

Lastly, there is a more severe constraint to take into account. Yoga is a practice of experience and self-reflection and is orientated towards self-inquiry, non-attachment and internal change. To strengthen a performance-oriented attitude or develop a dependency on outsourced feedback, any technology that measures and enhances performance may be used. Otherwise, AI systems can end up encouraging people to lose track of inner understanding, commercialize spiritual tendencies, or shadow conventional teachers and traditions. These problems contribute to the necessity to engage in the consistent dialogue with yoga experts, ethicists, and practitioners. We need to make sure that the philosophical and ethical origins of Yoga are non-expressed with technological advances.

REFERENCES

Agarwal, V., Sharma, K., & Rajpoot, A. K. (2022). AI based Yoga Trainer - Simplifying home yoga using mediapipe and video streaming. *2022 3rd International Conference for Emerging Technology, INCET 2022*. DOI: 10.1109/INCET54531.2022.9824332

Anand Thoutam, V., Srivastava, A., Badal, T., Kumar Mishra, V., Sinha, G. R., Sakalle, A., Bhardwaj, H., & Raj, M. (2022). Yoga Pose Estimation and Feedback Generation Using Deep Learning. *Computational Intelligence and Neuroscience, 2022*, 1–12. Advance online publication. DOI: 10.1155/2022/4311350 PMID: 35371230

Anuradha, T., Krishnamoorthy, N., Kumar, C. S. P., Prasad, L. V. N., Chunduru, A., & Moorthy, U. (2024). A Method for Specifying Yoga Poses Based on Deep Learning, Utilizing OpenCV and Media Pipe Technologies. *Scalable Computing: Practice and Experience, 25*(2), 739–750. Advance online publication. DOI: 10.12694/scpe.v25i2.2590

Aydın, V. A. (2024). Comparison of CNN-based methods for yoga pose classification. *Turkish Journal of Engineering, 8*(1), 65–75. Advance online publication. DOI: 10.31127/tuje.1275826

Bansal, R., Sharma, R., Jain, P., Arora, R., Pal, S., & Vishal, . (2024). DeepYoga: Enhancing Practice with a Real-Time Yoga Pose Recognition System. *Engineering. Technology and Applied Science Research, 14*(6), 17704–17710. Advance online publication. DOI: 10.48084/etasr.8643

S Bhat, G., IL, S., Hariharan, H., & Swamy, H. (2023). Yoga AI Assistant with ReactJS. *INTERANTIONAL JOURNAL OF SCIENTIFIC RESEARCH IN ENGINEERING AND MANAGEMENT, 07*(04). DOI: 10.55041/IJSREM18878

Bolpagni, M., Pardini, S., & Gabrielli, S. (2024). Human centered design of AI-powered Digital Therapeutics for stress prevention: Perspectives from multi-stakeholders' workshops about the SHIVA solution. *Internet Interventions : The Application of Information Technology in Mental and Behavioural Health, 38*, 100775. Advance online publication. DOI: 10.1016/j.invent.2024.100775 PMID: 39314669

C, H. B., & Kumari, S. (2022). Yoga Ai Trainer Using Tensorflow. Js Posenet. Www .Irjmets.Com @*International Research Journal of Modernization in Engineering, 503*(02).

Chatterjee, A., & Prinz, A. (2022). Personalized Recommendations for Physical Activity e-Coaching (OntoRecoModel): Ontological Modeling. *JMIR Medical Informatics*, *10*(6), e33847. Advance online publication. DOI: 10.2196/33847 PMID: 35737439

Garg, A. (2025). AI-Powered Yoga Pose Detection and Feedback System. *International Journal for Research in Applied Science and Engineering Technology*, *13*(5), 6224–6230. Advance online publication. DOI: 10.22214/ijraset.2025.70581

Garg, S., Saxena, A., & Gupta, R. (2023). Yoga pose classification: A CNN and MediaPipe inspired deep learning approach for real-world application. *Journal of Ambient Intelligence and Humanized Computing*, *14*(12), 16551–16562. Advance online publication. DOI: 10.1007/s12652-022-03910-0

Gayakwad, M. (2024). Web Service Implementation "AI Yoga Trainer Using Human Pose Estimation" for Web Discovery. *Journal of Electrical Systems*, *20*(2), 2167–2176. Advance online publication. DOI: 10.52783/jes.1985

Jo, B. J., & Kim, S. K. (2022). Comparative Analysis of OpenPose, PoseNet, and MoveNet Models for Pose Estimation in Mobile Devices. *TS. Traitement du Signal*, *39*(1), 119–124. Advance online publication. DOI: 10.18280/ts.390111

Joshi, A., Kiran, R., Raj, R., & Agarwal, R. (2020). Stress management of engineering students through deep breathing yoga. *International Journal of Work Organisation and Emotion*, *11*(2), 140. Advance online publication. DOI: 10.1504/IJWOE.2020.110625

Kirk, M. A., Taha, B., Dang, K., McCague, H. P., Hatzinakos, D., Katz, J., & Ritvo, P. (2022). A Web-Based Cognitive Behavioral Therapy, Mindfulness Meditation, and Yoga Intervention for Posttraumatic Stress Disorder: Single-Arm Experimental Clinical Trial. *JMIR Mental Health*, *9*(2), e26479. Advance online publication. DOI: 10.2196/26479 PMID: 34499613

Kumar Mishra, A., & Mishra, K. (2024). YogaSiddhi: AI-Powered Pose Analysis using MoveNet for Yoga Refinement. *Article in International Journal of Computer Applications, 186*(8).

Labde, S. (2025). Real Time Yoga Posture Recognition and Correction. *International Journal for Research in Applied Science and Engineering Technology*, *13*(5), 4922–4927. Advance online publication. DOI: 10.22214/ijraset.2025.71355

Chi Lee, A. (2018). Acceptance and Commitment Therapy: A Mindfulness and Acceptance-Based, Value-Driven Approach to Human Flourishing With Christian Spirituality Considerations. *Acceptance & Commitment Therapy: A Mindfulness & Acceptance-Based, Value-Driven Approach to Human Flourishing With Christian Spirituality Considerations*.

Loughnane, C., Laiti, J., O'Donovan, R., & Dunne, P. J. (2025). Systematic review exploring human, AI, and hybrid health coaching in digital health interventions: trends, engagement, and lifestyle outcomes. In *Frontiers in Digital Health* (Vol. 7). DOI: 10.3389/fdgth.2025.1536416

Lu, H. B., Ma, R. C., Yin, Y. Y., Song, C. Y., Yang, T. T., & Xie, J. (2024). Clinical Indicators of Effects of Yoga Breathing Exercises on Patients with Lung Cancer after Surgical Resection: A Randomized Controlled Trial. *Cancer Nursing*, *47*(3), E151–E158. Advance online publication. DOI: 10.1097/NCC.0000000000001208 PMID: 36716034

Luo, C., Chu, X., & Yuille, A. (2018). Orinet: A fully convolutional network for 3D human pose estimation. *British Machine Vision Conference 2018, BMVC 2018*.

Mitsea, E., Drigas, A., & Skianis, C. (2023). Digitally Assisted Mindfulness in Training Self-Regulation Skills for Sustainable Mental Health: A Systematic Review. In *Behavioral Sciences* (Vol. 13, Issue 12). DOI: 10.3390/bs13121008

Narayanan, M. M. (2025). Yoga AI - Integrating artificial intelligence with yoga and therapy for personalized healthcare. *Annals of Geriatric Education and Medical Sciences*, *11*(2), 68–70. Advance online publication. DOI: 10.18231/j.agems.2024.015

Narimani, M., & Naeim, M. (2025). Artificial intelligence in mental health: Integrating opportunities and challenges of multimodal deep learning for mental disorder prevention and treatment. *Annals of Medicine and Surgery (London)*, *87*(9), 5757–5761. Advance online publication. DOI: 10.1097/MS9.0000000000003624 PMID: 40901142

Omotoyosi Adeyemi, J. (2024). Enhancing Elderly Wellness through AI-Powered Yoga and Exercise Support Systems. *Biomedical Journal of Scientific & Technical Research*, *54*(4). Advance online publication. DOI: 10.26717/BJSTR.2024.54.008579

Rajgure, E. G., & Patidar, R. (2025). The Scientific Analysis on Effective Yoga Posture Recognition Techniques. *Lecture Notes in Electrical Engineering, 1211 LNEE*. DOI: 10.1007/978-981-97-4359-9_13

Saini, N. (2024). Exploring The Synergy Of Ai And Yogic Practices: A Future-Oriented Approach For Holistic Wellbeing. *Educational Administration: Theory and Practice*, *30*(5), 15412–15420. DOI: 10.53555/kuey.v30i5.9101

Sinha, N., & Sinha, R. K. (2024). Harnessing the Potential of Artificial Intelligence in Yoga Therapy. *International Journal of Yoga*, *17*(3), 242–245. Advance online publication. DOI: 10.4103/ijoy.ijoy_124_24 PMID: 39959510

Sinpichetkorn, T., Chaunchaiyakul, R., Yang, A. L., Lin, Y. Y., & Masodsai, K. (2022). Effects of Vinyasa Yoga on Stress and Health Benefits in Office Workers. *Journal of Exercise Physiology Online*, *25*(4).

Swain, D., Satapathy, S., Acharya, B., Shukla, M., Gerogiannis, V. C., Kanavos, A., & Giakovis, D. (2022). Deep Learning Models for Yoga Pose Monitoring. *Algorithms*, *15*(11), 403. Advance online publication. DOI: 10.3390/a15110403

Talaat, A. S. (2023). Novel deep learning models for yoga pose estimator. *SN Applied Sciences*, *5*(12), 341. Advance online publication. DOI: 10.1007/s42452-023-05581-8

Vivekanandha, S., Bhargavi, N., Srinivas, I., Harika, K., & Raju, K. (2025). Enhancing Yoga with AI: Accurate Pose Detection Using Machine Learning. *International Journal of Computer Techniques, 12.*

Yadav, R., Chaudhary, R., Istwal, S., Kumar, S., Bohra, M., & Kumar, I. (2023). Development of an AI Enabled Yoga Posture (Aasans) Prediction System Using Deep Neural Network Model. *2023 International Conference on Sustainable Emerging Innovations in Engineering and Technology, ICSEIET 2023.* DOI: 10.1109/ICSEIET58677.2023.10303586

Yadav, S. K., Singh, A., Gupta, A., & Raheja, J. L. (2019). Real-time Yoga recognition using deep learning. *Neural Computing & Applications*, *31*(12), 9349–9361. Advance online publication. DOI: 10.1007/s00521-019-04232-7

Yenishettil, S., Karajkhede, G., & Panat, L. (2024). Virtual Yoga Teacher with AI Model for Yoga Posture Correction for Good Health. *2024 ITU Kaleidoscope. Innovation and Digital Transformation for a Sustainable World, ITU K, 2024*, 1–8. Advance online publication. DOI: 10.23919/ITUK62727.2024.10772930

Chapter 4
Artificial Intelligence-Based Yoga Guidance and Health Monitoring System

Meenakshi Sajwan
http://orcid.org/0009-0009-0437-5575
G.B. Pant Institute of Engineering and Technology, Pauri, India

Pushkar Praveen
http://orcid.org/0000-0002-3288-5128
G.B. Pant Institute of Engineering and Technology, Pauri, India

Hannan Akhtar
http://orcid.org/0009-0000-6874-8785
G.B. Pant Institute of Engineering and Technology, Pauri, India

Tanishq Negi
G.B. Pant Institute of Engineering and Technology, Pauri, India

Kriti Uniyal
G.B. Pant Institute of Engineering and Technology, Pauri, India

Agya Ram Verma
G.B. Pant Institute of Engineering and Technology, Pauri, India

ABSTRACT

The integration of traditional yoga practices with modern Artificial Intelligence technologies represents a significant step toward advancing holistic healthcare solutions. Yoga, with its long-standing history of promoting physical, mental, and emotional well-being, gains enhanced effectiveness when combined with AI-driven systems capable of real-time analysis, personalized feedback, and continuous health monitoring. The proposed Artificial Intelligence Based Yoga Guidance and Health Monitoring System demonstrates how intelligent technologies such as computer vision, machine learning, and wearable sensors can transform conventional fitness practices into interactive and data-driven experiences. By ensuring accurate posture guidance and monitoring vital health parameters, the system addresses

DOI: 10.4018/979-8-3373-7625-7.ch004

both preventive and corrective aspects of healthcare. This is particularly relevant in today's fast-paced world, where lifestyle-related health issues are increasingly common (Esteva et al., 2019).

A. INTRODUCTION

Modern human life has quietly made sedentary habits and chronic stress in the normal days. One may argue that sedentary life and increased stress have become a normal part of the lives of modern urban dwellers. Their consequences – reduce mobility, stress on the cardiovascular system, disrupted sleep, and increased anxiety – have been thoroughly studied. Regular engagement in yoga helps to counter all of these factors. It is not just an exercise trend since decades of research prove its ability to improve both motor functions and overall physical condition. The role of yoga as an ancient activity that helps one improve physically, mentally, and spiritually is well recognized by Field T. (2016). Even though there are numerous benefits associated with yoga, some people face problems with doing it correctly due to lack of professional guidance. However, the problem here does not lie in knowledge about yoga practices' advantages but in access to professional instruction and accuracy while doing the exercises. When practicing on one's own, people tends to build up their bodies incorrectly, this leads to painful sensations later. As discussed by Thoutam A. et al. (2022), incorrect posture while engaging in yoga can lead to pain and muscle damage as well as other long-lasting health problems, thus defeating the purpose of the exercises themselves. Such a situation presents the issue at hand.

Fortunately, thanks to modern technological developments, the analysis of body movements has become feasible with the use of computer vision and machine learning techniques. For example, Borthakur et al. (2023) showed how extracting data on joint angles and using it to train classifiers helped in recognizing yoga postures with an accuracy of more than 91%. Furthermore, following up on previous findings, Desai and Mewada (2023) investigated the efficiency of using BlazePose to recognize yoga postures, analyzing the postures using 33 keypoints per frame. Altogether, recent advances in technology indicate the readiness of AI-powered yoga postures recognition solutions to be implemented in practice. Finally, the modern wearable sensors record heart rate, blood oxygen levels, respiratory rate, and physical activity data, which could be processed by ML techniques to detect health conditions (Shajari et al., 2023).

In the context of yoga, this is important because both exertion intensity and cardiovascular responses can differ greatly from person to person and even between individual sessions. Sabry et al. (2022) point out that ML-enabled wearables offer particular value in settings where continuous passive data collection through clinical means is impractical — which describes home-based yoga practice almost exactly. Currently used systems usually separate these two processes and do not integrate them into one complete system that can provide real-time corrective feedback for unsupervised yoga training. In this regard, this chapter aims to introduce a novel AI-Based Yoga Guidance and Health Monitoring System which will combine real-time yoga posture estimation along with continuous physiological data monitoring. Specifically, the yoga tracking system will be used to provide postures correction feedback, monitor effort levels, and provide real-time feedback while training at home without any guidance (Irfan et al., 2025).

B. RELATED WORK

In general, the adoption of technology in healthcare and sports has significantly progressed during the last ten years owing to innovations in AI, sensor technologies, and data analysis. In particular, AI, including machine learning and computer vision, shows promise in evaluating human actions and providing feedback. In this way, smart health technologies become feasible and can help users to maintain physical fitness and monitor well-being in real-time mode (Esteva et al., 2019).

Yoga as a health-oriented practice has already been widely analyzed in connection with its positive effects on both physical and psychological well-being (Tripathi, S. M., 2021). In this regard, studies show that regular practice can positively impact stress levels, heart health, flexibility, and balance (Woodyard, 2011). Meanwhile, typical yoga classes usually involve experienced trainers who monitor learners' movements and correct their mistakes if any. In this case, without a trainer's supervision, users can make errors that do not allow them to receive all the benefits of yoga or even harm their health. As a result, recent researches examine the application of computer vision approaches to pose estimation that is the basis for building AI-based yoga guidance solutions. Such technologies as OpenPose and MediaPipe provide the possibility to detect body keypoints from images or video frames and analyze users' movements (Cao et al., 2017). Many researchers have come up with systems that compare user poses to ideal models and provide suggestions for improvement. It means that there is an opportunity to create virtual trainers that simulate real training classes and offer appropriate instructions for learners.

In addition to that, there is a trend to wear monitoring devices for tracking vital signs and users' activities. They can track various physiological characteristics of users, including heart rate, physical activity, and sleeping cycles. In general, wearable technology has been successfully implemented in mobile apps to help with preventative healthcare (Patel et al., 2012). The combination of wearable sensors and algorithms of AI makes it possible to conduct in-depth data analyses and generate appropriate recommendations for improving health. On the one hand, some projects try to implement health monitoring features in their yoga guidance technologies. In particular, there are smart fitness solutions that estimate postures and also track users' health status. On the other hand, many systems lack personalization, feedback accuracy, or health monitoring parameters integration, which means that there is still a gap in the field. It can be stated that previous researches reveal great opportunities offered by AI to revolutionize the field of fitness. At the moment, there are some challenges concerning pose detection and health tracking.

C. RESEARCH GAP

Though numerous papers have already explored the combination of AI, wearable sensors, and yoga poses, there are still several significant gaps in the development of an effective guidance and health monitoring system. Namely, most existing systems focus on posture detection or monitoring health parameters but not both. Thus, for example, Patel and Sharma (2022) explore AI-assisted posture correction; yet, their solution does not include health tracking or personal recommendations based on it. The study by Kumar et al. (2021) focuses on health tracking and recommends solutions for building health tracking models with wearable sensors but lacks intelligent adaptive yoga guidance features and real-time corrective feedback.

The second gap noted in previous studies is the lack of adaptive yoga guidance based on the current state of users. Most existing solutions provide standard yoga poses and training instructions regardless of health status, age, level of stress and/or fatigue, and any other individual factors. As was noted by Singh and Verma (2023), current AI-powered solutions use little to no algorithms for adapting poses and creating customized sessions according to results of training. It negatively impacts the effectiveness of yoga practice as a means of preventive healthcare and may lead to reduced user motivation in the long run. Finally, few systems can provide real-time correction and monitoring at once. Although some camera-based detection models prove efficient in laboratory settings, they often underperform in real-life situations due to the variety of interfering factors including light conditions, sensor errors, and complicated poses. As was shown by Rao et al. (2020), many vision-based detection methods cannot offer real-time correction and tend to be delayed while monitoring poses. Besides, wearables-based solutions often have synchronization issues between physiological readings and activity detection.

Another gap lies in the fact that most current solutions focus only on basic physiological parameters (heart rate, temperature, etc.). In addition to them, stress levels, oxygen saturation, breathing rate, fatigue rate, and even emotional condition need to be monitored for better effectiveness. As was noted by Chatterjee and Bose (2022), predictive healthcare analytics and yoga therapy combination remains underexplored despite high potential in preventive healthcare. Last but not least, privacy, affordability, and availability of devices are also important. Most of current solutions are costly and require significant computing capacity, which makes them unavailable for the majority of people. Furthermore, privacy is often a concern in dealing with sensitive health data retrieved from wearables. Secure, accessible, and inexpensive solutions should be designed in order to increase AI-based healthcare adoption rates, especially in developing countries. As was noted by Gupta et al. (2021), it is particularly relevant now. Therefore, it is important to develop an effective solution that would include pose detection, health monitoring, and intelligent feedback to promote yoga practice as preventive care. To achieve the aim, the current study seeks to build an Artificial Intelligence–Based Yoga Guidance and Health Monitoring System combining pose recognition, adaptive guidance, continuous health monitoring, and feedback provided based on AI algorithms and wearable technology. Table 1 below provides an analysis of previous studies in the area in terms of five criteria. Though most studies can detect poses, no system currently offers all four aspects mentioned above (real-time vital monitoring included). Adaptive recommendations based on individual characteristics remain an issue too.

Table 1. Comparison of Existing Systems with Proposed Work

References	Pose Detection	Vital Monitoring	Corrective Feedback	Adaptive Learning
Kishore et al. (2022)	MediaPipe	None	Yes	No
Thoutam, V. A. et al. (2022)	OpenPose + MLP	None	Yes	No
Upadhyay et al. (2021)	BlazePose + XGBoost	HR	Yes	No
Desai & Mewada (2023)	BlazePose	None	Yes	no
Borthakur et al. (2023)	BlazePose + XGBoost	None	Yes	No
Proposed System	BlazePose + XGBoost	HR, SpO_2, Temp	Yes	Yes

D. SYSTEM ARCHITECTURE

The proposed system is designed with a scalable architecture, where computer vision algorithms, machine learning techniques, and health monitoring via wearable sensors have been combined. Posture training and health monitoring are not considered separately but as a part of a single system, whose modules interact among each other providing efficient data transfer throughout the whole process.

1. **Data Acquisition Layer:** This layer is the first stage of processing in the system. A camera records video demonstrating users in specific yoga positions, and sensors measure physiological characteristics such as heart rate, body temperature, and SpO_2. The combination of two types of information allows getting a more comprehensive picture of user activities (Patel et al., 2012).
2. **Preprocessing Module:** At this stage, raw data are converted into a form suitable for subsequent analysis. In particular, the images are captured, resized, and normalized as input to the pose model. Sensor data are also subject to preprocessing in order to eliminate distortions and noises.
3. **Pose Estimation and Analysis Module:** This module is the central element of data processing. The pose recognition framework used is BlazePose, as it is known for high accuracy of detecting 33 body key points in each frame that allow constructing a skeleton in real-time. As noted by Desai and Mewada (2023), this number of points is enough to catch even small differences between postures. After the user's pose is calculated, a comparison with pre-saved reference poses from the system's database takes place according to an algorithm based on XGBoost classifier, which evaluates postures, balance, and joints and identifies the deviations from the correct one. According to Borthakur et al. (2023), angle-based feature extraction system ensures classification accuracy above 91%.
4. **Feedback and Guidance Module:** In case there is something wrong with the pose that needs to be corrected, the user receives immediate guidance. The instruction can be delivered by several means, including videos, text comments, and verbal commands (e.g., about excessive knee bend or incorrect arm position). The goal of this module is to provide the user with the same feedback an experienced trainer would do.
5. **Health Monitoring Module:** At the same time when the pose is being analyzed, another module constantly monitors users' physiological metrics by employing data from wearable sensors. This information is then analyzed using machine learning models to evaluate user's condition. According to Shajari et al. (2023), AI-powered sensors are perfectly fit for such tasks in non-clinical settings. The user is informed if any abnormalities in heart rate and signs of exhaustion are detected.
6. **Data Storage and Management:** A central database collects all the information related to user posture, health parameters, and exercise history allowing tracking his/her progress. Cloud storage expands system scalability and makes it available on any device (Kumar et al., 2025).

7. **Personalisation and Recommendation Engine:** Personalization develops over time. Using the results of previous exercises and performance, machine learning algorithms make adjustments to tasks' complexity, posture, and feedback. According to Sabry et al. (2022), machine learning adjustment is beneficial especially in cases such as personal yoga session at home with high levels of individuality.
8. **User Interface Layer:** Design of the interface is aimed at simplicity and user-friendliness regardless of his/her technological skills. Currently, the interface presents users with data on their poses, health indicators, previous exercises, and progress reports, thus helping keep them focused on the activity itself rather than software.

As a whole, these eight modules form a system designed to overcome the shortcomings mentioned in the problem statement. Additionally, the modularity of the system makes sure that each module can be improved separately from the rest of the application, especially considering the fact that both AI models and sensors are constantly evolving.

E. YOGA POSE RECOGNITION USING AI

Recognition of yoga poses using artificial intelligence (AI) is based on the integration of AI, computer vision, and machine learning techniques to identify and analyze yoga poses in real-time. This process makes use of a camera to record bodily movements while analyzing anatomically critical points such as shoulders, elbows, hips, and knees in order to recognize yoga poses. The popular AI architectures like MediaPipe, OpenPose, and TensorFlow enable pose recognition and postural analysis. These technologies provide users with real-time feedback, help correct posture mistakes, and ensure better learning experience when practicing yoga. They prove to be especially useful when dealing with beginners who practice yoga at home.

A variety of yoga poses are used to train machine learning models, thus ensuring high-quality results regardless of lighting, inter-individual differences, and camera position. Although there are certain difficulties connected to using AI for pose recognition, modern technologies are still making great strides in terms of their effectiveness. Thus, Recognition of Yoga Poses Using AI can be considered a pioneering method which makes yoga practice smart, safe, and convenient.

1. Pose Estimation Techniques (Skeleton Mapping)

Pose estimation is one of the basic building blocks in identifying yoga poses. In this regard, it involves detecting significant anatomical points such as joints and limbs from images or video feeds. Modern computer vision techniques leverage deep learning algorithms to come up with a skeletonized version of the human body which is referred to as skeleton mapping. The Figure given below shows the different types of yoga position for skeleton mapping.

Figure 1. Cobra Pose

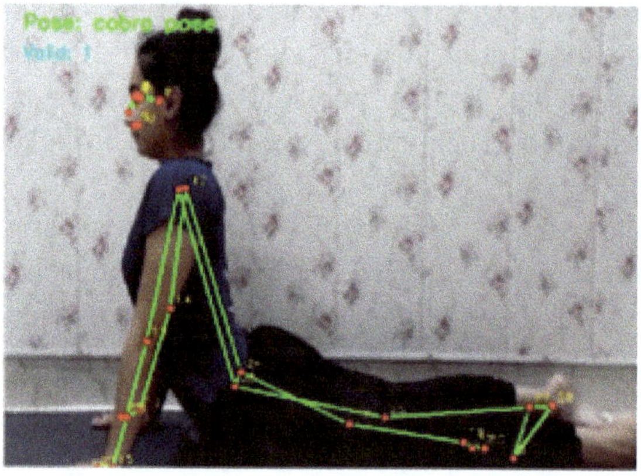

Figure 2. Uttanpadasana (Raised Leg Pose)

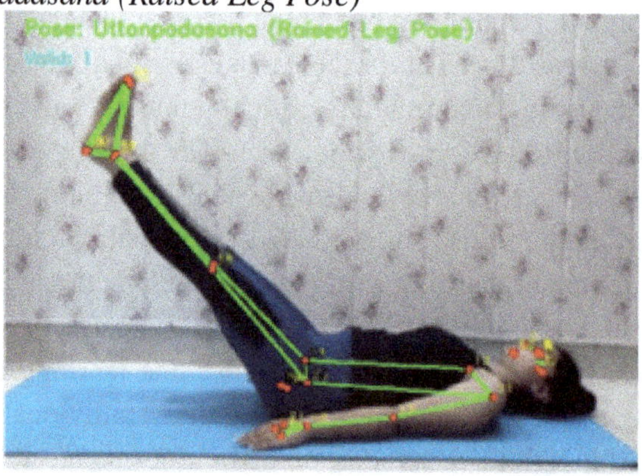

Figure 3. Paschimottanasana (Seated Forward Bend)

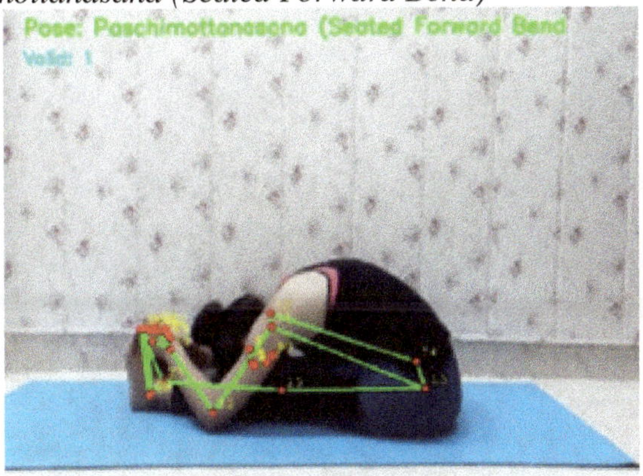

Figure 4. Ubhaya Padangusthasana (Both Big Toe Pose)

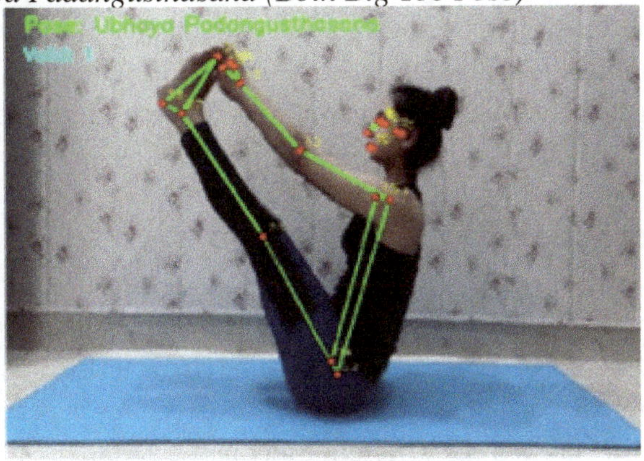

Figure 5. Adho Mukha Svanasana (Downward - Facing)

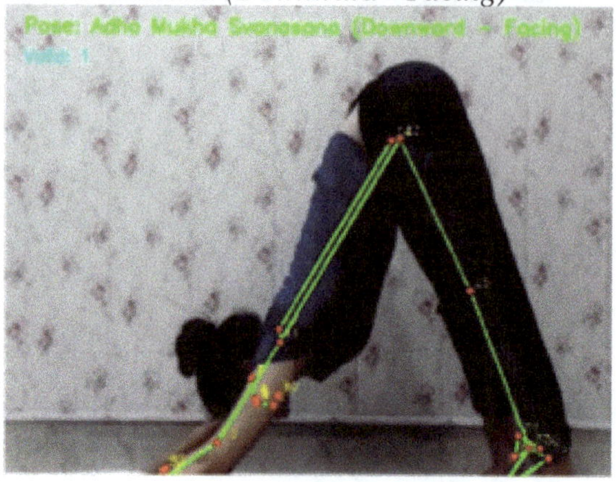

The well-known architectures that are used widely for pose estimation include OpenPose and MediaPipe, among others. Such platforms are capable of detecting specific landmarks on the human body and encoding them in such a way as to define the overall posture of the individual (Cao et al., 2017). Through the technique of skeleton mapping, the complicated input image is converted into coordinates, which is useful for posture analysis.

2. Feature Extraction

After developing the skeletal structure, the next step is feature extraction. This step entails the extraction of the most distinguishing characteristics using the obtained keypoints to model the yoga pose accurately. These features generally include joint angles, the distance between the different body parts, and the relative positions of various body parts. For example, joint angles made at the hips, knees, and ankles could help in determining the correctness of certain postures such as the lunges or squats. Also, the position of the legs and arms would give a sense of how balanced the particular pose is. The extracted features help the computer model to understand the data in a more coherent way (Zhang et al., 2020). More sophisticated models might even have temporal features while dealing with a sequence of poses.

3. Model Classification (CNN, LSTM, and Hybrid Models)

Once relevant features are extracted, various classification models are used to recognize the type of the yoga pose and check whether it was performed correctly. The following models based on deep learning can be used in this phase:

- Convolutional Neural Networks (CNNs): As an efficient technique for processing images and extracting spatial features, CNNs are useful in the case of yoga pose recognition where they can be directly used on pictures or heat maps created by pose estimation methods in order to classify postures. The use of this method is very efficient when dealing with pictures (LeCun et al., 2015).
- Long Short-Term Memory Networks (LSTMs): LSTMs refer to a type of recurrent neural network that is used for analyzing sequences of data. Due to the ability to deal with time series, this model is helpful in the case of sequential information like yoga pose sequences. The use of this algorithm allows capturing temporal relationships and detecting transition errors (Hochreiter & Schmidhuber, 1997).
- Hybrid Models (CNN + LSTM): This hybrid approach uses both CNNs and LSTMs in order to incorporate both spatial and temporal features. In this way, CNNs process pictures one by one while LSTM analyzes their sequence.

It should be noted that classical algorithms, such as SVM or random forest, can also be used as classifiers for extracted features. However, they are usually less accurate because of the inability to detect more complicated relations. In that case deep learning models generally provide higher accuracy due to their ability to learn complex patterns from large datasets. In the study published by Parashar et al. (2023) presented a refined methodology of yoga pose detection by adopting the integration of MediaPipe and MoveNet in the context of deep learning. The researchers increased accuracy and efficiency by developing such an AI-driven detection system.

4. Pose Evaluation and Feedback

Once the pose is categorized, the next step in the system is the evaluation of the correctness of the pose through comparison with pre-defined standards. If there are any abnormalities in the joint angles and body posture of the user, then the user is given corrective feedback.

F. HEALTH MONITORING INTEGRATION

By incorporating the function of health monitoring in an AI-assisted yoga guidance system, it significantly enhances the capabilities of the system through merging health monitoring and physical exercises. The health monitoring section of the system helps to continuously monitor various health-related information such as heart rate, stress level, and breathing pattern. The process of analyzing the data obtained from the above health information helps the system in guiding the users on how to perform yoga poses safely and effectively.

1. Heart Rate Monitoring:

The tracking of heart rate is one of the most essential aspects of health monitoring in fitness systems since it provides useful information regarding the activity of the cardiovascular system and assists in measuring the intensity of exercise performed by individuals. Modern wearable devices like smartwatches or fitness bands can monitor heart rate using PPG sensors.

In regard to yoga practices, heart rate measurements help estimate whether the individual performs exercises at the appropriate rate. Considering that yoga involves controlled and moderate activities, any rapid heart rate increases or other anomalies could be attributed to the fact that an individual either exerts too much effort or breathes improperly during exercise (Patel et al., 2012).

2. Stress Detection

Stress detection forms an essential component of health monitoring systems. Current AI-based systems utilize physiological parameters such as HRV, skin conductivity, and respiration rates to measure stress. Indeed, changes in HRV have been shown to be highly correlated with the body's stress response (Zhu et al., 2024).

By implementing stress detection features, the state of mind of the individual practicing yoga will become evident. In cases where increased stress levels are detected, relaxation-based poses and breathing activities may be recommended. Such an approach is congruent with the objective of yoga, as yoga aims at both physical and psychological well-being (Selye, 1956). Increasingly, wearable sensors and AI have been used together to perform affective state monitoring (Kumar & Srivastava, 2023).

3. Breathing Pattern Analysis

Breathing serves a crucial purpose in yoga, and the proper breathing techniques or pranayama are critical for gaining maximum benefit from it. The system has the ability to track breathing patterns using wearable sensors, chest belts, or even computer vision technology which tracks movements of the thorax. Inadequate or improper breathing is likely a sign of poorly executed yoga or low effectiveness of the exercise. By tracking the breathing patterns, the system will be able to advise the user to maintain a healthy breathing rhythm. This, in addition to improved respiratory rate, improves concentration and helps relax (Jerath et al., 2015).

4. Purpose of Health Monitoring Integration

The primary purpose of health monitoring as part of yoga guidance system implementation is to develop an overall and personalized solution for health improvement. Unlike conventional yoga teaching systems that focus solely on postures, the proposed system combines considerations of physical exercise and physiological processes within the body. Integration of health monitoring helps in:

- Providing personalized guidance based on the current health condition and level of fitness of a user.
- Ensuring safety through detection of deviations in physiological parameters and preventing overtraining.
- Improving user's performance by helping maintain proper heart rate and breathing.
- Promoting preventive healthcare practices through detection of early signs of stress or fatigue.

In this way, the proposed system enables the use of modern AI technologies within the framework of yoga practices to create an integrated and adaptive system for health improvement. By introducing such health monitoring into a regular yoga guidance system, we transform it from an elementary tool to a more sophisticated and intelligent health and wellness platform. This means that besides correct performance of exercises, users can monitor their physiological condition.

G. WORKING METHODOLOGY

Working methodology of the Artificial Intelligence Based Yoga Guidance and Health Monitoring System explains the process of interaction between the system and user, posture analysis, provision of feedback on real time basis along with simultaneous health monitoring. This system operates in a repetitive cycle in order to provide accurate guidance and effective health monitoring. The workflow of the methodology can be easily understood through the flow chart shown in figure 6.

1. User Session Initialization

The first step involves the initiation of the yoga practice through a web-based application or a mobile phone. At this stage, the user can choose the specific yoga practice or exercise that matches his/her fitness path. The data concerning the posture required, health parameters, and other thresholds can be obtained from the system.

Individual data such as age and fitness levels can be taken into consideration too. (Esteva et al., 2019).

Figure 6. AI-based yoga guidance and health monitoring system

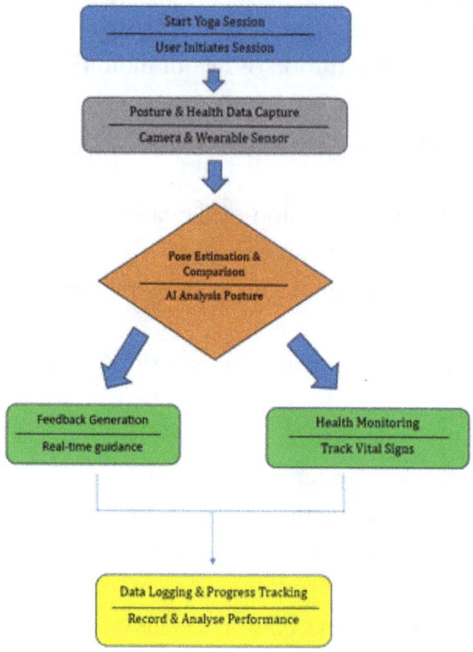

2. Posture Capture

Once the process starts, the system operates the camera to capture real-time video or images of a person performing yoga poses. Synchronously, physiological data such as heart rate and breathing patterns are collected by wearable devices. To ensure continuous monitoring of the user's movements, captured visual data is processed frame by frame.

3. Pose Estimation and Comparison

The data is passed through a pose estimation model, which identifies key body points and generates a skeletal representation of the user's posture. These key points are analysed with stored relevant data representing ideal yoga poses.

The model measures variables such as body alignment, joint angles, and positional differences to differentiate how closely the user's pose matches the ideal pose. Any differences are identified and quantified, allowing the system to evaluate the precision of the performed posture (Cao et al., 2017).

4. Feedback Generation

The comparison that serves as the basis of the system allows generating feedback aimed at helping the user. The feedback can be transmitted to the user via various means, such as visual signs, sounds, or even written directions. If the body posture of a user is not correct, the system can provide him/her with feedback, such as "adjust your body position." Thus, feedback generation will ensure the correction of mistakes and improve efficiency.

5. Monitoring Physiological Parameters

Apart from posture, some other health-related parameters will also be monitored by the system. These parameters will include a heart rate, breathing frequency, and the intensity of exercises. In case there are abnormalities in terms of these factors (a high heart rate or abnormal breathing), the system can generate an alarm or suggest adjusting certain variables, such as reducing intensity or resting. In this way, the safety of the exercise will be provided.

6. Data Storage and Analysis

The data generated in terms of accuracy of postures and other parameters are stored in order to monitor a user's performance and his/her progress. Moreover, using the accumulated data, the machine learning model can make certain suggestions aimed at improving the results in the future.

Specifically, one way to do this would involve progressively increasing task complexity or suggesting postures related to a particular level of progression of the user. Taken together, the outlined approach combines posture recognition and health tracking in order to create a fun and interactive yoga coaching application.

Figure 7. Proposed AI based System

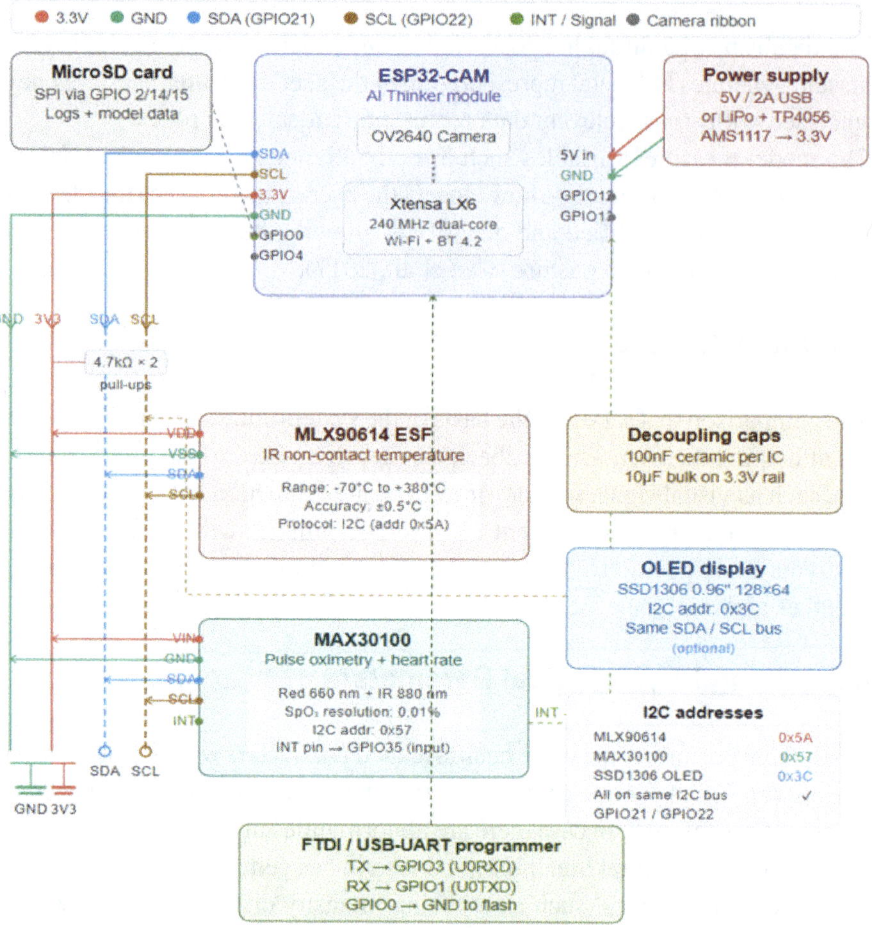

H. ADVANTAGES OF THE PROPOSED SYSTEM

The AI-based Yoga Guidance and Health Monitoring System present many benefits in bringing together the principles of yoga and modern technology. Additionally, it improves the user's experience, provides greater access, and makes yoga practice safer and more effective.

1. Personalized Yoga Training

However, the main benefit of the system is that it allows for individualized yoga classes. Unlike previous approaches that have used general recommendations for all, the current AI system takes into account personal requirements based on the analysis of correct postures, physical activity, and health-related habits. Based on such information, it is possible to suggest different types of yoga poses, as well as change their complexity. This way, better learning opportunities are provided (Esteva et al., 2019).

2. Reduced Dependency on Instructors

This system helps in minimizing the dependency on professional trainers. There is a good population who cannot join physical classes because of time, money, or location problems. The application of artificial intelligence technology allows them to get instant feedback and improve without having their instructors around all the time. As such, yoga becomes easy but very accurate and safe when it comes to executing yoga poses.

I. FUTURE SCOPE

This technology-based yoga and health monitoring system is only the first step towards an evolutionary transformation. With advancement in technology, this system will transform itself into a complete automation system that will support an individual's fitness regime very closely.

1. Immersive Training with AR and VR:

The model combines immersive techniques in tandem with guidance via displays instead of being solely based on the latter. In particular, the use of Virtual Reality (VR) technology allows one to train in yoga in a serene virtual setting guided by a personal tutor. Moreover, the usage of Augmented Reality (AR) makes it possible to guide users' bodies for posture adjustment. The outlined methodology helps ensure greater interactivity, precision, and effectiveness of the whole process.

2. Emotion-Aware System:

In yoga techniques, mental and physical elements have been taken into account; thus, emotion detection becomes a constituent of the system development. The use of face expressions and voice tones to detect the user's emotions (stress, fatigue, or anxiety) leads to offering the user some advice on breathing and yoga techniques that may result in his/her relaxation.

3. Personalized Therapy and Well-being:

The system goes beyond regular health-related apps in terms of offering personalized advice to individuals. By means of constant analysis of the health metrics and performance level of the user, the system operates as a digital physical therapist. If the system detects that someone has back pain or stress, it recommends certain exercises and yoga classes aimed at treating these health issues or stabilizing health indicators (e.g., blood pressure).

4. Interaction with Medical Doctors:

The system works as a link between home exercises and medical doctors because the health information gathered can be sent to healthcare professionals and used in remote control of patients' health status. It will be particularly convenient for those patients whose rehabilitation process is going on but who do not have access to health facilities (Tunduny & Shibwabo, 2026).

5. Adaptive and Self-Learning Technology:

In addition to that, the system continuously evolves through an adaptive learning algorithm. User input is analyzed and used as a basis for improvements. Therefore, the system continuously changes training programs according to user progress, which can be achieved through increased intensity or reduced speed.

J. CONCLUSION

Combining traditional techniques used in yoga with artificial intelligence offers a major innovation in the field of health and wellbeing research. Traditionally, yoga seeks to synchronize cognitive and bodily functions; through the use of AI, a balance of these functions is attained more easily because the personalization process is simplified.

This is achieved by using AI tools like health monitoring in providing feedback about how the body responds to exercises. In addition to improving exercise technique, the system provides suggestions based on the analyzed data that match the users' needs. The application of sophisticated AI technology like computer vision and intelligent sensors shows how digital platforms can be used to find solutions beyond simply tracking the activities of users. Apart from the benefits that users will gain, the impact on society from the use of this technology is very significant. The problem of inadequate healthcare due to remoteness can be tackled through encouraging physical activities and identifying health problems in time.

REFERENCES

Borthakur, D., Paul, A., Kapil, D., & Saikia, M. J. (2023). Yoga pose estimation using angle-based feature extraction. *Health Care, 11*(24), 3133. DOI: 10.3390/healthcare11243133 PMID: 38132023

Cao, Z., Simon, T., Wei, S. E., & Sheikh, Y. (2017). Realtime multi-person 2D pose estimation using part affinity fields. In *Proceedings of the IEEE Conference on Computer Vision and Pattern Recognition (CVPR)* (pp. 7291–7299). https://doi.org/DOI: 10.1109/CVPR.2017.143

Chatterjee, S., & Bose, R. (2022). AI-based predictive healthcare monitoring using wearable devices. *International Journal of Medical Informatics, 164*, 104812. DOI: 10.1016/j.ijmedinf.2022.104812

Desai, M., & Mewada, H. (2023). A novel approach for yoga pose estimation based on in-depth analysis of human body joint detection accuracy. *PeerJ. Computer Science, 9*, e1607. DOI: 10.7717/peerj-cs.1152 PMID: 37346636

Esteva, A., Robicquet, A., Ramsundar, B., Kuleshov, V., DePristo, M., Chou, K., Cui, C., Corrado, G., Thrun, S., & Dean, J. (2019). A guide to deep learning in healthcare. *Nature Medicine, 25*(1), 24–29. DOI: 10.1038/s41591-018-0316-z PMID: 30617335

Field, T. (2016). Yoga research review. *Complementary Therapies in Clinical Practice, 24*, 145–161. DOI: 10.1016/j.ctcp.2016.06.005 PMID: 27502816

Gupta, H., Arora, P., & Malhotra, S. (2021). Privacy and security challenges in AI-driven healthcare monitoring systems. *Journal of Information Security and Applications, 58*, 102765. DOI: 10.1016/j.jisa.2021.102765

Hochreiter, S., & Schmidhuber, J. (1997). Long short-term memory. *Neural Computation, 9*(8), 1735–1780. DOI: 10.1162/neco.1997.9.8.1735 PMID: 9377276

Irfan, M., Ali, A., & Rehman, A. U. (2025). Integrating artificial intelligence with naturopathy and yoga for chronic disease management: A systematic review. *Journal of Integrative and Complementary Medicine, 31*(2), 115–134.

Jerath, R., Edry, J. W., Barnes, V. A., & Jerath, V. (2015). Physiology of long pranayamic breathing. *Medical Hypotheses, 85*(5), 486–496. DOI: 10.1016/j.mehy.2015.07.004 PMID: 16624497

Kishore, D. M., Bindu, S., & Manjunath, N. K. (2022). Smart yoga instructor for guiding and correcting yoga postures in real time. *International Journal of Yoga, 15*(3), 254–261. DOI: 10.4103/ijoy.ijoy_137_22 PMID: 36949838

Kumar, D.. (2025). *Federated learning with explainable AI for disease prediction.* ScienceDirect.

Kumar, R., & Srivastava, S. (2023). Wearable sensor data for stress and affective state monitoring: Challenges and opportunities. *Sensors (Basel)*, *23*(4), 2215. DOI: 10.3390/s23042215 PMID: 36850813

Kumar, S., Mehta, A., & Joshi, V. (2021). Wearable sensor-based health monitoring systems using Internet of Things and Artificial Intelligence. *Journal of Healthcare Engineering*, *2021*, 1–12. DOI: 10.1155/2021/9983652

LeCun, Y., Bengio, Y., & Hinton, G. (2015). Deep learning. *Nature*, *521*(7553), 436–444. DOI: 10.1038/nature14539 PMID: 26017442

Parashar, D., Mishra, O., Sharma, K., & Kukker, A. (2023). Improved yoga pose detection using MediaPipe and MoveNet in a deep learning model. *Revue d'Intelligence Artificielle*, *37*(5), 1197–1202. DOI: 10.18280/ria.370511

Patel, R., & Sharma, P. (2022). Artificial intelligence techniques for yoga posture detection and correction. *International Journal of Advanced Computer Science and Applications*, *13*(4), 210–218.

Patel, S., Park, H., Bonato, P., Chan, L., & Rodgers, M. (2012). A review of wearable sensors and systems with application in rehabilitation. *Journal of Neuroengineering and Rehabilitation*, *9*(1), 21. DOI: 10.1186/1743-0003-9-21 PMID: 22520559

Rao, K., Prakash, M., & Iyer, S. (2020). Real-time human pose estimation and yoga monitoring using computer vision techniques. *Procedia Computer Science*, *171*, 1450–1459. DOI: 10.1016/j.procs.2020.04.155

Sabry, F., Eltaras, T., Labda, W., Alzoubi, K., & Malluhi, Q. (2022). Machine learning for healthcare wearable devices: The big picture. *Journal of Healthcare Engineering*, *4653923*, 1–25. Advance online publication. DOI: 10.1155/2022/4653923 PMID: 35480146

Selye, H. (1956). *The stress of life*. McGraw-Hill.

Shajari, S.. (2023). The emergence of AI-based wearable sensors for digital healthcare applications. *Sensors (Basel)*, *23*(23), 9498. DOI: 10.3390/s23239498 PMID: 38067871

Singh, D., & Verma, N. (2023). Machine learning approaches for personalized yoga recommendation systems. *International Journal of Intelligent Systems and Applications*, *15*(2), 45–56.

Thoutam, V. A.. (2022). Yoga pose estimation and feedback generation using deep learning. *Computational Intelligence and Neuroscience, 4311350*, 1–12. Advance online publication. DOI: 10.1155/2022/4311350

Tripathi, S. M. (2021). Yogic theory of consciousness and its neuroscientific correlates: Chitta, vritti, and the default mode network. *Journal of Consciousness Studies*, *28*(5–6), 112–145.

Tunduny, T., & Shibwabo, B. (2026). Explainable AI approaches in federated learning for healthcare. *JMIR AI*, *5*, e69985. DOI: 10.2196/69985

Upadhyay, A., Basha, N. K., & Ananthakrishnan, B. (2023). Deep learning-based yoga posture recognition using the Y_PN-MSSD model for yoga practitioners. *Health Care*, *11*(4), 609. DOI: 10.3390/healthcare11040609 PMID: 36833142

Woodyard, C. (2011). Exploring the therapeutic effects of yoga and its ability to increase quality of life. *International Journal of Yoga*, *4*(2), 49–54. DOI: 10.4103/0973-6131.85485 PMID: 22022122

Zhang, J., Li, W., Ogunbona, P., Wang, P., & Tang, C. (2020). RGB-D-based action recognition datasets: A survey. *Pattern Recognition*, *60*, 86–105. DOI: 10.1016/j.patcog.2016.05.019

Zhu, X., Li, X., & Liu, S. (2024). Predicting mental health from physiological signals: A review of machine learning approaches using wearable data. *PLOS Digital Health*, *3*(1), e0000312. DOI: 10.1371/journal.pdig.0000312

Chapter 5
AI-Guided Meditation Techniques:
Focus, Awareness, and Deep Relaxation

Sandeep Kumar Singh
http://orcid.org/0000-0002-1741-7254
Jindal Global Business School, O.P. Jindal Global University, Sonipat, India

Ravi Tomar
http://orcid.org/0000-0002-3712-6702
Department of Chemistry, SRM Institute of Science and Technology, Delhi NCR, India

Shafiul Haque
Department of Nursing, College of Nursing and Health Sciences, Jazan University, Saudi Arabia

ABSTRACT

The chapter presents how the proposed paradigm shift in meditation applications is going to utilize a bio-responsive, and fully interactive artificial intelligence. It will move away from the passive nature of all meditation applications currently on the market by utilizing a wide variety of non-invasive physiological sensors (i.e. EEG and HRV) to fully understand the users' internal state during real time as they are practicing yoga. The proposed system will be able to provide the users with intelligent, real-time feedback as they go through the classical yogic states of Dhāra ā (concentration), and Dhyāna (meditation). Also, the proposed system will be able to allow the users to reach a deep state of relaxation using techniques such as Yoga-

DOI: 10.4018/979-8-3373-7625-7.ch005

Nidra. Through establishing the ethical framework of the AI system (based upon the Yamas and Niyamas), it will be ensured that the AI system promotes the growth of self-awareness and inner stillness, rather than promoting digital dependency.

1. INTRODUCTION

Research into the use of artificial intelligence to aid meditation has grown as a distinct area of study for about ten years. The rise in mental health problems and the need for low-cost and effective treatments have caused this area to grow (Yu et al., 2025) (Mitsea et al., 2023). Traditionally, meditation courses were held in classrooms and involved traditional forms of meditation and yoga. Today, many meditation courses include new forms of therapy such as AI, virtual reality and other digital treatment methods (Shamekhi & Bickmore, 2015) (Kaprekar et al., 2024). This evolution has expanded the number of people who are able to experience the benefits of meditation and has improved participants' comfort levels, relaxation levels and ability to focus and control their emotions during sessions (Mitsea et al., 2024) (Singh & Kaunert, 2024). The growing burden of global mental health issues demonstrated by increasing levels of anxiety and stress, makes the objective of the research described in this paper to explore a method for developing well-being through the utilization of AI and meditation for the general population (Adebisi et al., 2025) (Luo, 2025).

However, there are several limitations to overcome in terms of developing AI applications to meditations; primarily, they include personalization, cultural binding and ongoing user engagement with the application (Shankar et al., 2025; Fonseca et al., 2025; Divino, 2024). Current available digital meditation modalities fail to meet the requirements of interactivity, immediacy and contextual relevance necessary to maximize the operational enhancement of focus and deep relaxation (Yu et al., 2025; Khan et al., 2025; Ayub et al., 2025). There are also questions surrounding the effectiveness of achieving a truly meditative state using computer and the ethics of using technology for mindfulness (Tripathi, 2025; Keny, 2025). Furthermore, there exists "knowledge gaps" regarding the use of AI in awareness training of various demographics and in conjunction with holistic practices such as yoga (Narayanan, 2025; Sinha & Sinha, 2024; Walia, 2024). If these knowledge gaps remain unaddressed, they may impede the development of inclusive and culturally sensitive meditative modalities and limit their therapeutic potential (Divino, 2024; Luo, 2025).

Conceptually, AI Guided Meditation brings together for the user, the elements of Machine Learning, Natural Language Processing and Biofeedback to facilitate a Mindfulness intervention that promotes enhanced meta self-knowledge, emotional regulation and cognitive clarity (Shankar et al., 2025) (Singh et al., 2022) (Pandey et al., 2022). As these technological components function synergistically with the Immersive Environment and Physiological Monitoring, it allows the user to acquire the self-regulatory skills required to promote deep relaxation (Wieczorek et al., 2025) (Barton et al., 2024) (Kumar et al., 2024). The conceptual framework provides a bridge between AI's Adaptive capabilities and the long-term goals of Meditation, providing the user with the opportunity to establish Personal and Contextual Meditative Practices to enhance not only their mental, but also spiritual well-being (Marade et al., 2025) (Rosario et al., 2024).

The primary goal of this chapter is to explain the effectiveness of AI-Guided Meditations in the areas of Focus, Awareness Training, Deep Relaxation and Overall Mental Health in Various Demographics and Culture (Shankar et al., 2025) (Mitsea et al., 2023). This chapter will also not only synthesize the theoretical with practical aspects of AI-Guided Meditations, but will also examine the potential inclusion of Yoga in AI-Guided Meditations, for the enhancement of Holistic Health. Finally, the ethical implications of AI-Guided Meditations will be examined, concerning the likelihood of deleterious effects (Tripathi, 2025) (Narayanan, 2025). By synthesizing the previously mentioned gaps, this chapter is expected to contribute to the progression of Personalized and Culturally Competent AI Meditation Applications, in order to improve international Mental Health (Divino, 2024) (Luo, 2025).

2. SECTION 1: THE YOGIC FOUNDATION – FROM SENSE WITHDRAWAL TO MEDITATIVE ABSORPTION

To create an artificial intelligence capable of directing humans in the gentle pursuit of meditation, we need to have a broad understanding of the area that the AI is going to be navigating — namely, the interior landscape of the human psyche as described by the ancient Indian science of Yoga. In this section, we are going to lay out the philosophical and psychological foundation upon which our proposed system is based, specifically through reference to The Yoga Sūtras of Patañjali, a foundational text that describes both the philosophy and the scientific method of realizing one's own true nature. We will describe the Yogic structure of the mind (the citta); the fundamental dynamics of yogic practice (abhyāsa and vairāgya); and the gradual process of developing the internal limbs (antara ga yoga) of pratyāhāra, dharana and dhyāna. Our description of these concepts is not simply theoretical; they provide the fundamental "why" behind all aspects of the AI's development and operation.

2.1 The Mind's Architecture (Citta) according to Patañjali's Yoga

Patañjali defines Yoga at the opening of his treatise in a single sentence that has an enormous depth of meaning: yogaś citta-v tti-nirodha (Yoga Sūtra 1.2). As such, this definition can also be translated as "Yoga is the stopping of the modifications of the mind." Citta is a term that refers to the complete consciousness or "field of mind," composed of three different but interconnected mental faculties: manas (processing part of the mind); buddhi (discerning faculty of the mind); and aha kāra (the ego, or sense of self). These three faculties create the whirlpool-like or fluctuating processes of thought, memory, emotion and perception (v ttis) that are constantly occurring in all levels of consciousness. Yoga does not have the intention of eliminating or suppressing these fluctuations; rather, the purpose of Yoga is to develop a nirodha (state of perfect control or restraint) over them so that the true state of the observer, or Puru a (pure consciousness), may be seen clearly and without obstruction caused by the mental process.

Patanjali has a comprehensive strategy for achieving nirodha . He uses a dual strategy, which includes both abhyāsa and vairāgya (Yoga Sūtra 1.12). The first strategy, abhyāsa is the persistent and continuous effort to keep the mind focused. In order words it is the "do-ing" part of meditation. The second strategy, vairāgya is the practice of detachment or objective indifference, to release the attachments of desires, repulsions, and even the attachment to the practice of meditation itself. Furthermore, the central element of the meditative process contains a dualism. While the mind cannot be made to remain still using sheer will power (the rajasic type of effort), this only produces additional tension. Therefore, the mind must be "skillfully invited to peace", using a combination of persistence and peaceful surrender. This fundamental insight is embodied in the philosophical foundation of the AI. Thusly, the AI cannot operate as an authoritative force requiring attention, but rather as a knowledgeable and intelligent advisor capable of discerning when a soft suggestion is needed or when total silence is the best course of action.

However, the path to the mind being still is not devoid of challenges. Patanjali identifies nine major obstacles (antarāyā) or distractions (citta-vik epā) to the calming of the mind (Yoga Sūtra 1.30); including disease (vyādhi), mental lethargy (styāna), doubt (sa śaya), carelessness (pramāda), idleness (ālasya), sensual longings (avirati), false perceptions (bhrāntidarśana), lack of ability to maintain a state (alabdhabhūmikatva), and inability to maintain a condition (anavasthitatvāni). A bio-respondent AI, using the physiological indicators of each of the previously listed states; i.e., the lethargy of styāna, the agitation of avirati — can provide gentle and customized interventions to assist the practitioner to overcome some of the more frequent impediments to making progress.

2.2 Pratyāhāra: The Connection to the Internal Realm (Antaraṅga Yoga)

Pratyahara is the fifth of eight limbs in Patañjali's A a ga Yoga system that transitions us from the outer or active world of interaction and our physical body (Bahiranga Yoga), and into the inner world of meditation (Antaranga Yoga). Thus, it serves as a bridge between the outer or active world of the first four limbs (Yama, Niyama, Asana, and Pranayama), and the internal or meditative world of the last three limbs (Dharana, Dhyana and Samadhi). Pratyāhāra is usually translated as "the withdrawal of the senses". It is the process whereby the practitioner consciously detaches the senses (indriyas) from their external objects, and turns the flow of awareness inwards. As one commentary puts it, Pratyāhāra is like a turtle drawing its limbs within the shell, the shell being the mind, and the senses the limbs. This withdrawal is not by force, but by skillfully directing energy otherwise.

The yogic philosophy distinguishes several forms of this work. Prā a-pratyāhāra consists in the withdrawal of prā a (the vital life-force), and the control of prā a, the senses following the flow of prā a. When prā a is collected and centralised by the breathing or prā āyāma, (control of breath), then, the senses turning inwards. Mano-pratyāhāra is the process of withdrawing the consciousness itself from the senses, with conscious detachment of awareness of the stream of sensory input. The AI machine is regulated for this process, which helps the production of a condition of as few external stimuli as possible, and also turns the inward focus of the user spiritually to internal fixed points, like the breathing, so that the attention will tend to be turned inwards.

From a neurological point of view Pratyāhāra can be looked at from the standpoint of sensory gating, the neural process of filtering out unnecessary or unrecognized objects from the total flow of the continuous stream of sensory stimuli arising in the brain. Any effective sensory gating is quite essential for the maintenance of focus and avoiding of cognitive overload. While meditation was once assumed simply to mean that this process of filtering was increased, recent neuro-imaging work has shown a more complex position. It is found that the experienced meditators may perhaps have less sensory gating, so to speak, which means that they "hear" or register more sensory data with greater sensitivity. Yet, this is offset by increased ability to regulate their attention and emotional response to the inputs. This reacts perfectly to the Yogic position of Pratyāhāra being conscious redirection, and not grosser suppression. The practitioner does not make himself deaf or insensitive, but he is more exquisitely aware of sensory input, so that the mind is not "caught" by it, and the inner anchor of awareness kept.

2.3 Dhāraṇā: The Art of Single-Pointed Concentration

Having retracted the senses inward through Pratyāhāra, the practitioner is ready for the sixth limb, that of Dhāra ā. This state is defined by Patañjali (Yoga Sūtras 3.1): deśa-bandhaś cittasya dhāra ā, which translates as "Concentration is the binding of the mind to a single place". Dhāra ā is the foremost, voluntary and effortful act of concentrating the mind's focus upon a single object (*ālambana*) to the exclusion of all others. It is the first stage of deep meditation, that mental body-building which is necessary for the passive state of Dhyāna.

The Affective Neuroscience of Focused Attention (FA) Meditation gives us a very definite physiological response to the sensibility which accompanies the subjective position of Dhāra ā. The results of f.M.R.I. studies of the brains of practitioners engaged in FA meditation show a distinct increased activity in certain brain regions repeatedly, which areas have to do with areas of brain control of top-down attentional control and executive function. The parts of the brain concerned are the dorso-lateral pre-frontal cortex (PFC) and anterior cingulate cortex (ACC), which are concerned with working memory, goal maintenance and conflict monitoring. This type of brain-activity represents the conscious effort directed to the sustaining of attention and the inhibiting of distractions, and limbs of a neural signature which will clearly distinguish the active Doings of Dhāra ā from the passive Being of Dhyāna.

2.4 Dhyāna: The Uninterrupted Flow of Awareness

With the practice of Dhāra ā becoming more sustained as a result of continued practice, Dhyāna will naturally arise and emerge. Patañjali describes Dhyāna in the Yoga Sūtras as follows in 3.2: tatra pratyayaikatānatā dhyānam—"in that place (tatra), continuous, uninterrupted flow of cognition (pratyayaikatānatā) is meditation (dhyānam)". The state of Dhyāna is not an additional method or process to apply but rather the qualitative outcome resulting from the transformation of the mind's ability to concentrate without conscious effort, continuously, and completely absorbed in the experience of concentration.

The transition from Dhāra ā to Dhyāna is a highly subtle and critical shift in consciousness. When one is practicing Dhāra ā, one is still able to distinguish among three separate entities: the person doing the meditation, the subject of the meditation, and the act of meditating itself. One is still using conscious effort to keep the mind on the subject of meditation. As the practice continues to unfold into the state of Dhyāna, this separation dissolves. There is no longer a need for conscious effort to focus attention on the subject of meditation and one's awareness rests steadily upon the object of contemplation.

These subjective experiences of the shift from Dhāra ā to Dhyāna are reflected in very distinctive alterations in brain activity. While Dhāra ā involves the deliberate engagement of the prefrontal cortex to sustain focused attention, the state of Dhyāna is associated with a marked reduction in activity within the brain's default mode network (DMN). The DMN comprises several interconnected brain regions, including the posterior cingulate cortex and the medial prefrontal cortex, which are typically active during periods of rest and internally oriented cognition, such as mind-wandering, self-referential thinking, and rumination. The diminished level of activity in the DMN during Dhyāna signifies that the mind is no longer habitually wandering. Simultaneously, EEG studies show a change in the predominant frequency of brainwaves that occur during the two states of consciousness. Beta waves associated with active thought cease to dominate brain activity and are replaced by slower frequencies of brain activity, i.e., high amplitude, coherent alpha waves and the emergence of theta waves, both of which have been linked to deep meditative and hypnagogic states. This objective, neuro-physiological shift from a state of effort to a state of effortless flow is one of the primary markers that a sophisticated bio-responsive AI can be taught to detect so that it may alter its support strategy from active to passive, silent facilitation.

2.5 The Science of Stillness: Yoga Nidra and Śavāsana

The ability to cultivate these deep states of relaxation required by meditation and deep nervous system regulation can be achieved through two well-structured methods of relaxation: yoga nidra and savasana. Although both of these relaxation states have the potential to be very relaxing, they are also active processes that require the individual to remain awake and aware throughout the process of relaxation. According to classical yoga texts including the ha hayoga pradīpikā (1.32) and gheranda sa hitā (2.19), savasana has been described as a resting position that can eliminate fatigue, and provide the mind with a restful state. Savasana is used as the base for the more complex technique of yoga nidra.

Yoga nidra is a method of guided meditation designed to lead the practitioner through each layer of their being (the košas) to a state of extreme relaxation, similar to sleep; however, this state is different than sleep because the individual maintains awareness. Typically, there are multiple stages involved in practicing yoga nidra. They include: an initial relaxation, a sa kalpa (an intention or resolve), a systematic movement of the practitioner's consciousness through all parts of the body (sensory-motor mapping of the brain), an awareness of one's breath, experiencing opposites (i.e., feeling heavy and feeling light), and using visualizations to guide the practitioner. Ultimately, the purpose of the practice of yoga nidra is to allow the individual to become so relaxed, that their entire body falls into a deep sleep; however, the individual's mind will still remain alert, awake and detached.

The primary purpose of the practice of Yoga Nidra is to serve as a doorway or portal to accessing and experiencing what the Mā ūkya Upani ad identifies as the fourth state of consciousness, referred to as Turiya. Turiya is not a place to be reached, it is the always present, quiet and unchanged screen upon which all other experiences (awake, asleep, and dreaming) are projected. Through the practice of Yoga Nidra, individuals are given the opportunity to directly experience this field of consciousness. The "Yoga Nidra Navigator" feature of the proposed AI application is designed to provide users with the tools to successfully travel to these profound places of restoration, tailoring the pace and content of the practice to the individual's unique real-time responses to promote entrance into the deep relaxation states.

3. SECTION 2. THE TECHNOLOGICAL FRAMEWORK – A BIO-RESPONSIVE AI ARCHITECTURE

The philosophical and psychological ideals of yoga are rich, but they require a much more advanced technology to transform them into a functional (AI-based) system. This section describes the system structure, from abstract to tangible. A closed-loop, bio-responsive system will provide an accurate representation of the internal experience of the yogi; utilize sophisticated machine learning techniques to interpret this data; and provide feedback in a non-intrusive, adaptive form. This is an architecture built upon the concept of subtle, intelligent interaction and reflects the delicate interplay between abhyasa and vairagya.

3.1 Input Modalities: The Senses of the AI

In order to see and interpret the state of the practitioner, the AI must be provided with the set of non-intrusive "senses" capable of recording the physiological correlates of mental-emotional activity. The combining of a plurality of biosensor streams produces a rich, multi-dimensional picture of the internal world of the user, one that is considerably stronger and finer-grained than any single modality in isolation. The "sensor fusion" approach is required because it will allow the AI to unravel knotty states. As a single example, high levels of activity in the theta wave band will be indicative of both deep meditation as well as drowsiness; cross-checking this with the HRV and respiration streams will allow the AI to reach a superior classification (Zakaria et al., 2025).

3.1.1 Electroencephalography (EEG)

Wearable EEG sensors, typically incorporated in soft headbands, provide a direct readout of the brain's electrical activity, or brainwaves. Brainwaves are categorized based on their frequency and are strongly correlation with states of consciousness, making the EEG a rich source of information for a meditation AI (Attar et al., 2021) (Kim et al., 2014). The key frequency ranges to understand include:

- **Beta Waves (12-30 Hz):** Beta waves define our usual conscious state. We use these for active thought, solving problems and focus on what is going on around us. When you meditate and see a lot of beta waves, this indicates your mind is busy, ruminating or wandering off at will.
- **Alpha Waves (8-12 Hz):** The alpha band defines the relaxed wakeful state. The strongest alpha activity occurs when you are relaxing with eyes closed and looking inward instead of outward. Alpha amplitude and stability are therefore the primary physiological correlates of a successful meditative state which is an internally-focused and calm but still alert awareness.
- **Theta Waves (4-8 Hz):** As you go deeper into relaxation, the brain typically shifts from alpha to theta wave activity. The frequencies of theta have been related to deep meditation, increased creativity, decreased anxiety and the hypnotic state - that area of consciousness between being awake and being asleep. If there is a strong theta wave during Dhyana (or other meditation), this may suggest the person is very absorbed and is entering a deep state of concentration. Similarly, if there is a strong theta wave during Yoga Nidra (relaxation), this could mean that the person has entered a very deep relaxation state, and is resting (as opposed to merely sleeping).
- **Delta Waves (0.5 Hz):** The delta range represents the lowest of the brainwaves and is found in the deep phases of non-rapid eye movement (NREM) sleep (dreamless). Very rarely is the delta wave considering the target of meditation, however, its emergence is useful as an indicator that the person has gone to sleep and is no longer fully conscious. It would also be useful for the AI to remind the user that they need to awaken.
- **Gamma Waves (30-100 Hz):** The highest of the brainwaves, gamma waves are associated with the highest order cognitive processes such as insight, and peak performance. Although the specific role of gamma in meditation is complex, there are studies indicating that gamma is related to higher levels of non-dual awareness and insight in more advanced meditators, yet gamma waves are not the primary focus of the current guidance system.

3.1.2 Heart Rate Variability (HRV)

HRV refers to the variation in the time interval between successive heartbeats. In a healthy individual, the heart does not beat at a perfectly constant rhythm; instead, the intervals between beats naturally fluctuate. These variations reflect the activity of the autonomic nervous system. The autonomic nervous system consists of two main branches: the sympathetic nervous system (SNS), which regulates the body's "fight-or-flight" responses, and the parasympathetic nervous system (PNS), which controls "rest-and-digest" functions (Park et al., 2022).

- **Low HRV:** A low, metronomic HRV is a marker that the SNS is dominant. This is the physiological marker of stress, anxiety, cognitive load, and fatigue. The body is under high alert, and it is less adaptable with decreased capacity to recover.
- **High HRV:** High, irregular HRV implies that the PNS dominates. This is a mark of relaxation, stress hardiness, as well as cardiovascular health. The body recovers readily as it is capable of managing stressors.

In the case of the meditation AI, the HRV is a strong, real-time indicator of stress and relaxation. The device will track the HRV to gauge the user's baseline stress state and monitor their improvement in shifting the ANS to a parasympathetic-dominant state, the main objective of the yogic breathing and relaxation exercises.

3.1.3 Galvanic Skin Response (GSR)

GSR detects subtle fluctuations in skin's electrical conductance caused by physiological responses. The conductance is contingent on the state of moisture of the skin, as regulated by the eccrine sweat glands. Notably, the hands' palms as well as the feet' soles contain sweat glands that are highly responsive to emotionally elicited stimulation. As such, the GSR is a very sensitive as well as direct indicator of sympathetic nervous system arousal (Zakaria et al., 2025).

- **Function:** Upon the occurrence of an emotionally significant idea, a state of anxiety, or even a startle reaction, the SNS is triggered and produces a brief, typically imperceptible, ramp-up of the sudoriferous gland secretion. This creates a noticeable increase in the skin conductance.
- **Usage:** The GSR will be used by the AI to recognize instances of physiological or emotional arousal that could disturb the state of meditation. The sudden spike in GSR can be indicative of a distracting idea or anxiety wave that usually occurs prior to the practitioner's consciousness. On the other hand, a

continuous drop in GSR throughout the session is a clear indicator of relaxation and emotional peace that continues to deepen.

3.1.4 Respiration Sensors

Breath (Prana) represents the physical relationship with consciousness that is central to the practice of Yoga and thus monitoring a person's breathing pattern is fundamental to the function of the device. In this regard, strain gauges with the ability to detect contact may be able to capture a person's breathing patterns via a thoracic strap (e.g., Soni & Muniyandi, 2019). Additionally, contactless technology such as a cell phone camera could be used to detect slight movements in pixels that correspond to expansion/contraction of the thorax due to breathing activity.

Based on this information, the AI will track the following three breathing parameters.

- **Rate:** The number of breaths taken per minute. When you slow your breathing rate through meditation, the parasympathetic relaxation response is activated.
- **Depth:** The amount of air inhaled during each breath. Shallow chest breathing, which is typical of stressful states, contrasts sharply with diaphragmatic breathing, which is characterized by greater volumes of air being inhaled into the lungs when relaxed.
- **Rhythmicity:** The consistency of breathing cycles. A steady, consistent breathing cycle is a good indication that the user's mind is both calm and focused.

In addition to its role as an input metric related to the user's current state, breath also plays the role of primary focus of the AI device. As such, the AI device can utilize either auditory or haptic feedback to provide gentle encouragement toward establishing a slower, deeper, and steadier breathing pattern while simultaneously providing positive reinforcement toward promoting relaxation and concentration.

3.2 The AI Core: A Learning, Adaptive Brain

The raw data is generated by the biosensors; however, it has no value without a sophisticated central processing unit (or “core”) that can interpret the data and apply the findings. The “brain” or central nervous system of this system will be a highly complex, multi-layered machine learning based central processor, which will have two major goals: to identify accurately, the user’s present mental status; and to establish the most effective way for the system to assist the user. As such, the system will grow from a basic, rudimentary biofeedback device to a total artificial intelligent assistant.

3.2.1 The Closed-Loop Biofeedback System

In a general sense, the overall design operates as a closed-loop biofeedback system. This is in complete contrast to the open-loop nature of traditional meditation apps. An open-loop system (such as playing a pre-recorded sound file) provides a fixed output no matter what the user's response may be. A closed-loop system, on the other hand, produces a dynamic and ongoing loop of interaction:

- **Sense:** Input channels (EEG, HRV, GSR, Respiration) obtain real-time data about the user's psychophysiological condition.
- **Interpret:** This multi-modal data is interpreted by the AI core to infer the mental state of the user (e.g., 'focused', 'distracted).
- **Guide:** Based on this interpretation, the machine learning model recognizes and issues a short, adaptive prompt through one of its output channels.
- **Sense Again:** The system immediately identifies the user's physiological response to the guidance and hence restarts the process iteratively.

This ongoing loop of feedback allows the AI to function at a level of responsiveness and delicacy that would never even become available in a static system, so that direction is at all times timely, pertinent, and personalized.

3.2.2 Classification of Mental States (Supervised Learning)

The "Interpret" step in the feedback loop is performed by a supervised machine learning model.1 Supervised learning entails an algorithm learning to map inputs to outputs based on a vast number of labeled examples.

- **Training Phase:** A data set will be generated in developing the classifier by gathering multi-modal biosensor data from hundreds of users who will take part in meditation sessions. Concurrently, these users will also give labels that translate to their mental state at intervals that will be chosen (e.g., by pressing a button when they notice that they have begun mind-wandering). This produces a rich data set in which specific patterns from the aggregated EEG, HRV, GSR, and respiration data are associated with accurate, subjectively signaled mental states such as 'focused,' 'mind-wandering,' 'agitated,' or 'drowsy.'

- **Inference Phase:** This supervised algorithm, in this case, a deep neural network, gets trained on this labeled set of data. It learns to recognize complex, high-dimensional bio-signal patterns correlated with each of these mental states. Once trained, the model can be deployed in real-time applications. It takes the real-time stream of sensor data as input and produces a probabilistic output of the user's current mental state and provides the interpretation needed to allow the guidance system to perform optimally.

3.2.3 Personalized Guidance Strategy (Reinforcement Learning)

Knowing that a user is distracted is one thing; figuring out the very best way to shift their attention elsewhere is quite another, and this is where the system's "intelligence" becomes truly personalized. This function is achieved through Reinforcement Learning (RL), a branch of machine learning where an "agent" comes to have the capability to make the very best decisions by interacting with an environment and experiencing consequences in the form of reward or punishment for its actions.

- **The Reinforcement Learning Paradigm:** In this paradigm, the "agent" becomes the artificial intelligence itself. The "environment" consists of the state of meditation in the user. The agent's possible "actions" consist of the possible types of direction that it could give (e.g., generating a chime, giving a voice prompt, giving a haptic feedback pulse, or doing nothing). The "reward" consists of a positive signal that arises upon the user's biosensors registering a return to the desired meditative state (e.g., an increase in the activity of alpha waves or an increase in heart rate variability coherence).
- **Learning a Policy:** What the RL agent hopes to learn is a "policy"—a set of decision-making rules that tell it which actions to take to maximize its total reward in the long run. At first, the agent may try all these actions haphazardly. If it gives a verbal stimulus and the HRV of the user increases (positive reward), it learns that this action works in this situation. If it gives a haptic stimulus and the GSR goes up (stimulation, a negative reward), it learns to refrain from that in the future.
- **Deep Personalization:** After several sessions, the RL agent builds a very personalized policy per individual user. It learns that **User A** needs subtle sound cues when they go off-task, and **User B** prefers to receive a gentle haptic prompt. It learns the very "minimum effective dose" of intervention that will get a user back on track with minimal intrusiveness. This two-part intelligence—applying supervised learning to respond to "What is happening?" and reinforcement learning to respond to "What is the wisest thing to do about it?"—is what transforms the system from sensor to intelligent guide.

3.3 Output Modalities: The Voice of the AI

The last part of the architecture deals with how the artificial intelligence presents its instructions to the user. Such presentation modalities have been made to be non-disturbing, non-obtrusive, and efficient and give a set of options that could be customized by the reinforcement learning agent.

3.3.1 Adaptive Auditory Cues

Generative sound is used instead of pre-recorded sounds/music. Generative sound is able to dynamically respond to the user's experience, creating an ever-changing dynamic sound-scape, and therefore able to extend the subjective state into a continuous, smooth experience.

For example, if a user selects a gentle rain auditory environment; upon AI detecting a user is "mind-wandering" - characterized by increased beta EEG and decreased HRV - the gentle rain may grow slightly louder, become more complex. Once the user becomes aware again, the rain returns to a gentle rhythmic pattern. The above is a non-verbal continuous feedback loop that promotes awareness and does not burden the brain with language based information processing. As such other variations could be made in the pitch of a singing bowl, the complexity of an ambient drone, the rate of soft chime.

3.3.2 Personalized Verbal Guidance (Natural Language Processing)

Although the system will need to use verbal cues if necessary; it must do so as gently and efficiently as possible. A natural language processing (NLP) model, in conjunction with voice generation models, can enable the system to provide users with simple, timely, and contextually aware cues.

- **The timing principle** guides how the system uses its verbal instruction to reinforce the user's understanding, because these are used with restraint. That is, they are only used when other methods are ineffective or when direct guidance is required (i.e., in the case of yoga nidra).
- **Generative Voice:** Advanced text to speech technologies are capable of producing extremely realistic, soft spoken, and emotionally intelligent voice recordings. These can provide you with an extensive library of voices and based on your user's feedback, it can determine which tone, pitch and rhythm works best for each individual and can adjust accordingly.
- **Sophisticated NLP Methodologies:** Verbal cue content can also be improved using advanced NLP and hypnotherapy techniques. By applying "pacing and

leading" (wherein the user is aligned with their current state and then gently guided toward a new location), and embedded command (using permissive language such as: "you may easily…") the verbal cue becomes more hypnotically effective while becoming less directive and therefore more effective.

3.3.3 Haptic Feedback

Within a loop for pure non-auditory non-visual feedback, it would seem that a system could utilize haptics. These would be a form of feedback carried out by a vibration motor in a mobile phone or wearable device. Haptics have an extraordinarily potent potential for individualized feedback as a form of entrainment of awareness.

- **Used In Breath Guidance:** This equipment would generate smooth rhythmic pulsations that match the user's desired breathing rhythm (a resonating comfortable breathing rhythm, generally around 5-6 breaths per minute). These pulsations would lead the user to awareness of the rhythm and allow them to entrain their breathing to this comfortable rhythm very easily since the awareness yet again flows into breathing with no cognitive action required through the introduction of guides or label of counting or utterance of sounds through auditory means.
- **Application As a Nudge:** A gentle but immediate short vibration would be an "innocent tap on the shoulder" by the artificial intellect so to speak. It could become an implication that the attention has been led elsewhere and the now needs to be revisited. Experimental research has made evident that in some instances feedback which was given in the form of haptics alone was found to be more calming in the individual than auditory feedback alone and therefore potentially a better medium for a mind to feel reduced stress and so on. It therefore is a greatly efficacious part of the tool supply of the artificial intellect. Using a variety of multi-modal influences and an advanced artificial intelligence core and various subtle outputs, this technological system has a probable and resilient shape for the evolving of a truly bioresponsive and empathetic companion for meditation of the artificial intellect nature.

4. SECTION 3: PRACTICAL APPLICATIONS – THE AI AS A MEDITATION GUIDE IN ACTION

In this section, we present an illustration of how the theoretical frameworks and technical tools discussed in previous sections can be applied practically. We present the specifics of how the Bio-Responsive Yoga AI would function as part of each of the three modes of its operation. Each mode illustrates a different dimension of the practice context and the user's purpose for using the AI, and together they show the great flexibility of the AI. These are narratives that describe how the Bio-Responsive Yoga AI would function in real-time; from the level of theoretical principles to the lived experience of the practitioner.

4.1. The Dhāraṇā Trainer: Cultivating Single-Pointed Focus

The Dhāra ā Trainer is designed for beginners with meditative practice or for individuals that would like to enhance the fundamental ability to sustain focus on a single point for extended periods of time. The app provides an interactive but very subtle coach to assist users in building the "mental muscle" required for concentration. Many apps labeled with similar names to this app will essentially provide timed concentration or act as reminders, however there is no interactive (dynamic) response from the app to assist the user in developing concentration.

4.1.1. User Profile and Setup

This individual has little to no experience in meditating with what can best be described as a "monkey mind". This user wants to perform a 15-minute session using the specific ālambana of the sensation of the breath at the top of the nostril. Additionally, the user has worn an EEG headband and a wrist mounted device to monitor HRV, GSR. Finally, the user has identified a "Soft Stream" generative soundscape as their preferred auditory feedback method.

4.1.2. Session Walkthrough:

4.1.2.1. Session Start and Baseline

The session begins, the AI performs its first action to determine a user's physiological baseline. The AI evaluates the user's baseline condition: high levels of beta activity in the EEG indicates an active mind; low turbulence in the HRV shows minimal stress; fluctuation in the GSR indicates moderate nervousness. A soft, almost imperceptible stream of sound is presented by the soundscape.

4.1.2.2. Initial Focus Achieved

Immediately after the first audio cue for the user to "begin by focusing on the sensation of your breath", the user has directed his or her attention. The AI's classifier detected the associated physiological changes in the bio-signals, specifically the decrease in Beta wave amplitudes, the emergence of Alpha waves primarily in the frontal lobe area, the slowing and regularization of the users' breathing, as well as an increase in HRV Coherence. The AI classified this as "Initial Focus." No intervention occurred at this time, and the volume of the stream sound remained low.

4.1.2.3 Mind-Wandering Detected

About ninety seconds into the session, the user experienced a mental distraction regarding an impending work deadline. The user's attention shifted away from the breath and toward this internal narrative. The AI's sensor fusion model detected the physiological response to this distraction: the alpha wave pattern disappeared and Beta waves returned to the higher frequency ranges; HRV Coherence dropped precipitously; and a slight, but discernible spike in GSR indicated a brief, minor surge in emotional arousal (i.e., anxiety regarding the impending deadline). The classifier output changed from "Focus" to "Distraction (Cognitive)".

4.1.2.4. Minimum Effective Dose of Guidance

Having learned through previous sessions that this particular user could be successfully guided using relatively subtle, non-verbal interventions, the AI reinforcement learning policy made its first intervention. Utilizing the principle of "Minimum Effective Dose," the AI increased the complexity and quantity of the generative stream soundscape. Specifically, the stream sounds were modified so they would be attention grabbing but not startling. A faint, but notable turbulence was added to the stream soundscape.

4.1.2.5. Focus Re-Established

The user became aware of the change in the stream soundscape due to the AI's intervention. The user recalled their original intention and returned to the feelings associated with their breath. Upon this transition, the AI immediately perceived the effects of this transition on the physiological data: the Beta waves retreated, the Alpha wave intensified, and HRV coherence began to rise.

4.1.2.6. Diminishing the Intervention

Upon triggering a return to the "Focus" state, the AI terminates its intervention. The stream soundscape diminishes in intensity and returns to its soft, base-line level. This action of diminishing the intervention is important; it allows the user to utilize their own self-regulatory abilities. The AI had served as a temporary scaffold for the user who then regained their balance as the scaffold was removed. This dynamic continues throughout the remainder of the session, with the AI acting as a stationary, observational partner; making intermittent interventions as required and always with the least amount of force possible.

Figure 1 illustrates this complete feedback cycle, mapping the specific sequence from the physiological detection of distraction to the application of the 'minimum effective dose' of guidance. This visualization demonstrates how the AI serves as a temporary scaffold, intervening only when necessary to support the user's return to single-pointed concentration.

Figure 1. The AI-Assisted Dhāra ā Feedback Loop – From Distraction to Refocusing

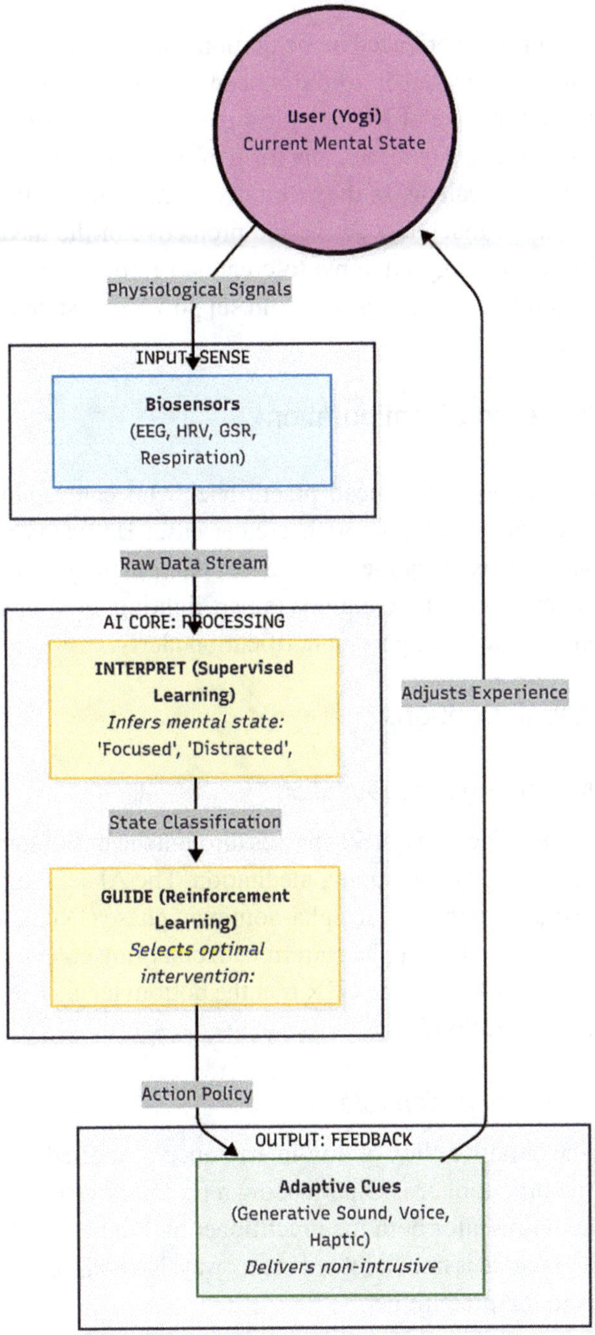

4.2. The Dhyāna Facilitator: Supporting Effortless Absorption

As the practitioner is experienced in meditation, the facilitation role of the guide changes. The challenge is no longer to hold concentration, but to help the practitioner progress further into the state of Dhyāna (absorbed concentration), which is spontaneous and uninterrupted. Therefore, any form of intervention (even the slightest) could disturb the delicate balance of the meditative state, and the facilitative Dhyāna role of the guide will be much less active and protective of the meditation space.

Virtual Reality technology attempts to create an immersive environment, but lacks the biological intelligence to protect and support a true state of Dhyāna without intrusion.

4.2.1. User Profile and Configuration

The practitioner is an experienced practitioner who can retain a Dhāra ā for relatively extended periods of time with greater ease. He wants to move further into the absorptions. He is using the same sensor equipment, but he configures the AI to use the environmental interventions (smart lighting, etc.) or a single pre-set chime tone on only the most important notification alerts.

4.2.2. Session walkthrough:

4.2.2.1. Quickly entering the meditation

The session begins. The user quickly passes through the initial startup phases due to his extensive experience in practicing meditation. The AI sees the normal neurophysiological progression: the initial alpha-dominant phase (Dhāra ā) transitions to a highly-stable, high-amplitude alpha pattern with emerging coherent theta activity. The HRV is high and stable, and the GSR is at the bottom level. The AI defines this state as "Dhyāna (Absorption)".

4.2.2.2. The passive guardian role

At this point the default policy of non-interference is applied by the AI. The AI recognizes that the practitioner is experiencing a profound level of self-sustaining focus. The AI should monitor both the practitioner and the environment to ensure that the practitioners' state is not disrupted in any way. No auditory, verbal, or tactile feedback is given to the practitioner.

4.2.2.3. Identifying and mitigating subtle agitation

20 minutes into the session, a car horn is sounded outside of the user's window. The AI detects a small almost instantaneous physiological reaction: a small spike in GSR and a short desynchronization of the brainwaves. The user's conscious awareness may not have even been aware of the sound; however, the user's nervous system was reacting. The AI's classifier calls this “Subtle Agitation”.

4.2.2.4. Intervention with environmental stimuli

The AI does not provide a direct alert to the user, as it would simply increase the degree of disturbance; rather the AI provides intervention in another way. The AI sends a command to the user's home automation system to activate a previously selected white noise machine. As a result, all other external background noise is muffled and the integrity of the user's meditation space remains intact. The user's physiological state returns to a state of deep Dhyāna immediately, their immersion is unbroken.

4.2.2.5. Preventing drowsiness

Later in the session the AI determines that there has been a major change in the user's physiological state. The alpha waves are decreasing, and the theta waves are slowing down and becoming intermixed with emerging delta waves. Additionally, the user's acceleration (measured by the wearable's accelerometer) indicates a decrease in movement. These indicators represent a significant transition from a state of conscious meditation to a state of unconscious sleep. At this point, the AI must intervene to maintain the continuity of the practice.

4.2.2.6. Minimum cue to arousal

The AI follows its predetermined procedure for preventing drowsiness. The AI produces a single clear, low volume chime. The chime is sufficient to awaken the user's consciousness from delta/theta sleep, returning the user to the alpha/theta state of meditation, while remaining below the threshold of full wakefulness (beta). The user's consciousness is regained, but the state of Dhyāna continues.

To visualize the system's protective function, Figure 2 maps the decision-making logic of the Dhyāna Facilitator. This flowchart illustrates how the AI differentiates between external disturbances, which trigger environmental masking to preserve immersion, and internal drowsiness, which necessitates a direct auditory cue to restore alertness.

Figure 2. The Dhyāna Protection Protocol – Passive Monitoring vs. Active Intervention

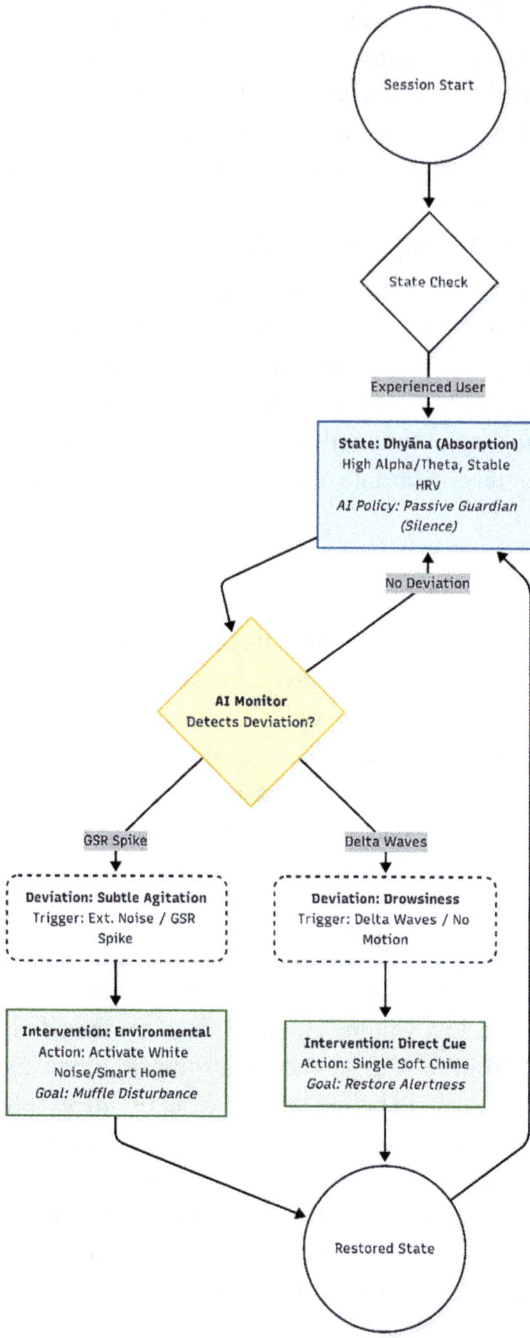

4.3. The Yoga Nidra Navigator: Customizing Deep Relaxation

The Navigator mode of Yoga Nidra is a therapeutic use that will lead the customer through the systematic stages of the yogic sleep in order to achieve deeper psycho-physical relaxation, stress release, as well as healing. Whereas there are many apps that give guided recordings of Yoga Nidra, they are completely static in nature and cannot be adjusted to the nervous system reaction that each individual possesses. The Navigator adapts the experience in real-time, so it is a much stronger and effective device.

4.3.1. User Profile and Setup

The user is very stressed and employs the practice to aid sleep improvement. The user is in the recumbent position of Śavāsana with the full set of sensors. The AI will issue instructions with a generative NLP voice.

4.3.2. Session Walkthrough:

4.3.2.1. Establishing the Saṅkalpa (Intention)

The practice opens with the calm, generative voice of the AI prompting the user to construct a sa kalpa—a concise, affirmative statement of intent. The AI waits until the user's physiology settles (marked by the deceleration of breath and the increase of HRV) before continuing, so the intention is seeded in a receptive mind.

4.3.2.2. Personalized Body Scan (Rotation of Consciousness)

The AI starts to lead the user's consciousness through various regions of the body. This is the core of the personalization. As the AI states, "Bring your awareness to your right shoulder," it simultaneously tracks the user's GSR. If it recognizes a consistently high GSR reading that correlates with that part of the body, its internal model assumes the accumulation of stored physical or emotional tension. The AI then responds with the NLP engine adjusting the script dynamically. It may introduce the phrase "Allow the shoulder to feel heavy... releasing and letting go... breathing into any tightness you might find there." It will stay on this point for one or two additional breaths, waiting to see the corresponding decrease in the GSR signal prior to proceeding. A pre-recorded recording would simply proceed regardless of the state of the user.

4.3.2.3. Bio-Responsive Visualization

The AI places the user in a visualization, such as imagining a warm, golden light spreading throughout the body. The AI monitors the user's HRV response most carefully. If the visualization creates a strong parasympathetic effect (a strong increase in HRV), the AI reinforcement learning model notes this as highly effective in this user. The AI may then slightly intensify the imagery with some additional sensory descriptions: "Feel the warmth of the light. see the gentle glow of the light. a feeling of deep peace spreading with the light." However, if a particular visualization had resulted in a stress reaction (a loss of HRV), the AI learns this and transitions smoothly to a more neutral or previously-successful visualization.

4.3.2.4. Navigating the Hypnagogic State

The AI's ultimate goal is to hold the user in the deeply restorative theta-wave state, the threshold between wakefulness and sleep where the subconscious mind is highly receptive. The device utilizes your live EEG signal as an indicator for where you are in your state of consciousness. When the device senses that the person is drifting away from the alpha wave pattern and moving closer to the beta wave pattern (i.e., becoming too alert), the guidance will gradually soften and become more repetitive to bring the person back to a place of relaxation. Conversely, when the device detects that the person has slid down into the delta wave pattern (i.e., fallen completely asleep), the voice will gradually increase in clarity and definition, or the introduction of a soft background sound will help to keep the user aware that they are still connected to their conscious awareness. The use of this real-time, on-the-fly navigation of brainwave states is essential to providing a high-quality, effective Yoga Nidra session, so that the user can receive the full benefit of a deep rest while still maintaining the critical aspect of awareness.

These practical implementations demonstrate a new paradigm in wellness technology. With the change from a static, non-bio responsive content delivery paradigm to a dynamic, bio- responsive paradigm, the AI transforms from a mere tool to a personalized, intuitive and adaptive guide to achieving personal peace.

5. CONCLUSION: A PARADIGM SHIFT TO HOLISTIC WELL-BEING

The transformational capacity of AI-assisted meditation was demonstrated by a "paradigm shift" from static, open-loop applications to dynamic, bio-responsive systems which support yogic goals of concentration and deep relaxation. The transformation from maximizing engagement on standard wellness apps to a "minimum effective dose" philosophy (where AI serves as a non-invasive, ethical guide to assist users in becoming self-sufficient in their own wellness) is illustrated in Table 1. Through the integration of real time physiological data with the traditional contemplative practices of Eastern philosophies and religions, these holistic interventions have provided new avenues for users to achieve personalization in their stress management and emotional regulation; they are also transforming the way we approach mental wellness in the digital age.

A great deal of innovation has been seen in the area of AI-assisted meditation; however, a number of substantial barriers remain, many of which relate to issues of accessibility (inclusiveness), ethics and effectiveness over time. A number of current applications of AI-assisted meditation have limited cross-cultural validity and do not adequately address the needs of older adults or neurodiverse populations. To fill this gap in our understanding, Table 2 presents a number of key areas of focus for future research, including the conduct of longitudinal studies to identify optimal "dosing" of AI-assisted meditation and developing strong, inclusive systems to set the standards for how AI-assisted meditation is used ethically (and protect user privacy). Developing scalable and accessible solutions to benefit under-served populations will also be an important factor in addressing the limits of current AI-assisted meditation applications. Ultimately, for AI guided meditation to reach its full potential for transformation, there is a need for developers to create evidence-based applications that utilize rigorous methodologies and that exhibit cultural sensitivity in the design of the tools, so that they may be developed into supportive and respectful resources for mental health across the globe.

Table 1. A Paradigm Shift in Digital Wellbeing

Feature	Standard Wellness Apps (e.g., Calm, Headspace)	Bio-Responsive Yoga AI
Guidance Method	Static, pre-recorded audio/video. Open-loop.	Dynamic, bio-responsive. Closed-loop feedback.
Personalization	Based on user-selected preferences and history.	Real-time adaptation to psychophysiological state.
Core Metric of Success	User Engagement (Time in app, sessions completed).	User Self-Reliance (Decreasing need for intervention).
Design Philosophy	Engagement-Maximization (Gamification, streaks, notifications).	Minimum Effective Dose (Intervene as little as possible).
Ethical Foundation	Standard Corporate Ethics, GDPR/ HIPAA compliance.	Yogic Virtue Ethics (*Yamas* & *Niyamas*).
Data Architecture	Centralized cloud storage.	Decentralized, user-sovereign (on-device processing).

continued on following page

Table 1. Continued

Feature	Standard Wellness Apps (e.g., Calm, Headspace)	Bio-Responsive Yoga AI
Ultimate Goal	User retention and subscription.	User liberation and system obsolescence.

Table 2. Research Gaps and Potential Directions for Future Studies

Research Gap	Brief Description	Potential Research Directions	Rationale
Longitudinal Efficacy and Dose-Response of AI-Guided Meditation	Most studies lack long-term follow-up and detailed dose-response analysis of AI-guided meditation effects on mental health and cognitive outcomes.	Conduct large-scale longitudinal studies with varied session lengths and frequencies to establish sustained benefits and optimal dosing of AI-guided meditation interventions.	Long-term adherence and sustained benefits are critical for clinical and practical adoption; current evidence is limited to short-term or pilot studies (Shankar et al.,2025) (Wieczorek et al.,2025) .
Ethical Frameworks and User Privacy in AI Meditation	Ethical considerations, including data privacy, algorithmic transparency, and risks of over-dependence on AI in meditation, remain underexplored in empirical research.	Develop and empirically test ethical guidelines and privacy-preserving AI architectures tailored for meditation and mindfulness applications. Investigate user perceptions and societal impacts of AI-mediated contemplative practices.	Addressing ethical concerns is vital to build trust, prevent misuse, and ensure responsible AI deployment insensitive spiritual and mental health domains (Tripathi,2025) (Kumar & Singhal, 2024) (Divino,2024) .
Personalization Algorithms for Complex User Needs	Current AI personalization often relies on limited physiological or behavioral data, insufficiently capturing complex mental states, preferences, and neurodivergent profiles.	Develop multimodal AI models incorporating physiological, psychological, and contextual data to enhance personalization, especially for neurodivergent and special needs populations.	Enhanced personalization can improve engagement and efficacy but requires richer data and adaptive algorithms beyond current capabilities (Khan et al., 2025) (Fonseca et al., 2025) (Singh et al., 2022) .
Scalability and Accessibility of AI Meditation Technologies	High costs, technological complexity, and digital literacy barriers limit widespread adoption of immersive AI meditation tools, especially among older adults and low-resource settings.	Innovate low-cost, user-friendly AI meditation platforms with voice-based and wearable interfaces; evaluate usability and effectiveness in underserved populations.	Accessibility is key to democratizing AI meditation benefits; current technologies often exclude vulnerable or less tech-savvy users (McCarren & Kuoppamäki, 2024) (Ghosh et al., 2025) (Ezer et al., 2024) .

REFERENCES

Adebisi, E., Balogun, S. T., Oguntuase, S. B., & Olajide, F. O. (2025). Leveraging artificial intelligence (ai) for stress management in peak athletic performance: An integrative review. *Scientific journal of engineering and technology., 2* (2), 94-106. DOI: 10.69739/sjet.v2i2.999

Attar, E. T., Balasubramanian, V., Subasi, E., & Kaya, M. (2021). Stress Analysis Based on Simultaneous Heart Rate Variability and EEG Monitoring. *IEEE Journal of Translational Engineering in Health and Medicine, 9*, 1–7. DOI: 10.1109/JTEHM.2021.3106803 PMID: 34513342

Ayub, F., Gul-E-Sehar, Javed, M. M., & Iqbal, H. H. (2025). Mindfulness and focus in AI based learning platforms: A cognitive behavioral analysis. *The critical review of social sciences studies, 3* (3), 778-796. DOI: 10.59075/zpy09450

Barton, A. C., Do, M., Sheen, J., & Byrne, L. K. (2024). The restorative and state enhancing potential of abstract fractal-like imagery and interactive mindfulness interventions in virtual reality. *Virtual Reality (Waltham Cross), 28*(1), 53. Advance online publication. DOI: 10.1007/s10055-023-00916-7

Divino, F. (2024). From meditation to techno-mindfulness: On the medicalization of contemplative practices and future prospects. *Histories, 4*(1), 125–143. DOI: 10.3390/histories4010008

Ezer, T. S., Giron, J., Erel, H., & Zuckerman, O. (2024). Somaesthetic meditation wearable: Exploring the effect of targeted warmth technology on meditators' experiences. DOI: 10.1145/3613904.3642557

Fonseca, A. A., Espinosa-Parra, I. M., Dávalos, M. B. M., & Montoya, C. D. C. R. (2025). Exploring experiences: A qualitative study on ai-enhanced mindfulness for neurodivergent individuals. *Journal-health education and welfare*. https://doi.org/ DOI: 10.35429/JHEW.2025.9.16.4.1.7

Ghosh, S., Chanda, D., & Mukhopadhyay, C. (2025). Efficacy of wearable AI driven mindfulness practices in the management of stress. *Advances in computational intelligence and robotics book series*, 85-120. DOI: 10.4018/979-8-3373-0467-0.ch004

Kaprekar, H., Thakurta, A. G., & Shirsekar, S. S. (2024). Virtual reality makes mindfulness accessible. https://doi.org/DOI: 10.58532/V3BDSO24P1CH1

Keny, V. (2025). Can artificial intelligence experience spirituality?. *Journal of advances in science and technology, 22* (2). DOI: 10.29070/3t5w4a12

Khan, M. N. H., Creswell, D., & Albert, J. O'CONNELL, P., Fallon, S., Polowitz, M., Xu, X., &Islam, B. (2025). Mindfulness meditation and respiration: Accelerometer-based respiration rate and mindfulness progress estimation to enhance app engagement and mindfulness skills. *Proceedings of the ACM on interactive, mobile, wearable and ubiquitous technologies, 9*, 95:1-95:32. https://doi.org//arxiv .2507.17688DOI: 10.48550

Kim, D.-K., Rhee, J.-H., & Kang, S. W. (2014). *Reorganization of the brain and heart rhythm during autogenic meditation.* https://www.frontiersin.org/journals/integrative-neuroscience/articles/10.3389/fnint.2013.00109/full

Kumar, A., Sankhyan, S., Tripathi, K., Rao, A. K., Bhavsar, A., & Dutt, V. (2024). Vrzm: Exploring the psycho-physiological benefits of zen meditation in immersive environments. DOI: 10.1109/ISMAR-Adjunct64951.2024.00063

Kumar, A., Sankhyan, S., Tripathi, K., Thakur, S., Bhavsar, A., & Dutt, V. (2024). Vrzm: Exploring the effect of zen meditation on eeg patterns in immersive environments. DOI: 10.1109/SMC54092.2024.10831479

Kumar, N., & Singhal, D. (2024). Empowering mental well-being: Ai-guided self-recognition and support. *International research journal of computer science, 11* (05),465-470. DOI: 10.26562/irjcs.2024.v1105.06

Luo, Y. (2025). How AI transforms mental wellness: From applications to essential questions. https://doi.org/DOI: 10.59350/mn6az-tfm26

Marade, A., Suvarna, K., Chaudhari, P., & Bhandiwad, P. V. (2025). Spiritual.ai: An ai-driven platform for enhancing mental, emotional, and spiritual well-being. *International Journal for Research in Applied Science and Engineering Technology, 13*(4), 4211–4216. DOI: 10.22214/ijraset.2025.64703

McCarren, L., & Kuoppamäki, S. (2024). The use of a voice-based digital mindfulness app to facilitate self-perceived bodily and emotional well-being among older adults: A mixed method study. DOI: 10.2196/preprints.67533

Mitsea, E., Drigas, A., & Skianis, C. (2023). Digitally assisted mindfulness in training self-regulation skills for sustainable mental health: A systematic review. *Behavioral Sciences (Basel, Switzerland), 13*(12), 1008. Advance online publication. DOI: 10.3390/bs13121008 PMID: 38131865

Mitsea, E., Drigas, A., & Skianis, C. (2024). Artificial intelligence, immersive technologies, and neuro-technologies in breathing interventions for mental and emotional health: A systematic review. *Electronics (Basel), 13*(12), 2253–2253. DOI: 10.3390/electronics13122253

Narayanan, M. (2025). Yoga AI - integrating artificial intelligence with yoga and therapy for personalized healthcare. *Annals of geriatic education and medical sciences, 11* (2),68-70. https://doi.org/DOI: 10.18231/j.agems.2024.015

Pandey, P. K., Gupta, P., Chaudhary, S., Miyapuram, K. P., & Lomas, D. (2022). Real-time sensing and neurofeedback for practicing meditation using simultaneous eeg and eye tracking. https://doi.org/DOI: 10.1109/TENSYMP54529.2022.9864414

Park, C., Youn, I., & Han, S. (2022). Single-lead ECG based autonomic nervous system assessment for meditation monitoring. https://www.nature.com/articles/s41598-022-27121-x

Rosario, C. D. P. D., Fernández, L., Agustin, V. A., Centeno, C. J., Mangrobang, M. B., &Cortez, D. M. A. (2024). Ai-powered intelligent mindfulness-based cognitive therapy companion for emotion recognition and context-aware therapy. DOI: 10.1109/ISAS64331.2024.10845635

Shamekhi, A., & Bickmore, T. (2015). Breathe with me: A virtual meditation coach. DOI: 10.1007/978-3-319-21996-7_29

Shankar, R., Devi, F., & Xu, Q. (2025). Mindfulness-based interventions using artificial intelligence: A systematic review protocol. DOI: 10.1101/2025.06.20.25329981

Singh, B., & Kaunert, C. (2024). Augmented reality and virtual reality modules for mindfulness. *Advances in medical technologies and clinical practice book series*,111-128. https://doi.org/DOI: 10.4018/979-8-3693-1123-3.ch007

Singh, S., Pandey, P. K., Chaudhary, S., Miyapuram, K. P., & Lomas, J. D. (2022). Towards the development of personalized and generalized interfaces for brain signals across different styles of meditation. DOI: 10.1145/3571600.3571656

Sinha, N., & Sinha, R. K. (2024). Harnessing the potential of artificial intelligence in yoga therapy. *International Journal of Yoga*, *17*(3), 242–245. DOI: 10.4103/ijoy.ijoy_124_24 PMID: 39959510

Soni, R., & Muniyandi, M. (2019). Breath Rate Variability: A Novel Measure to Study the Meditation Effects. *International Journal of Yoga*, *12*(1), 45–54. DOI: 10.4103/ijoy.IJOY_27_17 PMID: 30692783

Tripathi, R. L. (2025). AI meets mindfulness: Redefining spirituality and meditation in the digital age. https://doi.org/DOI: 10.53032/tvcr/2025.v7n1.03

Walia, A. (2024). Integrating classical yoga and modern psychology: Insights from neuroimaging and AI on mind transformation. *International Journal for Multidisciplinary Research, 6*(5), 27627. Advance online publication. DOI: 10.36948/ijfmr.2024.v06i05.27627

Wieczorek, A., Pintz, F., & Wagner, M. (2025). Physiological and psychological health effects of a mobile vr-based mindfulness breathing meditation with integrated biofeedback: A replication study. *Virtual Reality (Waltham Cross), 29*(4), 152. Advance online publication. DOI: 10.1007/s10055-025-01235-9

Yu, A., Lee, G., Liu, Y., Zhang, M., Jung, S. E., Park, J., Rhee, J., & Cho, K. (2025). Development and evaluation of an immersive metaverse-based meditation system for psychological well-being using llm-driven scenario generation. *Systems, 13*(9), 798–798. DOI: 10.3390/systems13090798

Zakaria, T. M., Langi, A. Z. R., Nazaruddin, M. S., & Anshori, I. (2025). Artificial Intelligence (AI) in Neurofeedback Therapy Using Electroencephalography (EEG), Heart Rate Variability (HRV), and Galvanic Skin Response (GSR): A Review. *IEEE Access : Practical Innovations, Open Solutions, 13*, 133078–133112. DOI: 10.1109/ACCESS.2025.3582805

Chapter 6
From Asana to Algorithm: Reimagining Holistic Wellness Through Yoga-Informed AI

Sohom Saha
http://orcid.org/0009-0006-9438-1554
Lakshmibai National Institute of Physical Education, India

Mahendra Kumar Singh
http://orcid.org/0000-0001-9989-9420
Lakshmibai National Institute of Physical Education, India

Awesh Khati
http://orcid.org/0009-0009-9090-1593
Lakshmibai National Institute of Physical Education, India

Komal Komal
http://orcid.org/0009-0007-1415-6857
Lakshmibai National Institute of Physical Education, India

ABSTRACT

The intersection of AI and yoga represents a paradigm shift in technology-supported holistic wellness. Current AI yoga applications focus narrowly on posture correction, neglecting yoga's multidimensional essence encompassing mental clarity, emotional resilience, and spiritual development. This chapter introduces Yoga-Informed AI, a framework where classical yogic principles from the Yoga Sutras, Bhagavad Gita, and Hatha Yoga Pradipika meaningfully shape AI models and user experiences. We examine how AI systems can support mental stillness (citta-vritti-nirodhah), guide concentration and meditation (dharana and dhyana), and enhance awareness of breath and inner experience. The chapter analyzes current limitations, proposes comprehensive design blueprints, addresses ethical and cultural considerations,

DOI: 10.4018/979-8-3373-7625-7.ch006

and projects future research directions. Yoga-Informed AI bridges ancient wisdom with computational capabilities, making holistic well-being accessible across socioeconomic, cultural, and geographical barriers.

1. INTRODUCTION

The use of artificial intelligence in the global wellness sector has seen an unmatched growth in the use of AI in the interaction between people and health tracking, behavioral change programs, and personalized coaching (Gonem et al., 2020). At the same time, yoga has developed into a global movement with millions of believers, who have been attracted by a yoga discipline that started in ancient India more than 5,000 years ago, but which has since evolved into a spiritual discipline whose benefits are geared towards physical fitness, clarity of mind, and elimination of stress (Woodyard, 2011). The overlapping paths provide a fertile ground on the new model of integrated digital wellness that goes beyond the constraints of current technological solutions.

The introduction of artificial intelligence into yoga therapy can be considered as the so-called paradigm shift in the holistic health management, as it was defined by the researchers (Sharma and Yadav, 2024). The new developments in AI have made it possible to monitor and respond to users in a customized way in real-time during yoga sessions, providing unprecedented personalization and effectiveness. Yoga therapy interventions can be expanded to virtual assistants powered by AI and telehealth platforms that would increase accessibility and inclusivity (Sharma and Yadav, 2024). However, this has seen most of its developments being concentrated towards the physical aspects of the yoga practice especially in correcting asana (posture) but with very little emphasis on the entire philosophical and experiential context that makes up the true yogic practice.

This chapter introduces a new direction called Yoga-Informed AI, according to which classical yogic principles significantly influence the AI models, algorithms and user interfaces. Instead of viewing yoga as a data-based workout program, this framework makes AI an ally of the overall change namely as a concept of technology in support of the mental, emotional, and energetic transformation that is envisaged in the classic literature on yoga. The aim is not to oust human teachers or to start measuring yoga but to develop smart systems that honor and advocate the multidimensional experience of yogic practice. The importance of such undertaking goes beyond technological innovation. The studies have always revealed that yoga interventions are capable of delivering positive outcomes in a variety of health areas, such as pain management, mental wellbeing, heart activity, and life quality (National Center for Complementary and Integrative Health, 2024).

In a 2018 Agency for Healthcare Research and Quality report, a trial of yoga in the treatment of low-back pain has been assessed and resulted in yoga relieving pain and improving functioning in both short and intermediate terms, but with similar effects as exercise (Skelly et al., 2018). Meta-analyses have suggested positive use of yoga on conditions like arthritis up to cancer related symptoms (Bussing et al., 2012). With the creation of AI systems that are inspired by yogic philosophy, we can potentially make these advantages available to the population that lacks access to qualified teachers or conventional yoga groups. The chapter has the following structure: 2 will discuss the history of yoga and its cultural development and meet the modern wellness technology. The limitations of the existing AI-based yoga applications are critically examined in Section 3. Section 4 introduces the theoretical background of Yoga-Informed AI, in the form of classical texts of yoga. Section 5 presents the blueprint of the design of Yoga-Informed AI systems. Section 6 touches on ethical and cultural issues. Section 7 is a research direction into the future and Section 8 provides a close on implications to practice and policy.

2. HISTORICAL AND CULTURAL CONTEXT

2.1 The Evolution of Yoga from Spiritual Discipline to Global Wellness Phenomenon

The historic timeline of yoga is more than 3000 years of history where yoga existed as an esoteric practice shared between guru and disciple schools of thoughts, to its present-day form of a globally accepted health and well-being method. The classic manual of classical yoga, Yoga Sutras of the sage Patanjali (c. 400 CE) does not depict yoga as a physical practice but as a disciplined way to the end of the mind and mind changes and ultimate freedom (Bryant, 2009). The well-known text of the Sutra 1.2, which is the yogas citta-vrtti-nirodhah (yoga is the cessation of the impurities of the mind), sets the main goal as the psychological and spiritual change instead of bodily well-being.

Yoga Sutras outline an eight-fold practice (ashtanga yoga) including moral restraints (yama), practices (niyama), postures (asana), relatively breath control (pranayama), withdrawal of senses (pratyahara), concentration (dharana), meditation (dhyana), and absorption (samadhi) (Feuerstein, 1998). In this holistic context, physical postures are only a part of a whole holistic program to develop bodily awareness, mental clarity, emotional control, and spiritual clarity. Swatmarama wrote the Hatha Yoga Pradipika in the fifteenth century and it is one of the most effective texts on hatha yoga, detailing practices such as postures, breath control, energetic locks (bandhas) and seals (mudras) (Muktibodhananda, 2006). This reading insists on the fact that hatha yoga practices prepare the body with the higher levels of consciousness: "The work contains 389 verses (shlokas) that are organized in four chapters describing such topics as purification, posture, breath control, spiritual centres in the body (chakra), kundalini, energetic locks, energy (prana), channels of the subtle body (nadi) and energetic seals (Mallinson and Singleton, 2017).

The text describes physical practices as a preparation of raja yoga, the royal path of meditation to samadhi. Yoga became a world sensation in the twentieth century, especially after the work of T. Krishnamacharya, B.K.S. Iyengar, and Pattabhi Jois, who invented and popularized different styles that focused on physical exercise (Singleton, 2010). It was also the time when the scientific community started to be more interested in the health benefits of yoga, and studies were done on the impact of yoga on cardiovascular health, respiratory health, mental health, and the management of chronic diseases (Bussing et al., 2012). The yoga practice adopted by modern culture in the West tends to focus more on physical fitness and alleviation of stress rather than on the philosophical and spiritual aspects upon which the traditional practice focused.

2.2 The Rise of AI in Health and Wellness

In line with the globalization of yoga, artificial intelligence has become a revolutionary concept in healthcare and wellness. Within the last 10 years, the field of AI and machine learning tools in the medical field has seen a boom of interest due to advances in the development of deep neural networks that can take multi-faceted input data and give classifications, similar to those provided by human professionals (Gonem et al., 2020). Its use in respiratory medicine, e.g. has shown AI uses in the interpretation of thoracic imaging, lung pathology and processing of physiological data such as pulmonary functional tests. The business sphere of personal health and sports performance-tracking technologies is growing, comprising of smart watches, bracelets, clothing, and patches with sensors, as well as portable devices and mobile apps (Peake et al., 2018).

Wearable health gadgets have facilitated parsimonious tracking of vital signs and new biofeedback services in insidious ways, as body sensor networks have photoplethysmography sensors, electrocardiogram sensors, and noninvasive blood pressure sensors to make constant physiological measurements (Wang et al., 2011). Mindfulness-based interventions that are provided via smartphone apps have been shown to have a therapeutic effect on a variety of psychological disorders, and systematic reviews can find positive results in repetitive negative thinking, attention regulation, and psychological decentering (Gal et al., 2024).

Research has revealed that even a comparatively short-term use of meditation apps may result in such effects as less depression, anxiety, and stress, and better sleep symptoms (Creswell and Goldberg, 2025). The mentioned advances indicate that the potential of AI-assisted wellness interventions is huge, but it also brings up the question of how to maintain the richness and authenticity of contemplative practices in the digital form. Weaknesses of the existing AI-based applications of yoga. Although there is an increasing interest in using AI in yoga, its existing applications are marked by a high level of limitations that limit their capacity to aid in the real practice of yoga. The critical analysis shows that there are some spheres which need significant improvement.

3. LIMITATIONS OF CURRENT AI-BASED YOGA APPLICATIONS

Most yoga applications based on AI are primarily concerned with correcting and recognizing postures, and they use computer vision and deep learning as methods to analyze body positions.

3.1 Overemphasis on Asana Biomechanics

Studies have found that deep learning-based architectures such as OpenPose, PoseNet, and MediaPipe can be very accurate in estimating yoga poses, and that some of these architectures can be up to 99 percent accurate in estimating yoga poses (Mohan et al., 2022). Nonetheless, this technology feature covers the surface aspect of yoga practice. Research has investigated various ways to classify yoga poses with the help of convolutional neural networks, posture estimators to identify the property of yoga asana through images and use these properties to measure the accuracy of poses (Yadav et al., 2019). Although these systems can be used to determine whether warrior pose of a practitioner is similar to a reference picture, it fails to measure the qualitative aspects of practice experienced teachers believe are critical: the quality of attention, the correlation between the breath and movement, a distribution of effort and ease, or the experience of a practitioner.

Thoutam et al. (2022) note that improper position may pose a threat to their health, leading to acute and chronic problems. The AI systems that should be used to promote this issue offer great safety features, but the reduction of yoga to biomechanical perfection is also at odds with the classical concept that asana should be mostly used to ready the organism to the state of meditation and pranayama. The Hatha Yoga Pradipika notes that asanas form firmness of body/mind, disease-lessness and flexibility as a preparation to higher practices, not in themselves.

3.2 Lack of Breath-Centered Modeling

Pranayama (breath control) is one of the essential aspects of Japanese yoga but is very inactive in the AI-based yoga applications. Classical literature has stated that pranayama is a key towards regulating fine energies and aligning the mind to meditation. In the Hatha Yoga Pradipika, whole a chapter is devoted to techniques of pranayama and it is said that pranayama is practised in order to increase the size of prana in the subtle body (Muktibodhananda, 2006). Although AI and machine learning have been used in respiratory monitoring in clinical settings, where wearable devices can continuously track respiratory rates and detect abnormal breathing instances (Manoni et al., 2020), the technologies have not been used in any meaningful way applied to yoga.

Studies have established that machine learning models are capable of identifying the breathing patterns with high accuracy and that neural network models can be used to stress detection and health monitoring by analyzing the breathing patterns (Applied Sciences, 2023). The needs of the breathing practices taught in yoga, however, in terms of regulation of inhalation and retention ratios and exhalation ratios; of nostril alternation; and breath co-ordination with bandhas are not addressed.

3.3 Minimal Attention to Internal States and Subtle Energies

Classical yoga defines a subtle body (sukshma sharira) that is made of energy channels (nadis), energy centers (chakras), and vital energy (prana) which are not visible to the external sensors. The Hatha Yoga Pradipika teaches methods of opening kundalini energy and channeling it via the central channel (sushumna nadi), techniques through which internal experiences cannot be detected by computer vision systems. The existing AI applications do not have the system to measure or assist awareness of internal states.

Although physiological markers like cardiac variability of heart rate, skin conductance, and electroencephalogram can be used as indirect measures of autonomic nervous system activity and brain conditions, these are measures of correlates of internal experience but not of the subjective awareness that is the core of the practice of yogi. The studies have detected similarities between neurofeedback and mindfulness in terms of mental states training, where the mindfulness practices are found to positively influence the brainwaves of the practitioners instantly (Drigas and Karyotaki, 2019). Nevertheless, applying such results to the effective support of the subtle energy awareness is a rather considerable challenge.

3.4 Weak Ethical Grounding in AI Design

Ethical aspects of AI development have become an increasingly important subject in healthcare settings, and researchers state that they employ fairness, accountability, transparency, and ethics (FATE) during AI development (Chen et al., 2024). AI systems may cause inequalities in healthcare provision, which means that these systems are less accurate in their diagnosis and treatment results among demographic groups (Abramoff et al., 2023). Research has discovered that dermatology artificial intelligence systems were not as accurate with dark-skinned people than with light-skinned people, which shows that unbiased training data could yield unfair results (Adamson and Smith, 2018).

Existing AI-driven yoga solutions are not often concerned with these ethical aspects. Algorithms fairness questions, whether systems can be equally effective with different body types, different age groups, abilities, and cultural backgrounds, have not been properly investigated. Furthermore, commercialization of yoga by AI platforms is a topic that is associated with cultural appropriation and commodification of spiritual traditions, which is an issue that requires ethical consideration.

3.5 Cultural and Philosophical Misalignment

This is, probably, the most basic reason why the current AI applications are philosophically not very suitable to the traditional functions of yoga. Yoga developed as part of the Indian philosophical traditions which comprehend human experience in ways fundamentally unlike the Western scientific materialism. Ideas of karma, dharma, the gunas (qualities of nature), and the kleshas (afflictions causing suffering) give explanatory schemes of psychological experience and prescriptive advice to practice which do not have analogues in other more common AI architectures.

Bhagavad Gita, in its turn, presents three ways of spiritual liberation: jnana yoga (knowledge), karma yoga (action), and bhakti yoga (devotion), and each of these ways is appropriate in various temperament and circumstances (Easwaran, 2007). The article expounds on the idea of nishkama karma, selfless deed which we give without being tied to the outcome as one way of achieving mental equanimity and spiritual liberty. These teachings cannot be optimized to algorithms, where it requires a great deal of philosophical translation but such translation has not been generally undertaken in contemporary AI applications.

4. THEORETICAL FOUNDATIONS OF YOGA-INFORMED AI

To create AI systems that will be informed by a yogic philosophy in real sense it is necessary to work seriously with the classical texts and translate the knowledge they contain into the computation formats. In this section, the investigator will explore the major ideas in the classical yoga texts and how they can be applied in the creation of AI.

4.1 Citta-Vritti-Nirodhah: Stilling Mental Fluctuations

The definition of yoga as citta-vritti-nirodhah (the stilling of mental fluctuations) by Patanjali is the basis of a principle of Yoga-Informed AI. According to the Yoga Sutras, there are five kinds of vrittis (mental modifications) correct perception, misperception, imagination, sleep, and memory which are afflicted or non-afflicted (Bryant, 2009). Yogic practice is not a process of forcibly shutting down the activity of the mind but a process of developing a witnessing consciousness that will not be disturbed by these variations. The modern neuroscience offers some confirmation to this ancient model.

The studies of the default mode network (DMN) have shown that this network is activated in the process of self-referential thought, mind-wandering, and rumination, which are the activities that can be referred to as vrittis as described in the yogic texts (Brewer et al., 2011). Research indicates that more established meditators are able to decrease the DMN activity considerably, which results in less self-referenced thought and more relaxed state of perceiving (Farb et al., 2007). AI systems that facilitate citta-vritti-nirodhah may thus include the elements of neurofeedback, which assists practitioners with becoming aware of and diminishing the activation of DMN, which feeds a person with real-time feedback throughout the meditation practice.

The development of ekagrata (one-pointedness), which is the concentration before the process of meditation, could also be enhanced by AI systems with the help of adaptive attention training. The studies of mindfulness apps have shown that digital interventions can help manage attention and decrease repetitive negative thinking (Gal et al., 2024). With systems to monitor the metrics of attention and give a personalized feedback, Yoga-Informed AI may prove to be helpful in assisting the practitioners in achieving the sustained focus that the classical texts call the key to further practice.

4.2 Dharana and Dhyana: Concentration and Meditation

According to the Yoga Sutras, there is a distinction between dharana (concentration), dhyana (meditation), and samadhi (absorption) as the increasingly deeper forms of the mental focus. Dharana is the process of stabilizing the mind so as to concentrate on one thing; continuity of concentration up to a state where the meditator loses his consciousness and the only object of meditation is attained is samadhi (Feuerstein, 1998). Dharana can be developed with help of AI systems, which may involve biofeedback technologies. The studies have shown that mindfulness training assisted by neurofeedback can enable a practitioner to reach the states of consciousness that a practitioner might otherwise need to practice over an extended period of time (Drigas and Karyotaki, 2019).

EEG headband devices like the Muse headband have been paired with meditation apps to give users feedback on their brain states in real-time to allow users to understand when their attention was lost and when they were in focused states. The problem of AI assistance in dhyana and samadhi is more serious because these two states imply the gradually less external activity and the more subtle experiences. Nevertheless, the AI systems may provide the conditions of these states by optimizing the practice settings, scheduling practice sessions throughout the circadian rhythms and personal patterns, and give relevant advice at various levels of practice. Algorithms of machine learning that are trained with longitudinal data of already experienced meditators may extract patterns related to deeper states of practice and make a personalized recommendation on how to facilitate meditation progression.

4.3 Yukta and Nishkama Karma: Balanced Action and Desireless Action

Bhagavad Gita is a book that presents ideas that are directly applicable to the philosophy of AI design. The state of nondisjunctive, balanced action that does not take to extremes of either asceticism or indulgence is called yukta: "Yoga does not belong to him who eats excessively, or him who eats insufficiently; it does not belong to him who sleeps excessively, or him who sleeps insufficiently (6.16). Such a principle of moderation implies that Yoga-Informed AI needs to encourage balanced use, versus overuse or addiction. Nishkama karma or selfless action carried out without attachment to the outcome offers a guide to practitioner involvement as well as designing the system.

There is a study on how the notion of nishkama karma as stated in the Bhagavad Gita could be useful in coping with modern situations in which the practice of developing an attitude of not caring about outcomes yields a clean and stable mind (Harmonist, 2024). In the case of AI systems, this principle implies that it should be designed in a way that encourages internal engagement, not external rewards manipulation, and it should not use gamification techniques to make someone addicted to the results instead of being able to stay in the present moment. Samatva (equanimity), the state of keeping the mind at peace in pleasure and pain, success and failure, is also described in the Gita. Systems based on AI and designed on the principle may include emotional regulation assistance, allowing practitioners to detect reactive order and develop equanimous reactions. The studies have also established that mindfulness applications can enhance emotional regulation and stress reactivity (Walsh et al., 2019), which means that AI-guided samatva development is possible.

4.4 Pranayama and Subtle Energy Systems

The Hatha Yoga Pradipika gives specific ways of practising pranayama that are used in order to cleanse the channels of energy and activate dormant spiritual energy. It explains that when pranayama is done properly, it destroys all the diseases and karma whereas improperly, it brings such diseases as headaches, asthma and pains in the ears (Muktibodhananda, 2006). This attention to technique and the slow development of the process has direct consequences on the design of AI systems. The AI that is informed by yoga must have advanced respiratory monitoring to facilitate the practice of pranayama. It has been shown that machine learning algorithms have the opportunity to highly classify the respiratory behavior and offer real-time feedback about the breathing patterns (Applied Sciences, 2023).

Body sensor network based wearable respiratory biofeedback systems have been demonstrated to be effective at respiratory training, whereby, paced respirations at abdominal level with the same inhaling and exhaling ratios have been shown to adequately reduce sympathetic arousal and enhance parasympathetic activity (Wang et al., 2011). It is difficult to realize breathing monitoring and address the needs of the yoga breathing in particular. Classical pranayama includes very specific ratios of inhaling, holding and releasing; synchronization with bandhas (energy locks), and focusing of the fine sensations of pranas flow. To implement pranayama AI systems would have to monitor these parameters and give advice based on the level of experience and the condition the practitioner is in. Design Blueprint: Yoga-Informed AI. Relying on the theoretical platforms provided above, the following section will provide an elaborate design blueprint of the Yoga-Informed AI systems. The framework includes multimodal sensing, machine-learning models, human interfaces, privacy practice, and adaptive learning systems.

5. DESIGN BLUEPRINT FOR YOGA-INFORMED AI

Based on the theoretical foundations outlined above, this section presents a comprehensive design blueprint for Yoga-Informed AI systems. The framework encompasses multimodal sensing, machine learning models, human-centered interfaces, privacy-focused practices, and adaptive learning systems.

5.1 Multimodal Sensing Systems

To be able to think effectively about AI in Yoga, one should consider a combination of sensing modalities since the world of yoga includes several dimensions to be taken into account. Sensing architecture will comprise:

Computer vision and deep learning of visual sensing of posture. A study has shown that like MediaPipe, the accuracy of the pose estimation has high scores with a minimal number of cameras (Mohan et al., 2022). Nevertheless, the Yoga-Informed AI needs to employ posture sensing as a tool not only to measure the correctness but to contribute to more comprehensive models of practice quality.

Wearable or contactless respiratory sensing. Respiratory impedance plethysmography (or similar technologies) can be used to offer respiratory monitoring of the body sensor networks (Wang et al., 2011). Non-contact techniques based on camera surveillance of chest movement or thermal monitoring of nasal airflow can provide alternatives to practitioners who want to use minimal equipment.

Physiological detection such as heart rate variability (HRV), electrodermal activity (EDA) and possibly electroencephalography (EEG). It has been shown that the signals can be used to detect stress and infer emotional state with the help of machine learning models (Peake et al., 2018). The HRV specifically gives an insight into the balance of the autonomic nervous system that is related to meditation.

Contextual sensing of the environmental conditions (time of day, ambient conditions) and behavioral patterns (quality of sleep, activity levels, practice history). Studies of just-in-time adaptive interventions have shown the usefulness of contextual information in personalization (Yom-Tov et al., 2021).

5.2 Machine Learning Models Trained on Yogic Parameters

A machine learning architecture of the Yoga-Informed AI must include models that are tailored to learn yogic parameters and qualities:

Models of practice quality that do not just measure biomechanical correctness, but such attributes as taught in the traditional teaching: stability (sthira) and ease (sukha) in postures; fluidity and continuity of transitions; coordination of breath with movement; and the right progress according to the session and session-to-session.

Breath-body coordination models which follow the relationship between respiratory cycle with posture and internal muscle interactions. The classic vinyasa practice is based on alignment of breath and movement which is the major aspect of the pose recognition systems that are currently being developed.

Models of internal state inference who approximate psychological and energetic states by using accessible physiological and behavioural data. Although one cannot directly observe subjective experience, machine learning models can be trained to associate observable variables with self-reported variables, which allows it to make approximate predictions of dimensions of interest in practice, like focus, relaxation, and energy level.

Progression models, which trace the progression of development in the various dimensions of the practice of yoga over time. These models are supposed to reflect not only physical flexibility or strength improvement but also the changes in the breathing capacity, meditation stability, and ability to regulate oneself.

5.3 Human-Centered Interfaces Encouraging Mindful Engagement

The interface design of the Yoga-Informed AI must pay attention to enabling and not interrupting mindful interaction. The studies of digital mindfulness interventions have found that the traditional designs of apps with a strong focus on measurements and gamification, as well as on frequent notifications, can create the opposite effect of the contemplative elements that such interventions are designed to promote (Lukoff et al., 2018).

Yoga-Informed AI interface design principles should entail: There is minimal distracting during practice with feedback through mechanisms that facilitate instead of interrupting attention. Audio signals can be better than visual ones that attract attention to screens; haptic feedback is yet another form of non-obtrusive instructions. The right timing of feedback and recommendations, since various stages of practice need various kinds of support. Online correction in the face of difficulty is not the same as reflection on practice patterns after the sessions.

The agency of the users in deciding the role of AI support, whether to provide minimum tracking to the experienced practitioner and more significant guidance to the novice. The system should be flexible to suit the users instead of having standardized interactions. Reflective aesthetics that bears out the characteristics desired in practice. The elements of interface design such as colour palette, typography, image, and sound design must convey yogic principles of simplicity, harmony and presence.

5.4 Privacy-Focused and Ethically Aligned Data Practices

The Yoga-Informed AI systems record personal information regarding the bodies of the practitioners, their actions, and possibly their psyches. Such information is to be rigorously secured based on the regulatory aspect and ethical considerations. The studies of AI ethics point to the importance of fairness, accountability, transparency, and ethics, which have to be considered attentively to provide responsible application and protect the well-being of individuals (Chen et al., 2024).

In the case of Yoga-Informed AI, these principles are converted into the following requirements: Minimization of data that only gathers data needed to run the system, and justification provided on the basis of each data item. Practitioners ought to be informed of the data that is being gathered and the purpose of doing so. On-site processing wherever possible, retention of sensitive information in user devices instead of sending the data to central servers. The strategies of edge computing allow advanced AI to be done without centralizing data. Openness of the algorithmic decisions allowing the practitioners to learn the way the recommendations are made.

Model reasoning can be revealed through explainable AI techniques. Equity auditing to guarantee the equitable functioning of systems in varied groups. Data used in training must reflect different body types, ages, capabilities and cultural differences and performance differences should be regularly tested. Consent and control that allows practitioners to access, edit and destroy their data. The systems must offer substantial control within data use instead of only notifying users of nontransparent practices.

5.5 Adaptive Learning Systems

AI, which is informed by yoga, ought to respond to the needs, capabilities, and development of individual practitioners. Studies of customized digital health interventions have shown that the reinforcement learning algorithms can be used to customize the intervention based on the individual characteristics and reactions (Yom-Tov et al., 2021; Aguilera et al., 2024). The essential adaptive Yoga-Informed AI capabilities are: JIT adaptation which changes instructions based on present condition and situation.

It has been shown that digital interventions based on reinforcement learning are capable of changing their adaptation to changes in daily activity, preferences, and attitudes (Yom-Tov et al., 2021). The long-term progression model which follows the growth of an individual in the course of weeks, months, and years, and modifies the practice recommendations to sustain the growth. The traditional yoga acknowledges that proper practice differs significantly according to the level of experience and according to personal constitutions.

Multi-dimensional personification that takes not only physical abilities into account but also psychological behavior, life limitations, spiritual orientation. The various practitioners might find it useful to focus on various aspects of practice at various times. Teacher integration which will allow human yoga teachers to look through AI suggestions and give feedback that will result in system adjustment. Yoga-Informed AI needs not to take the place of teachers but amplify their advice.

6. ETHICAL AND CULTURAL CONSIDERATIONS

The creation of Yoga-Informed AI poses serious ethical and cultural concerns that have to be considered. In addition to the ethical standards of AI systems in general, there are yoga-related issues based on the cultural roots of the practice and spiritual aspects.

6.1 Cultural Authenticity and Appropriation

Yoga was introduced in Indian philosophical and spiritual traditions and its popularization around the world has often been carried out through decontextualization and commercialization which can often feel like appropriation to the traditional practitioners. These issues should be taken seriously in the development of AI that is informed by yoga. It involves genuine participation of practitioners and teachers in system design and evaluation with real meaning with the traditional lineages. It should not be a sense of tokenism in consultation but rather a sense of real collaboration where the traditional views guide the key decisions in designs.

The cultural roots and the philosophical context of yoga should be properly reflected in AI systems without introducing representations that facilitate the erase of traditional meaning or the false interpretation of yoga concepts. Revenue models need to take into account the ways of contributing to yoga communities and institutions in India and other countries. They were taught traditionally without fee in guru disciple relationships; although these commerce AI products work in different ways, some of the revenue could be used to fund traditional teachers, generations, or neighborhood centers.

6.2 Yama and Niyama: Ethical Foundations from Within Yoga

Interestingly, yoga itself offers a moral code that could be used in the AI development. The Patanjali ashtanga yoga of which the first two limbs (yama (ethical restraints)) and niyama (observances)) are the principles of ethical behavior that could guide Yoga-Informed AI design (Feuerstein, 1998). The five yamas include:

Ahimsa (non-harm): Systems based on AI must not harm their users or others physically, psychologically, or socially. This is applied to the need not to use manipulative design patterns, respect user autonomy, and effects of computational resources on the environment.

Satya (truthfulness): Systems are expected to give the correct information and do not deceive their offerings in terms of benefits or capabilities. Openness of algorithmic operation conforms with this principle.

Asteya (non-stealing): Traditional knowledge is respected by giving appropriate credit and proceeds with sharing the benefits. The information of the users must not be misused.

Brahmacharya (proper use of energy): Systems must be able to provide balanced and sustainable use, as opposed to encouraging addictive use patterns. Design must also save user focus and energy to significant practice instead of spending it to gauge of engagement metrics.

Aparigraha (non-grasping): Business models must not be over-monetized, which means they will take all the money without concern about whether the user gains or not. This principle might be better reflected in subscription models that are in line with real value delivered as opposed to aggressive monetization.

The five niyamas, purity, contentment, discipline, self-study, and surrendering oneself to a higher principle, also provide advice in the design of the system, as well as in the corporate culture of companies building Yoga-Informed AI.

6.3 Preventing Data Misuse and Ensuring Equitable Access

The personal information gathered by Yoga-Informed AI systems gives the possibility of misuse that needs to be prevented actively. Practice-based health-related inferences may have a possible impact on insurance, employment, or other areas as they are disclosed incorrectly. It should have strong data protection, strict limitations of use, and powerful protection. The other moral duty is equity in access. Studies have shown that the personalization approaches of machine learning are often not developed using the data of marginalized groups, which may constrain the effectiveness of the method in the case of ethnic and racialized minorities and low-income populations (Aguilera et al., 2024).

The proactive approach to the development of yoga-aware AI must include the representation of a wide range of data during the training process and the availability of AI in the workplace. This can involve deliberate design decisions that are cost-cutting or free of charge to economically marginalized groups. Components of the open-source may be able to adapt to different contexts. Community organization partnerships may also go beyond commercially viable markets.

7. FUTURE RESEARCH DIRECTIONS

The Yoga-Informed AI allows broadening the number of research directions at the crosspoint between computer science, contemplative studies, and health sciences. In this section, especially promising directions of future research are indicated.

7.1 Immersive Technologies for Yogic Experiences

Virtual reality (VR) and augmented reality (AR) promise to provide a chance to experience yogic experiences in an immersive setting, which cannot be done through existing flat-screen interfaces. Studies have started looking into AI-enhanced VR, meditation, and mindfulness, as platforms with virtual environments guiding relaxation and helping to control emotions (Brainz Magazine, 2023). Future studies could consider VR environments which have been made to assist in pratyahara (sense withdrawal) with the use of controlled sensory input that aids in inward focus. Delicate visual and auditory cues could be used to indicate where attention should be paid in the process of meditation, whereas the use of immersive versions of the practice setting could help in the process of adopting the cultural experience that home practice usually lacks. AR applications might provide guidance in alignment directly superimposed on the appearance of practitioners of their bodies, which might facilitate learning while still being in contact with the physical world. Bone conduction headphones based on audio AR might be able to deliver breathing cues without the user having to look at the screen.

7.2 AI for Energetic Mapping and Subtle Body Awareness

Though the existing technology is unable to directly measure the subtle energy systems that are mentioned in the writings of classical yoga, future studies may examine whether some form of consistent correlations can be found between anecdotal reports of subtle experience and the measurable physiological signals. Multimodal sensor fusion of EEG, HRV, respiratory patterns, and others may detect a signature that can be related to states which can be described in energetic terms by traditional practitioners. It is possible that machine learning models that are trained on the information about experienced practitioners sharing their experiences within the company can learn to predict subtle states based on their physiological patterns. There would be the need to design such research with keen methodological consideration not to reify phenomena that may not be physical and still be open to real correlations that could lead to support of practice. It would be necessary to join efforts of contemplative practitioners, neuroscientists and computer scientists.

7.3 Neuroscientific Correlates of Advanced Yogic States

Modern neuroscience is also starting to explore the brain states of meditation and they have discovered patterns relating to focused attention, open monitoring and non-dual awareness (Brewer et al., 2011). Future studies could build upon this study to investigate states contained in yogic texts, like those of different samadhis given as a list in the Yoga Sutras of Patanjali. This type of study would be useful in AI systems to help advance to higher levels by determining the neural phenotypes relevant to various stages of practice. Such signatures may be used to stabilize useful states with real-time neurofeedback, which practitioners can determine. But there is a caveat in this line of research in the fact that the spiritual experiences can be reduced to neural correlates. The connections between brain states and subjective experience are still an object of philosophical dispute and neural pattern should not be implicitly claimed by Yoga-Informed AI that will represent the reality that the traditional descriptions are primitive approximations to it.

7.4 Longitudinal Studies of AI-Supported Yoga Practice

Strict assessment of Yoga-Informed AI will involve longitudinal research studies of the effects in various areas of wellbeing. Although the existing research has proven it to be beneficial when applied to different health outcomes (National Center for Complementary and Integrative Health, 2024), the number of studies that specifically study AI-assisted practice is small. This study needs to be followed by other randomized controlled trials to compare AI-aided yoga with traditional education, self-directed education, and other digital wellness programs. Outcome measures are not to include just the physical fitness parameters, but also the psychological well-being and stress resilience, quality of life, and possibly some measures of spiritual development that align with different worldviews. Special concern should be paid to whether the AI support can improve the accessibility and compliance without disturbing the quality of practice. Studies may be done to examine the hypothesis that AI-assisted practitioners acquire the embodied knowledge and self-regulation skills inherent in traditional instruction, or the hypothesis that technological mediation unintentionally results in dependency that inhibits the ability to practice autonomously.

7.5 Cross-Cultural Adaptation and Validation

AI developed in yoga-informed ways in one cultural setting can need a lot of adaptation to work in other settings. Further studies need to be conducted on the effectiveness of systems in different populations and what amendments improve cross-cultural validity. The study is to involve working with the yoga communities in India and other parts of the world where the conventional practice is still thriving and whether the A.I. systems that have been created with mostly western practitioners in mind can serve those who have other cultural affiliations with yoga. The native research methodologies which focus on the perspectives of the community could prove useful in this research. The concept of language adaptation goes beyond translation to include the conceptual models on how practice can be known. The words such as energy, chakra, or mindfulness have different meanings in various cultures, and AI programs should not only accept the words but also the conceptual frameworks to meet the needs of various users.

8. APPLICATIONS OF YOGA-INFORMED AI

The above theoretical framework and design principles make it possible to have varieties of practical uses. In this section, I will explain the practical examples of the potential of Yoga-Informed AI.

8.1 Breath-Sensitive Meditation Trainers

The Breath-Sensitive Meditation Trainers were created by Michael and Anne in 1984 as a component of the Gestalt Psychotherapy program. Breath-Sensitive Meditation Trainers: Michael and Anne invented the Breath-Sensitive Meditation Trainers in 1984 as part of the Gestalt Psychotherapy course. Yoga-Guided meditations in the near future, Yoga-led AI can be developed by using meditation training applications based on yogic breath awareness. These applications would combine respiratory tracking with breathing instructions, which would give real-time feedback on breathing patterns besides aiding in the development of attention.

The system would monitor the respiratory rate, depth, regularity, and the ratio between the inhalation to exhalation identifying the patterns of calm and focused conditions compared to agitation or distraction. Physiological signature models of meditators with experience trained using machine learning could serve as standards to measure progress. The guidance would vary the sessions based on the present conditions of the practitioners, be shorter in case of agitation is spotted, or recommend particular breathing exercises to deal with the patterns in question.

The system would eventually be able to learn the overall pattern and successful interventions used by individual practitioners and will have the ability to provide more personalized support. It has been proved that even the short-term use of meditation apps can have quantifiable anxiety, depression, and stress effects (Creswell & Goldberg, 2025). To further benefit them, breath-sensitive systems may assist in offering more responsive and personalized guidance compared to what is currently being provided by applications.

8.2 Emotional Regulation Tools Based on Guna and Klesha Theory

Classical yoga psychology explains that there are three gunas (qualities of nature) sattva (clarity, harmony), rajas (activity, passion), and tamas (inertia, darkness) which are mixed in different proportions to create different mental states (Feuerstein, 1998). Psychological patterns that bring suffering are called the kleshas (afflictions), ignorance, ego, attachment, aversion, and fear of death. Yoga-informed AI software would be useful in emotion management by assisting yoga students in identifying the dominance of guna and activation of kleshas in their present state.

The physiological and behavioral data could show high levels of rajas (fast heart rate, irritable movement) or tamas (low level of activity, flat affect), making it possible to make specific recommendations. Upon identifying these klesha patterns say, aversion pattern signaled by avoidance behaviors or attachment pattern signaled by compulsive engagement, the system may provide practices that are traditionally advised to deal with these patterns. Practicing opposite thoughts (pratipaksha bhavana) as outlined in the Yoga Sutras could be the basis of interventions that may propose alternative ways of thinking when the presence of an afflictive pattern is identified.

8.3 AI-Guided Integrated Practice Routines

The whole yoga practice incorporates the use of asana, pranayama and meditation in a manner that suits needs and situations. Yoga-Informed AI may create tailored practice plans that suitably arrange these factors according to the available time, energy, goals of practice, and the state. The system would take into consideration circadian parameters, whereby it suggests energizing activities in the mornings and ones that relax in the evenings. It would adjust to the perceived stress levels, recommending restorative practices in case of a high level of stress.

Development would be monitored over sessions with the difficulty and duration of practice being changed to help maintain further growth without excessive strain. Notably, the system would take care of the relationships between the practice elements that are respected by traditional sequencing. Pranayama after asana, meditation after pranayama and special preparations before the more advanced methods would be included as per the traditional instructions and assessment of the individual readiness.

8.4 Digital Ecosystems Promoting Svadhyaya (Self-Study)

One of the niyamas that must be involved in yogic development is called Svadhyaya, which is more traditionally translated as study of sacred texts and self-observation. Yoga-inspired AI has the potential to build digital ecosystems that would facilitate this meditative self-inquiry with the help of journaling prompts, practice reflection tools, and custom-crafted educational materials. After practicing, the system may provide reflection prompts based on conventional wisdom that is applicable to the challenges or interests that the practitioner is facing.

A journaling tool may assist practitioners in keeping recordings regarding their experience over a period of time, and the analysis of AI may present new patterns that were previously unnoticed. The curation of educational contents would be based on personal interests and level of practice, whereby the introduction of philosophical concepts would be done when the practitioners are prepared to acquire a deeper comprehension. Instead of bombarding the beginner with abstract philosophy, the system would present concepts after experience in practice provides the occasion of intellectual comprehension.

8.5 Intelligent Lifestyle Guidance Aligned with Yogic Principles

The traditional yoga will include lifestyle suggestions that go far beyond the practice environment. Classical texts focus on diet, sleep, relationship, and daily routine as being supportive or hindering in the yogic development. Yoga-Informed AI may offer lifestyle advice based on the classical suggestions and be outfitted to respond to the modern realities. The idea of sleep optimization could be based on the yogic views on the proper rest and should be applied in the context of the modern sleep science. The diets provision can be based on the conventional ayurvedic laws and still meet the health needs and food supplies of the specific individual. The system would identify that lifestyle change must be done in a gradual and sustainable manner. Instead of applying idealized yogic ways of life, it would help in gradual changes that are suitable to the situation and motivation of each practitioner. It would be informed by the principle of yukta (balance) which would guide recommendations, which are not extreme and which promote sustainable well-being rather than unsustainable perfectionism.

9. IMPLEMENTATION CONSIDERATIONS

To convert the Yoga-Informed AI framework into effective systems, the theory will need to consider various implementation issues across the technical, organizational, and regulatory implementation areas.

9.1 Technical Infrastructure Requirements

AI systems that are informed by yoga would need a sound technical infrastructure to facilitate multimodal data processing, real-time data processing, secure data storage, and intelligent delivery of interventions. The most appropriate balance between privacy and capability requirements could be provided by edge computing architectures processing sensitive data locally with the ability to train models in the cloud. Interoperability standards that allow connection with various wearable devices and health platforms, practice management systems, etc. will improve adoption and usability.

Open APIs might also allow third-party developers to expand core abilities to unique populations or practice traditions. To improve the model on a continuous basis, infrastructure is needed to gather the feedback of the user, determine the performance problems, and implement the new models without causing the user a disturbance. Practices of MLOps adapted to wellness applications must respond to the specific needs of systems in which malfunctions can influence the health and well-being of users.

9.2 Organizational Capabilities

Institutions that create Yoga-Informed AI must have a wide range of skills in technology, meditation, and medical spheres. The development teams must also have not only software engineers and data scientists but also seasoned yoga teachers, researchers of contemplative practices and healthcare workers. The cultural competency training ought to equip the team members to approach the contextual backgrounds of yoga in a respectful manner. The cultural authenticity and proper representation can be achieved through advisory relations with traditional lineage and Indian yoga institutions. A user research methodology must be able to capture the experiential aspects of the yoga practice that a quantitative measure can not. In-depth interviews, phenomenological analysis, and participatory design that form part of qualitative research will be able to offer the insights that can be used to develop systems that can actually support practice.

9.3 Regulatory Compliance

Depending on the claims of the products and the population covered, yoga-informed AI systems can be regulated as digital health products. The regulatory framework of FDA of software as a medical device (SaMD) in the United States can be relevant to the systems that make therapeutic claims or treat clinical populations. Regulations on data protection such as GDPR in Europe and other state regulations in the United

States present requirements of data collection, data storage, and data use of personal information. In the United States, or other similar systems, health-related data may be given increased protection under HIPAA. The regulatory expertise needs to be involved early in the development of organizations so that development of compliance pathways is observed during system construction. Early consultation with regulators can assist in developing emerging frameworks of AI wellness application in a manner that can facilitate innovation without endangering users.

10. CONCLUSIONS

The transition between asana and algorithm is not only a technological breakthrough but also a rethinking of the whole idea of the ancient wisdom and modern technology working together to help human beings flourish. As defined in this chapter, Yoga-Informed AI provides a model of developing intelligent systems that maintain and promote the multidimensional nature of the yogic practice and apply its opportunities to the populations that otherwise couldn't have them. The shortcomings of existing AI-based yoga software, their excessive focus on physical exercises, the lack of attention to breathing and inner states, a poor sense of ethics, as well as the irrelevance to a specific culture, provide not only a challenge but also an opportunity. It is possible to create systems that underlie not just physical fitness but also mental clarity, emotional stability, moral growth and spiritual growth by taking the work of classical tradition of yoga seriously and translating what it has to say into the language of computation. The design blueprint hereof including multimodal sensing, yogic machine learning models, mindful interfaces, ethical data practices, and adaptive learning gives a path to development that respects the wisdom of the past and takes advantage of modern technological abilities.

Particular applications such as breath-sensitive meditation trainers, emotional regulation applications, integrated practice guidance, self-study ecosystems and lifestyle support demonstrate the practical potential of this framework. However, much is yet to be done. The areas of research in the immersive technologies, subtle body mapping, neuroscientific research, longitudinal outcome research, and cross-cultural validation should be maintained. Systems undergo ethical and cultural considerations which require constant attention as systems evolve between concept and implementation. The issues of implementation that are technical infrastructure, organizational capabilities, and regulatory compliance should be addressed. But, above all, the creation of the Yoga-Informed AI has to be developed with the appropriate humility.

The ultimate aspects of the yogic experience, the firsthand realization that the classical writings spell out as the ultimate goal of yoga may never be the one that is technologically aided. AI may possibly help to arrange the groundwork, eliminate impediments, and suggest directions on the way, but the process itself is too human to be reduced. However, the benefits that might be achieved are worth trying hard. Yoga-Informed AI can be used to add to the human well-being on large scale, respecting the ancient tradition, on which it is based, and by ensuring the practice of yoga is more accessible, offering an individualized support to a variety of practitioners, and offering tools in self-study and reflection of practices. The asana algorithm integration, when thought through and executed with great care, provides an idea of technology serving human flourishing that can have far more far-reaching implications than even the particular sphere of the yoga practice itself.

REFERENCES

Abràmoff, M. D., Tarver, M. E., Loyo-Berrios, N., Trujillo, S., Char, D., Obermeyer, Z., Eydelman, M. B., & Maisel, W. H. (2023). Considerations for addressing bias in artificial intelligence for health equity. *NPJ Digital Medicine*, *6*(1), 170. DOI: 10.1038/s41746-023-00913-9 PMID: 37700029

Adamson, A. S., & Smith, A. (2018). Machine learning and health care disparities in dermatology. *JAMA Dermatology*, *154*(11), 1247–1248. DOI: 10.1001/jamadermatol.2018.2348 PMID: 30073260

Aguilera, A., Hernandez-Ramos, R., Haro-Ramos, A. Y., Thapa-Chhetry, B., & Figueroa, C. A. (2024). A machine learning approach for personalized autonomous digital mental health interventions in underrepresented populations. *Journal of Medical Internet Research*, *26*, e59673. DOI: 10.2196/59673

Applied Sciences. (2023). Machine learning for respiratory behavior classification. *Applied Sciences*, 13(11), 6489. DOI: 10.3390/app13116489

Brewer, J. A., Worhunsky, P. D., Gray, J. R., Tang, Y. Y., Weber, J., & Kober, H. (2011). Meditation experience is associated with differences in default mode network activity and connectivity. *Proceedings of the National Academy of Sciences of the United States of America*, *108*(50), 20254–20259. DOI: 10.1073/pnas.1112029108 PMID: 22114193

Bryant, E. F. (2009). *The Yoga Sutras of Patañjali: A new edition, translation, and commentary*. North Point Press.

Büssing, A., Ostermann, T., Lüdtke, R., & Michalsen, A. (2012). Effects of yoga interventions on pain and pain-associated disability: A meta-analysis. *The Journal of Pain*, *13*(1), 1–9. DOI: 10.1016/j.jpain.2011.10.001 PMID: 22178433

Chen, R. J., Wang, J. J., Williamson, D. F. K., Chen, T. Y., Lipkova, J., Lu, M. Y., Saber, S., & Mahmood, F. (2024). Algorithmic fairness in artificial intelligence for medicine and healthcare. *Nature Biomedical Engineering*, *7*(6), 719–742. DOI: 10.1038/s41551-023-01056-8 PMID: 37380750

Creswell, J. D., & Goldberg, S. B. (2025). Mindfulness apps and health: Perspectives and prospects. *Annual Review of Psychology*, *76*. Advance online publication. DOI: 10.1146/annurev-psych-011624-025753

Drigas, A. S., & Karyotaki, M. (2019). A layered model of human consciousness. *International Journal of Recent Contributions from Engineering. Science & IT*, *7*(3), 41–50. DOI: 10.3991/ijes.v7i3.11117

Easwaran, E. (2007). *The Bhagavad Gita* (2nd ed.). Nilgiri Press.

Farb, N. A. S., Segal, Z. V., Mayberg, H., Bean, J., McKeon, D., Fatima, Z., & Anderson, A. K. (2007). Attending to the present: Mindfulness meditation reveals distinct neural modes of self-reference. *Social Cognitive and Affective Neuroscience*, *2*(4), 313–322. DOI: 10.1093/scan/nsm030 PMID: 18985137

Feuerstein, G. (1998). *The Yoga tradition: Its history, literature, philosophy and practice*. Hohm Press.

Gal, E., Irme, S., & Kube, T. (2024). Mechanisms of change in app-based mindfulness interventions: A systematic review. *Mindfulness*, *15*, 2105–2131. DOI: 10.1007/s12671-024-02426-w

Gonem, S., Sherif, M., Taylor, J., Lord, W., & Bafadhel, M. (2020). Applications of artificial intelligence and machine learning in respiratory medicine. *Thorax*, *75*(8), 695–701. DOI: 10.1136/thoraxjnl-2020-214556 PMID: 32409611

Lukoff, K., Yu, C., Kientz, J., & Hiniker, A. (2018). What makes smartphone use meaningful or meaningless? *Proceedings of the ACM on Interactive, Mobile, Wearable and Ubiquitous Technologies*, *2*(1), 1–26. DOI: 10.1145/3191754

Mallinson, J., & Singleton, M. (2017). *Roots of yoga*. Penguin Classics.

Manoni, A., Loreti, F., Radicioni, V., Pellegrino, D., Della Torre, L., Gumiero, A., Halicki, D., Palange, P., & Lukowicz, P. (2020). A machine learning approach for monitoring respiratory events during sleep. *MDPI Sensors*, *20*(20), 5785. DOI: 10.3390/s20205785

Mohan, V., Srivastava, S., & Kiran, M. (2022). Deep learning-based yoga posture recognition system. *International Journal of Engineering Research & Technology (Ahmedabad)*, *11*(5), 134–140.

Muktibodhananda, S. (2006). *Hatha yoga pradipika* (4th ed.). Bihar School of Yoga.

National Center for Complementary and Integrative Health. (2024). *Yoga: What the science says*. National Institutes of Health. https://www.nccih.nih.gov/health/yoga-what-the-science-says

Peake, J. M., Kerr, G., & Sullivan, J. P. (2018). A critical review of consumer wearables, mobile applications, and equipment for providing biofeedback, monitoring stress, and sleep in physically active populations. *Frontiers in Physiology*, *9*, 743. DOI: 10.3389/fphys.2018.00743 PMID: 30002629

Sharma, P., & Yadav, R. (2024). Artificial intelligence in yoga therapy: A transformative approach to holistic health management. In *Advances in computational intelligence for healthcare* (pp. 215–234). Springer., DOI: 10.1007/978-3-031-60542-7_11

Singleton, M. (2010). *Yoga body: The origins of modern posture practice*. Oxford University Press., DOI: 10.1093/acprof:oso/9780195395358.001.0001

Skelly, A. C., Chou, R., Dettori, J. R., Turner, J. A., Friedly, J. L., Rundell, S. D., Fu, R., Brodt, E. D., Wasson, N., Winter, C., & Ferguson, A. J. R. (2018). *Noninvasive nonpharmacological treatment for chronic pain: A systematic review* (Comparative Effectiveness Review No. 209). Agency for Healthcare Research and Quality. DOI: 10.23970/AHRQEPCCER209

Thoutam, V., Sai, A., Vyas, R., & Ghose, U. (2022). Yoga pose estimation and feedback generation using deep learning. *Computational Intelligence and Neuroscience*, *4311350*, 1–12. Advance online publication. DOI: 10.1155/2022/4311350

Walsh, K. M., Saab, B. J., & Farb, N. A. S. (2019). Effects of a mindfulness meditation app on subjective well-being: Active randomized controlled trial and experience sampling study. *JMIR Mental Health*, *6*(1), e10844. DOI: 10.2196/10844 PMID: 30622094

Wang, S., Zhou, G., Ma, Y., Hu, L., Chen, Z., Chen, Y., & Zhao, H. (2011). Wearable respiratory biofeedback system based on body sensor network. *Procedia Engineering*, *15*, 3296–3300. DOI: 10.1016/j.proeng.2011.08.618

Woodyard, C. (2011). Exploring the therapeutic effects of yoga and its ability to increase quality of life. *International Journal of Yoga*, *4*(2), 49–54. DOI: 10.4103/0973-6131.85485 PMID: 22022122

Yadav, S. K., Singh, A., Gupta, A., & Raheja, J. L. (2019). Real-time yoga recognition using deep learning. *Neural Computing & Applications*, *31*(12), 9349–9361. DOI: 10.1007/s00521-019-04232-7

Yom-Tov, E., Feraru, G., Kozdoba, M., Mannor, S., Tennenholtz, M., & Hochberg, I. (2021). Encouraging physical activity in patients with diabetes: Intervention using a reinforcement learning system. *Journal of Medical Internet Research*, *19*(10), e338. DOI: 10.2196/jmir.7994 PMID: 29017988

Chapter 7
AI-Enhanced Dharana and Dhyana

Anushka Banerjee
Ajeenkya D.Y. Patil University, India

Susanta Das
http://orcid.org/0000-0002-9314-3988
Ajeenkya D.Y. Patil University, India

ABSTRACT

Meditation studies have grown to provide a more concrete link between ancient yoga theories and modern neuroscience and smart devices to gain greater insight into organized mental training. Dharana (concentrated attention) and Dhyana (easy absorption of meditations) are considered to be consecutive, though different levels, characterized by distinct cognitive, neural, and physiological attributes. Empirical studies show that Dharana should be taken as active attentional regulation, but Dhyana should be described as stabilized mindfulness, neural coherence and predomination of parasympathetic activity. Recent developments in the field of AI provide even more opportunities to monitor multimodally in real time, provide adaptive feedback, and give personalized instructions without neglecting old meditative principles. The chapter explores conceptual underpinnings, neuroscientific data, AI-driven assessment instruments, and future research trends to frame technology-assisted Dharana and Dhyana as a solid framework of contemplative science and mental health studies development.

DOI: 10.4018/979-8-3373-7625-7.ch007

1. INTRODUCTION

Constant focus follows one step before complete stillness. Not so much ease, no, but to keep on holding on sinks back again into noise. Then, slowly, the grip fades. What follows is not impelled - it does not operate, but continues. When combat drifting stops being the object of the intensity, the drift is referred to as drift. Spectacles are long and wide and stretch. It is only after resistance has been exhausted by repetition that such state is attained. The effort is substituted with the continuity. The attraction of ideas is no longer as it used to be. One moment simply segues into the next, and is not separated. The transformation is manifested in the fact that the effort becomes still and this can be seen in the old teachings and how people view these teachings. The focusing strain is the setup to a stage and careless attention is the set-up to a higher stage - this is according to the new opinions (Tripathi & Bharadwaj, 2021; Thakur, 2025). Such stages, along with ideas, might be studied through observable variations of awareness. Such links of wisdom of the past and the existing research provide possibilities to realize well-being in more profound ways (Thakur, 2025).

This division can be proved today by science by means of the brain scan and the body tests which confirm the fact that the impressions of Dharana and Dhyana can be different on the nervous system. The readings of the brain waves recorded by the eLORETA and sLORETA instruments show that Dharana produces more alpha and theta waves in the frontal and top areas of the brain which is a sign of intensive mental activity. On the other extreme, Dhyana enhances the gamma activities between the regions associated with mind wandering and alertness describing a potentially smooth association as opposed to inner discourses. It is evidenced by scans of fMRI - in the state of Dharana, the upper part of the frontal lobe is activated, and the attention is narrowed. The area is quiet in the event of Dhyana, and the power is passed to other deeper areas like the back cingulate and insula to be extensively and broadly present. Definite lines also contain body signals - Dharana stabilizes the heart beat rhythm balancing the nerve systems. But Dhyana strengthens the calming nature of the nerves, slowing the breath, and reducing the blood pressure to an extent which is comparable to the action of a treatment of high blood pressure.

The intentional inhalation in working memory makes it better - consider Dharana, a of people who are alert, and yet, they occasionally pass out, mistakes reveal it. What comes next is perhaps the most shocking, there are those pauses between thoughts that are linked with capacity of an individual to handle distracters in a test. Deep calm conversely is synonymous with natural belly breathing in Dhyana and happens to make everything slower without trying to slow it very much. It is owing to this rhythm, the research work on Pragya Yoga reveals, that sleep is enhanced. This is where the emphasis is felt, since in any other place, it is possible to hear the stinging of the mind. These trends are also echoed in the operation of the immune system in connection with the different styles of yoga; there is one day without tension and the following days inflammation. These differences are critical than expected during emergencies of health including during pandemics - previously established defenses grow with training in focus, and elastic defenses grow in quiet intake. The joint pain research also suggests targeted exercises on the targeted regions with unique movement-breath patterns in comparison with more general, mental-physical effects of more advanced meditation (Biswas et al., 2025). As a result of this fact, researchers need to make sure that the two types are not mixed when carrying out experiments - it is necessary to be clear about the degree to which practice leads to what in mindfulness studies.

Science is better placed to understand the way the brains operate. Because of this fact, computers can help people to practice more attention and deep meditation than they did previously. The conventional methods depend on the traditional teachers who might be discriminatory or unreachable to a number of individuals. It is through machines that patterns of brain waves, heart pulses and signals on body showing the actual state of an individual are identified. They do not guess - they find out the extent of certitude of each reading. The forced attention and the calm awareness can be separated by some of the programs by tracking different kinds of brain waves. This helps in giving the appropriate advice at the right time and also one that differs according to how the individual is performing at that moment. The instructions in simulated conditions. In the simulated settings, guided watching exercises can be customized by means of live data. Plans that are developed individually minimize stress when it becomes overwhelming. Such installations are easy to multiply among big groups of people and are not lost in the process of this. Each step has its own progressive development founded on the changes that can be quantified, not on assumptions.

One of them is the personalization of the approaches: intelligent models show how they did it by showing how they reason, adjusting their approach to the brain patterns of rest like diet researched based on many data to make a guess about nutrient absorption (Sak & Suchodolska, 2021; Sengar et al., 2024). Instead of just pictures, ear-nose-throat and tumor examinations have also obtained scans with body signs; the intensity of meditation is also changed with live heartbeat and breathing rate, to calculate the time of the focus sessions, before deeper conditions (Demir et al., 2025; Saeidnia et al., 2025). A story of curing using emotional trauma with a context of attentiveness is possible antecedents of machines who testify to databases, a sense of subjectivity, and using codes in the issue (Hasan et al., 2025). Nevertheless, educating nurses or doctors, artificial intelligence creates an opportunity and learners familiarize themselves with how they read physical changes in conscious work (Rony et al., 2023; Sapci & Sapci, 2020). However, technology does not replace the tradition, but it is capable of facilitating the tradition, providing more regularity of the practices, but the development remains a matter of practice (Tripathi, 2025).

The combination of intelligent tools and intense focus practice opens up new opportunities - and they were tested in health research, but can be implemented in other destinations like India with small clinics (Basu-Ray et al., 2022; Nalbant et al., 2022). The latter is the mechanism, actual tests, clear-cut ways, concrete evidence. The old insight, however, is not replaced by machines, but only aids in passing it along.

Figure 1 displays the flow of chapter showing the topics that are discussed in the chapter, starting from the Classical Foundation of Dhayana and Dharma to Bibliometric Analysis showing the important keywords and the research on the topic.

Figure 1. Flowchart on the Chapter.

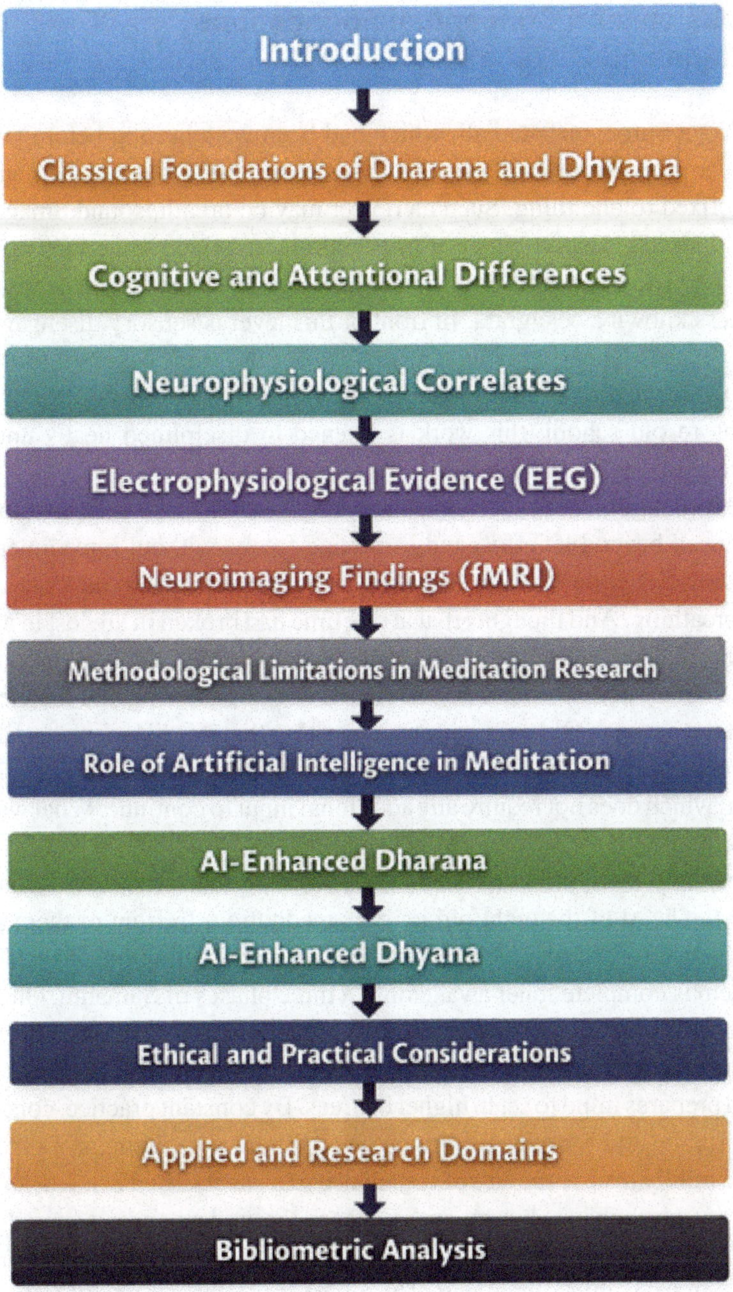

2. LITERATURE REVIEW

2.1. Classical and Conceptual Foundations to Dharana and Dhyana

The Yoga Sutras of Patanjali, which had been written long before our era, are steps, which proceed outwardly to inner hush. Sixth among them is Dharana - keeping the mind fixed to one thing. Such an object may be breath, sound, image, or even a candle flame. It is not a matter of just thinking and finding the focus since it has to be molded back time and time again when one loses thought. The aim? Single-mindedness known as ekagrata. In front of this level is sensory disengagement - a break of sound, vision, physical contact. Out of that, work becomes more refined. It requires repeated repetition to revert attention, to make a wild bird be perched. According to old school, this work is likened to disciplined heat - unchanging, gradual as it is, molding something soft into hardness.

A silent change occurs when concentration ceases to make such an effort. Attention is carried beyond its effort and is moving freely, without impediments, on its own rhythm. Not compelled, but floating as light over clear water - one deep note without breathing. And thoughts that at one time had broken in are lost in a pattering of knowing. Others refer to this phase as reflective, full of wordless inner-voice; others to entirely non-word moments. The viewer, the viewing and the viewed start to melt at the corners. Old manuals are suggesting that it is like pouring oil between vessels very gradually - no pauses, no foams, just continuity. Awareness is its own generator, which does not require any additional input to continue. What was distinct parted to meet until there is barely a definition.

Immediately after the outer steps are two important practices - Dharana and Dhyana - the heart of the eightfold journey meditation. In front of them are moral regulations, habits of mind, constant attitudes, breath regulation and self-shift and before them is complete inner awakening in three phases of Samadhi. One possible interpretation: Dharana is like a fire, purifying the mind by burning out the clutter in a stream of life force towards the central channel. This relaxes the five mind relations, and prepares mind to set in higher degrees. By constant practice, concentration becomes stable, and is no longer driven by agitation or excitement. Detachment is cultivated mildly to ease the sire of turbulence to have clarity. Then Dhyana spreads out - not by compulsion, but by rush - where the understanding spreads without possessing. This sustained release causes the inner walls to subside letting balance and knowing to manifest in unison. The ancient systems are useful today more so in the systems of wisdom in India that have a connection between focused training and smooth continuity. The sequence is reflected in current applications - a case in point being blood pressure management, where controlled focus transitions into the relaxed control of regulation without conscious focus.

From Dharana to Dhyana flows a flow that feeds the other Like breath to breath. The turn is often characterized by fourteen dozen consistent obsessions, in which gripping is substituted by a weightless sliding. Patanjali indicates this change - when the attention flows without interruptions, then it has entered Dhyana. This is not a success that is measured by force but the ease of strain dissipation. This route is constructed step by step, through practice, letting go without being on the alert, towards more profound states. Something of the same happens to trauma work - with its concentrated attention, space is made to soften, a sort of unbinding. Early tight control in body-based studies assists one in managing pain cues that will ultimately break into broader calm. Pragya Yoga is a mental practice that employs keen intellect to achieve profound stillness to enhance rest and sleep in the process.

Under these outdated ideals is the vivid dichotomy, one which pits concentrated trying against the flowingness. This is where science is able to intervene and make the ancient words relevant to modern thought but retain the original intent of the words. Suppose that the attention is the foundation, even and required; then the meditation is ascending, radiant and perfect. The same order is replicated in yoga texts, which provide a way that remains useful today even with brain research on awareness (Tripathi and Bharadwaj, 2021). The mind then proceeds to the bottom layers and ultimately releases itself. This structure stands firm when the tech is approaching and determines the way machines could help without disruption of the order.

This section talks about the progression from Dharana to Dhyana within the eightfold system of yoga sutras of Patanjali. Dharana involves focusing the mind on one particular object to improve concentration, or ekagrata. With proper practice, it naturally transforms into Dhyana where attention flows continuously without any control.

2.2. Cognitive and Attentional Characteristics

It is possible to regard Dharana as a concentrated grip, which is created with the help of conscious effort, whereas Dhyana is closer to flowing into and is effortless and smooth. Dharana instead of just holding the mind still, engages the mind with the force of will, as you do with your breath, it takes effort, energy, brain action. Research indicates that this type of concentration illuminates spaces that are associated with control, particularly in the process of avoiding distractions (Telles et al., 2016). It resembles that of dealing with duties that require continuous checkups, as thoughts become diverted and have to be drawn back to the spot. In this, the concentration is not constant - it is flickering, falling, resetting, betwixt purpose and insensibility. Next change to Dhyana: not sustained but driven on, nearly dragged along by its own beat. Less pushing, corrections, the experience is self-administered and minimal supervision is required (Telles et al., 2012). This condition does not keep the same mental muscles going since it is not strained but flows into an easy continuation.

It becomes more evident at every step what occurs in deep focus. In lieu of simply observing all things, Dharana teaches the mind to single out one item and surrender the background chatter - such as reducing the volume of the static in the background during meditation to allow individuals to perceive the body cues more easily in the case of joint pain (Biswas et al., 2025). Clinging to that single thread requires continual minor adjustments over the years; nonetheless, it is clear that when the work requires rapid decision-making, there are indications of distress with uneven reaction times. Mental storage space is spent in the work of maintaining focus on the target, repeating signals within oneself to including distracters, similar to the traditional concepts of ekagrata - continuous inner concentration preventing likeness of wandering thought (Thakur, 2025). Then there is Dhyana in which effort dissipates. The focus remains resolute without effort, fully awake, yet loose, and understanding comes of its own accord, free and uncontrived by the will (Telles et al., 2016).

These practices are different by what occurs in the mind. Mental work, sound and image systems in the brain, is actually what is required to hold focus on an object. When distractions strike, stress indicators increase - evidence of strain manifesting itself in body tests. Attention becomes more emphatic, mistakes are less frequent after practice, but it still requires effort, particularly when it comes to blood pressure and mental patterns assist in stabilizing the body reaction. The key feature here? Balancing conflicting impulses, switching gears - all to retain the focus in one spot, just like yoga practitioners who switch between color-word tests, which present conflicting information at a faster rate. Instead, meditation makes such a load lighter and distributes control rather than compelling it. The stability is maintained but more comfortable, ideas relate without falling apart but are in line with older conceptions of continuity in awareness aspects of some of the contemplative traditions.

When one observes closely, people with mental tasks have apparent patterns. When they train their Dharana during protracted focus drills, the former learners heed more objects, demonstrating reduced incidence of errors - however, the incidence of errors remains when distracted, which suggests that thoughts do drift under pressure (Telles et al., 2016). With the memory challenges such as the n-back test, their short-term memory recall improves with training but slower reaction predicts that additional mental effort has to be invested (Telles et al., 2012). Individuals who are immersed in Dhyana maintain steadfast attention with time, have little difficulty focusing, and perceive rapid changes without difficulty, and this is a sign of effortless resource allocation to the mind (Telles et al., 2016). Measures of various aspects of attention indicate that Dharana enhances control when there is a conflict between choice, but Dhyana enhances an early warning system and changes of direction - without overloading the higher control systems.

The healing process could be seen in terms of practice: yoga practices based on Dharana enhance focus in the times of the pandemic, which allows changing the experience of stress and body responses resulting in more profound relaxation in Dhyana that facilitate the stability of thinking (Basu-Ray et al., 2022). One of them is Pragya Yoga, which has very specific steps - the decision-making in the state of stress must be trained first, followed by the later stages based on Savita Dhyana, which help to maintain a calm and constant state of awareness and help to rest well (Yadav et al., 2025). The research in rheumatoid arthritis demonstrates that sharp, versus scattered, attention methods are more effective in terms of day-to-day functioning, whereas the former relates thoughts directly to coping with discomfort (Biswas et al., 2025). These echoes a way back to the Indian systems of the past, where the development of a powerful concentration in Dharana facilitates the natural clarity of Dhyana (Thakur, 2025).

Taking a closer look is the way around to changing our vision of things. Although the attention distance creates a small distance between the watcher and the watched, this distance assists people to deal with painful memories - such as a first step (Hasan et al., 2025). As one goes into deeper meditation, the distance disappears; the purpose of blending occurs without coercion. This foreshadows later in higher states. Due to these qualities, models must be able to approach them differently, one constructs mental structure, the other breaks it down on the way to stillness.

This section presents the difference between Dharana and Dhyana in terms of cognitive effort and psychological efforts. Dharana is described as an effortful and will-driven concentration helps in strengthening the focus but requires constant mental energy for support. Dhyana, on the other hand, represents transition to effortless and continued awareness.

2.3. Neurophysiological Correlates of Meditative States

According to brain research, Dharana and Dhyana influence the body in contrast to each other. In Dharana, the nervous system gets a compromise, not too alert or too relaxed. The patterning of heart rhythms becomes more adaptable due to the control of attention. This assists in eliminating noise in the head, maintaining thoughts on track. Indications of stress are decelerated; adrenaline releases are diminished. Meanwhile, the activity of nerves associated with respiration increases (observed in greater changes in the heartbeat during respiratory inhalation and exhalation). Entering into Dhyana, the body goes further down to rest mode. The relaxation division of the nervous system assumes the whole control. The variations of the heart rate increase significantly and tension indicators reduce sharply. It becomes more relaxed, and there are now long intervals without interruption. These changes are reflective of the yoga-based blood pressure interventions. Balance - balance comes first - Dharana. Then there comes the restorative calm, Dhyana fixes permanent rest, by even treading the nerves.

There are slight variations in the breathing styles. Stillness gives rise to a constant movement of the breath, slows down, full, between six and ten times a minute Dharana - deep belly movement will bring us here, to move the air well in a manner that maintains the level of carbon dioxide, making the awareness stand still (Telles et al., 2012). These heart rate checks force into a high breath rate, which slowly trains the body to relax the nervous system. Then, without any physical intervention, the rhythm becomes more soft - the breath becomes thin, possibly four to six breathing cycles per minute, almost none, the breath is extended, a manifestation of the body losing active control (Telles et al., 2016; Yadav et al., 2025). Pragya Yoga is one of such programs, or Savita Dhyana: the initial level of focus accuracy is used to remove stress, followed by breath shortages in later life (particularly in female followers) (Yadav et al., 2025). When the condition of stiff joints is closely observed, the question of a type of breath is important - a systematic Dharana practice modulates exacerbations by improving lung oxygenation, and in other cases a quiet pattern of Dhyana helps to heal the body as a whole (Biswas et al., 2025).

Attention decreases breathing, and body signals change when one is meditating during the initial stages. It is an initiation of a silent nervous system, which is determined by consistent patterns of breath that help to reduce the indications of stress gradually. Minor changes in the activity of the sweat glands show low arousal, although immune preparedness is enhancing behind the scenes. At later stages, it appears to be much more relaxed, with the eyes closing their eyes, and heating distribution on the skin becoming uniform. This step virtually muted the alert pathways leaving the recovery systems space to operate unimpeded. The variability of heart rhythm increases with practice, but another method is associated with different outcomes. The simple focus techniques elevate the heart rate fluctuation in an average way in weeks. Deep absorption practises take high-speed fluctuations way further and usually increase several folds of what had been obtained following consistent training. These transitions are similar to the development of breath control - intentional clearing of channels to automatic silence between breaths in and out. Previous patterns assist subsequent transitions with every layer building upon preceding, without compelling results.

The mind has never focused its senses as keenly as in Dharana - it makes what you listen to and feel sharper by shutting down some of the brain signals, and assists in maintaining the attention without spillage. It is not like withdrawing to silence intentionally, it is inseparable with deep inward withdrawal, which takes over towards the end of practice. It does not react but controls by high places damping to emotional stimuli making one point stable when tiny pulls are still there. When meditation becomes more intensive, the inner sensation becomes the primary one - body signals become less vivid, the sense of the gut becomes more developed, the external world transforms into silent humming without any effort. The sounds and touches, without efforts, cease to catch. Since focused attention at an early stage is a gate-way, subsequent stillness permits experience to unite beyond segregation, enabling painful memories to rise with a serene, untwisted clarity, without being mixed up with recent trauma.

The olden times have never found such an easy answer in modern science. Breathing slows. It is not that the body follows because it has to, but rather than because it can. Emphasis influences corporeal reaction - restrictiveness relaxes without pressure. Subsequently, more in-depth rest facilitates deviant immune conduct, cellular action gradients. One of the states is preparing the ground; the other is letting life wander freely under the earth. Body, breath, attention was considered to be threads in old structures. At first, stability and, then, where necessary, energy flows. The scientists are now able to measure the trace that is left by each phase. Aligning the old words with the new information assists in the clarification of what it happens - and why it is necessary to pay attention to the time. Clarification becomes achieved when observation is in agreement with tradition without rigor loss.

Dharana produces a state of balanced regulation with moderate awareness of the surroundings and controlled breathing (6-10 minutes per minute) while in Dhayana the body shifts into deeper parasympathetic dominance with slower breathing (4-6 breaths per minute).

2.4. Evidence of Electrophysiological

Studies of the brain waves demonstrate that there is a significant difference between deep meditation and focused attention. When the person focuses his or her mind on one thing, the brain activities increase in the frontal regions with more of theta waves - they have to do with mental effort. Rather than falling asleep, temporary bursts of quicker beta activity are periodically observed whenever distracted thoughts come to mind, and they serve to get oneself refocused again. That is equivalent to what ancient texts refer to as stable mind hold. When the state becomes more open-minded, another thing occurs: alpha rhythms become more intense behind the head and gamma signals connect far-off areas of the brain. This movement implies fewer pushing, more flowing, in which there is no strain in perception. These inner changes are mapped in definite electrical patterns.

Dharana enhances theta waves in focus and errors locales of the brain, as demonstrated by brain scan, which aids in stabilizing a concentration-lacking mind. This is an activity based on the front top section of the brain, which forms control and alertness. That picture is further refined in later analysis which reveals more left-side effort in practice as concentration ensues than in idle thoughts. Although Dharana heats up such areas, meditation triggers to Dhyana which is characterized by rapid gamma rhythms along inner midline areas. The daydreaming circuits are silenced by those patterns and the networks connected to now are reinforced. There are particular areas such as the upper back rear of the midbrain and right temple area where the mind becomes silent. With a shift of focus on goal-directed effort to an open flow, various hubs are brought into existence. The forehead position is softened as the sides towards the ears come in to take away the grip on meaning in order to see better.

This is where a change in brain activity takes place. As the concentration increases, the frontal and parietal lobes become the primary attentional focus advancing the neural rhythms, related to theta and alpha waves, to the cingulate and prefrontal areas - similar to how it becomes in some yoga practices or training to focus (Nalbant et al., 2022). The same areas become silent later on when deep meditation is attained. Rather, the signal flares between alpha and gamma rhythms in the back of the brain form smooth relayment states, as well as without pushing or trying, like the calm recovery modes of certain forms of meditation (Yadav et al., 2025). Comparing the two stages, one of them is indicative of what is mentally demanding - such as a greater beta over theta in frontal scans - the other demonstrates widespread alpha correlating with gamma, which today is associated with a reduction in the state of bodily inflammation as traced using EEG markers (Basu-Ray et al., 2022).

The shifts between the states can be monitored by the wave patterns in the brain responses. After focus practice, a major indicator in the midbrain region requires more time to reach its highest point, indicating slower early sound processing to enhance attention, and strong and later waves indicate active involvement of mental resources (Telles et al., 2012). Indications connected to hearing centers are lightly delayed, which indicates the halting of the relay stations such as the thalamus when focusing on the noises. In deep meditation, we can see that the first responses to sound become weak - one is approximately 100 milliseconds - and then even later processes become weaker; however, one of the waves accelerates in low-order regions, suggesting the possibility of effortless and smooth perception (Telles et al., 2016). Brain waves related to touch are no different: the focused concentration enlarges the distance between two responses, helping to suppress inappropriate sensations, and meditative awareness narrows this distance by spreading neural calmness, reducing the number of disruptions (Telles et al., 2012).

Calming down with attention is visualized as brainwave activity, as initial attention exercises provide a foundation to deeper meditative modes - observable in the literature of chronic joint pain (Biswas et al., 2025). Stress makes the mind retain sensory signals more, as though it acts as a gate that opens slowly; consequent stages release more quickly and the faster processing becomes possible (Hasan et al., 2025). The ancient processes of step-by-step mental training are now comparable to the activity of the brain, providing more visible map musings of how inner processes are carried out (Thakur, 2025).

2.5. Evidence of Neuroimaging and Higher Cognitive Processing

The fact that brain scans support previous electrical results by demonstrating that Dharana and Dhyana are distinct is weakened by the fact that they are quite different. One is lit up when concentration is required in working and the other when concentration is easy. Dharana involves upsurges of activity in the front regions of the brain- particularly the regions that are connected to decision-making and task-staying. These areas activate in a hard way when distractions are present as was the case with the rapid brain waves. Effort in this case is correlated to energy expended which is perceived in scan signals and in mental strain in separate locations. Activated brain circuits will only remain so long as the will allows. The more difficult the refocusing, the more fuel is burnt. The higher the signal the higher the load which is what was found to be the case with guided concentration tests. On the contrary, Dhyana silences such command centers. Rather, deeper midline positions awaken - those associated with body awareness and self-awareness. The fighting is less, inner distractions are less. The change of attention is not abrupt, but carried on by the

by perhaps a rhythm instead of by a push. These silent states are connected with smooth wave movements at the posterior of the head an indication of a stable perception. Sensory reactions become softer, reactions are dulled - not blocked, but merely unenhanced. True peace is not acquired by holding on, it is lost.

The process in the brain changes evidently in phases. Embracing attention illuminates regions such as the DLPFC, as in the case of making people better at remembering items sequentially, which is bound to specific brainwave activity that is observed in experiments (Telles et al., 2012). Areas of the left frontal part next to the temple and a point in the temporal lobe are useful in this stage when considering an idea because they establish network connections around the selected idea, forming more profound inner speech - this form of reflection narrows the focus on selecting what is important (Telles et al., 2016). In more profound flow, the speaking networks get silence; the PCC slows, silencing personal reminiscences and narratives, opening the way to the unfixed presence of a verb and a category - where words and classifications disappear (Tripathi and Bharadwaj, 2021). What follows is attention remaining even without effort, fewer distracting thoughts intrude, which is apparent when individuals remain on their vigil in extended periods (Telles et al., 2016).

The stages of alteration of brain patterns are associated with deep meditation. Attention areas connect when attention is shifted to enhance control over distractions and signals among frontal areas assist in silencing the mind, as breath and body balance variations in 2012 and 2021 literature. With increasing stillness, some circuits decelerate, and others become stronger, and central hubs synchronize in a manner that makes smooth awareness that is not connected to the ego - a state that is associated with high-frequency waves and restful domination of the nervous system in later studies. Further into the brain, early training consists of relay centers that narrow sense, movement loops that aid in the repetition of redirection, as well as, stability systems in association with breathing rhythms. During the longer flow, links between recollections and inner senses areas become stronger forming eternal perception, whereas zones to do with survival encourage deep relaxation, bent civilized senses into understanding, as demonstrated lately.

The scans of the brain indicate that meditation is useful in the treatment of high blood pressure - brain activity when focused on the front of the brain is the guiding force of initial nervous system balance, and then it is replaced by more intensive back-brain activity, which is the sustainment of long-term calming (Nalbant et al., 2022). When practicing rheumatoid arthritis, switching to the frontal networks that interpret discomfort and transitioning to default mode adaptations that further sustain overall endurance should be turned in inward (Biswas et al., 2025). When yoga is used in post-COVID recovery, periods of concentration engage memory-related regions to relieve stress, and deeper stillness silences areas of key hubs associated with immune adaptiveness (Basu-Ray et al., 2022). In a "so gentle with the trauma" mode, directing awareness makes control areas strong initially, which prepares the ground to a gentler letting go without any additional damage (Hasan et al., 2025).

Location guesses of theta activity - which is connected to DLPFC by eLORETA - and gamma sparks in the precuneus via sLORETA are cleared off when EEG is combined with fMRI, creating an effect of hard mental work being replaced by the smooth rhythm of the brain (Telles et al., 2012; Telles et al., 2016). In ancient Indian philosophy, this point is considered as the energy of the breath resting in clear consciousness, when concentration of attention creates the surface brain patterns and the deep meditation falls below the cortex (Thakur, 2025). Pragya Yoga is a practice that charts out such steps to enhance rest and resilience through switching on a particular circuit at each stage (Yadav et al., 2025). Collectively, these cumulative results bring science to finer models of mind states, indicating training attention and letting go as coupled steps prepared to digital assistance.

2.6. Objections to Traditional Meditation Research and Evaluation

The majority of research on meditation is not able to distinguish between focused attention and deep smooth awareness. Although there are patterns that have been mapped in the brain it is difficult to narrow down the time when one is trying hard or just being absorbed. These states are easily confounded by people in their personal reports due to gaps of memory, ambiguous words, or personal anticipation. Instruments that are supposed to be used to quantify mindfulness seldom record the small changes - such as alterations in brainwave activity associated with various states. Due to this, errors that occur during labeling mental states during practice are experienced. In practice, this confusion can confuse the results; a case in point is that the results of yoga programs during the pandemic were summed up in a group, so it was hard to detect whether the temporary alertness or permanent relaxation contributed to the immune reactions.

Even though the patterns of heart rate capture the overall trends such as SDNN or RMSSD (Standard Deviation of Normal-to-Normal intervals or Root Mean Square of Successive Differences), they do not capture such brief mental changes that happen moment-by-moment - the brief ECG samples overlook the small changes between brain activity and the response of the vagus nerve (Nalbant et al., 2022; Tripathi and Bharadwaj, 2021). The breathing measurements provide an overall picture but lack specific details on timing that would be important to distinguish between actual meditative breath control and fatigue, particularly in researching the state of inflammation (Biswas et al., 2025; Telles et al., 2016). The skin sensors or the size of the pupil can indicate a less aroused state, but these indicators drift out of control without considering what is actually attracting the mind - thus complicating the process of blood pressure trials as the phases mix together (Nalbant et al., 2022). In some cases, inner experience reports during mindful yoga are not associated with the heart rhythm data, and it is questionable how effective mindful yoga practices can be in the context of rest and stress recovery (Yadav et al., 2025).

People start to move, and it becomes more difficult to notice mental states. Under natural flow, lab tests by EEG or fMRI disrupt flow hence distorting the results. The wearable devices detect shaky signals as people take a walk or stretch themselves. Slices of information lack the component of transformation of a single individual with time. Late surveys are not able to detect rapid brain changes such as AEP patterns or FPCN clashes. Confusion of focus slips with consistent meditations occurs frequently. It is risky to observe the trauma in research. The personal scores ignore P300 waves which display blocked processing. Misplaced timing of exposure can do more harm than benefit. Loopholes in tracking make clear causes and effects of deep practice problematic. The Indian ways of antiquity emphasise the accuracy of steps. Existing techniques are not as accurate as they should be in seconds.

Ratings of the same behavior by different observers who view the behavior on video usually differ - particularly in times of slight changes in attention - and the discrepancy increases beyond reliability of 30 per cent, making large studies more difficult to reproduce. A trial could have breath work and a different one could have poses thus making the results messy when combining data. There has been a variable effect in the outcomes in the research on the effects of yoga on the joint disease due to the inconsistencies in the measurement of the important biological markers. The number of people involved in most experiments is less than twenty, as talented participants are difficult to locate, which means a low level of statistical strength when it comes to the measurement of brain processes related to deep meditation. The instruments created in the West are not always sensitive to the non-Western experience, which restricts the transferability of findings to a variety of health practices.

The point that researchers resort to AI is the fact that the old ways are not effective anymore. Machines have replaced the guesswork in order to sort signals based on brain waves, heart patterns, and breathing simultaneously. The most interesting is that these tools make states distinctly different in gauging their doubt. There are even systems that adapt to people without pooling personal information, due to joint training, albeit disjointed. This flexibility is an open door - such as custom-made treatment of blood pressure or immune response. Once the process of sorting mental states becomes automated, the distance between theory and hard evidence becomes narrow. Computation, in turn, is not additional - it is perfectly compatible with study practices in which reflection collides with measurement.

2.7. Artificial Intelligence in Meditation Research and Practice

By applying the artificial intelligence to the study of meditation, the way we view old practices is transformed. Researchers no longer have to be content with unreliable self-reports but have reliable tools that are fast and broad. These tools distinguish between forced focus and free flowing when practicing. Issues such as ambiguous emotions combined with body cues delay development. Quick change of mental stages is usually missed in body measurements. Research does not correlate due to diverse manner of doing things in each group. Machine learning works with sloppy data - pattern in brain activities or heart rate other algorithms miss. It evaluates states with more distinct margins than individuals are able to handle. It works more reliably as demonstrated by numbers. Yet the aim isn't replacement. Imagine that AI is the aid to individual observation and recurring training. It cleans awareness like a mirror protruded before the eyes, without usurping it. Advancement is always step by step - of making efforts to letting go. Instruments help, understanding develops internally.

One perspective - AI assists in structuring the impact of yoga on the state of health, particularly when it comes to examining large-scale research on such aspects as immune responses during pandemics. Concentration exercises, akin to Dharana, appear to arouse early defense mechanisms, whereas more profound meditation, approaching Dhyana, make long term responses persist. Other studies indicate that machines are capable of sifting through brain signals by use of special forms of networks: one type is capable of searching through space patterns in EEGs, whilst another one is able to track time-related changes. These tools detect rhythm enhancement advances in the frontal part of the brain at 4-8 Hz with practice of concentration, as well as enduring indicators of signal peaks of calm awareness associated with higher-frequency waves in the rear parts, occasionally more than 30 Hz. These marks when compared to mental modes have an accuracy rate of more than ninety percent. To interpret concealed decisions within intelligent algorithms, techniques such as SHAP or LIME point will directly indicate active points - such as a center of thought along the forehead which lights up when one is focused, or regions of inner awareness which coordinate when one is motionless. This is enough transparency to eliminate skepticism concerning the reliability of automated readings as is done elsewhere in scan interpretation.

Systems are less volatile when various body signals are combined. Rather than one measure, the integration of the changes in heart rate during breathing, the slightest movements of the sweats glands, and the patterns of rhythms provide more concrete reports. Models adapt with ease to situations in which individuals enter a new situation at varying levels of nervous system balance, by using the information of previous training running. Imagine making quiet mind tracks, on the basis of early recordings - such are what artificial setups achieve, by simulating deep focus stages, prior to the commencement of complete absorption. Similarly to the monitoring of the flow of nutrients in the blood using blood indicators, these instruments predict mental preparation stages. This work has been reviewed as such methods aid in bridging gaps where the data is limited primarily when dealing with advanced methods of meditation that are not common. In ear and throat experiments, even where slight brain responses to sound are involved, the method of obtaining the responses works equally well where applied to the responses of a study of timings in a state of inward stillness.

Learning algorithms are adapted into feedback devices that operate in the background and direct attention by making soft sounds in response to changes in the brainwave or by producing gentle vibrations that can be used to relax the breathing process. These arrangements automatically adapt to time to ensure that users are not adversely affected. An example is a virtual reality program named Otti, which has been tested in controlled studies, in which artificial intelligence is used to assist college learners meditate by altering the sense of immersion with respect to balance measures of the nervous system as measured through brain and heart signals. Findings reveal the evident reductions in tension, which may be utilized in the future in the field of medicine, such as the treatment of high blood pressure or joint pains. The custom plans are based on sorting initial measures of the activity of the brain and the heartbeat rate and dividing people into two categories, which respond better to focused effort than those who can easily enter deeper states. Every route receives its approach, and yoga sessions aimed at sleep and stress reduction among women groups are created. Smart simulation systems are used in the training of nurses to learn how to read the indicators of inner regulation, and to distribute skill access among the health teams, preparing to face the challenges of mind-body treatment.

Considering how meditation becomes deeper and more profound as distracters become fainter, now consider a computer being taught to detect cancer based on scans, along with signals in your body, as it learns. This mix intensifies the medical outcomes and reflects the inner calmness which is measured by the moments of uncertainty which are taken by hand. Schools are starting to educate future health laborers now to associate machine revelation and instructed yoga exercises and fold ancient tranquility into the current proof framework. Other tales put the concentrated attention as a gateway beyond the emotional traumas, where intelligent systems can detect changes in words without cause pain once again. Combined, these technological components can fill gaps in the past - it is now possible to repeat studies on large populations with ease, as the yoga tradition is honored, yet helping people stretch even in places with limited resources.

2.8. AI-Enhanced Approaches to Dharana

Detecting deep focus brainwaves such as frontal theta spikes, fading alpha waves, activity in areas of the brain of interest, and slowing P300 signals are measured using intelligent algorithms. Tagged brain scans teach machines to distinguish between sharp focus and wandering mind by models like the SVMs and neural nets with reported accuracy of more than 88 percent. HMDs are devices that will track multiple EEG channels, pupil size measurements, and eye trackers or eye movement measurements, which detect the stability of the eye gaze of the person wearing it by looking at tiny eye flickers and visual noise. These devices detect attentional dispersion in the daily activities, and borrowing techniques reminiscent of live diagnostics applied in ear-nose-throat monitoring. Silent slips, such as momentary increases in beta pattern against continuous flow of theta, are detected by pattern-learning systems that compare findings with scores on mental tasks performed on tests such as CPT and memory tests.

The effort involved in being focused intensifies depending on how one accounts it. Bifurcation of tasks in two allows one to know about the strain in the mind whereas the patterns of the brain waves on the left and right front can reveal how difficult the person is trying to be. When the rhythms of the heart are altered - become more active in the lower part - it is frequently proportional to what one has in the mind. These signals are added together to form one number depicting the level of toughness of self-control at the moment. Dubious results are captured by machines constructed with smart guessing of results and distinguishing between profound concentration and daydreaming or exhaustion. That is important when stable thinking is used to control the high blood pressure using the guidance of the brain. Performance of links depends on the period of holding effort without slipping, and curves are created which expose points of balance. Computer systems generate possible results depending on different practice time such as program that predicts meals but in this case applied to training attention.

Here is a change now - predictive models are employed by feedback loops within virtual spaces. Learning algorithms do not wait, but provide small cues which direct attention. You can imagine that sound keeps drawing your attention, or images, which blur as long as you remain still. The difficulty increases when there is increased clarity of brain signals, such as those P300 waves that are in line with theta waves. The latter trend became especially evident in the course of examinations known as Otti, during which pupils would construct mental support buildings throughout weeks. It occurs by tracking in real time with the help of devices attached to the body that monitor the duration that one remains in task mode. Curt momentary lapses come up here and there; any reduction in rhythm is tallyed by the minute. Clean signal flow across thinking zones in the brain is most important and in fact, measured at the source. Information accumulates on the ground, without clouds, creating fast-slow charts at months long. At these points of rarity of the concentration - known as ekagrata - the system unravels the higher places of experience. This is not a fun exercise - it assists individuals with sore joints in taking mind off safely. Excessive load destroys it and gates stay open only enough to reject noise. The artificial scenarios played by nurses during practice are influenced by live performance statistics. The strength of mind is developed gradually, reflecting the ancient concentrating exercises that became hospital floor exercises.

Over time, these practices can sustain the practices of abhyasa, and they have exit and entry points that are gradual, which develop the sense of self-direction and enable close supervision in case of studying stress when there are pandemics or exposure to traumatic events (Basu-Ray et al., 2022; Hasan et al., 2025). Knowledge of tech skills implies that the machine learning will be applied to consciously processed data, and the doors that were closed tight will be opened (Sapci and Sapci, 2020). Artificial intelligence is used to sharpen measures of effort in cancer research, which are associated with body outcomes, demonstrating that Dharana can be expanded without being lost (Saeidnia et al., 2025). Based on the tradition of ancient Indians, smart devices have become enhanced to focus, which preconditions the next stage of meditation, where brain science and inner clarity coincide (Thakur, 2025; Yadav et al., 2025).

2.9. Artificial Intelligence-Improved Dhyana

Such a state of mind quietness is detected by intelligent software monitoring brainwaves. Rather than strenuous effort, the system detects the situation where one is experiencing things such as gamma pulses getting into a rhythm at the back of the head. It also verifies timing during alpha waves as well, which are associated with activity within - near areas, which are associated with self-awareness. Trends extracted out of these readings assist in distinguishing between the mind-immobile stillness and the minimal strain mental activity. Sound hardly activating the brain reaction, and some networks working against each other on scans are clear indications that flow is underway. These signs are combined into special models with data that is mapped over the scalp, intercepting any attention shifts that may occur smoothly and do not fade away. Experiments in virtual environments verify the correspondence of inner experience and body cues that are monitored by variations in breath and heart rate. The absence of low chaos in breathing cycles, as well as the constant heart rhythms produced by the nerves, exclude the drowsiness simulation depth. Every piece of signal is joined together in such a way that what seems to be ease does not betray the real nervous composure.

Slow breathing pattern watching employs intelligent systems that are developed through learning. Such clues about the heart rhythm of the watch, such as breath-linked pulse changes, are tied to brain scan images of quiet and can tell when the body is starting to wake up once again with no poking or prodding. The presence of brain waves synchronization across areas and loss of touch sensitivity contributes to the image. Special models can construct probable courses of profound stillness based on initial information as in the case of food science instruments forecasting nutrient uptake. Such cues during rest (meditative) are a way of mapping the interaction between sleep and stress, and that that is as distant calm as it is possible to achieve without effort of the mind. Techniques that are imported to cancer imaging focus on results. In this case, the artificial way of thinking incorporates both sound-like indications and time information to identify the indications of mindbody equilibrium.

This is where there goes a humming, deep down hearing, to keep minds focused. Light also varies gradually, with the rhythm of the brain, maintaining attention constant. Every individual receives his/her rhythm without questioning. Soft signals through headphones remind that the focus has been lost and it is restored back. The system remains unobtrusive like a nurse that understands when to intervene. It takes ancient ways with modern means. With time, it recedes back to everyone becoming self-reliant. The goal? Unambiguous knowledge, achieved more easily, with less effort.

2.10. Ethical, Philosophical and Practical Implications

Mindfulness should be a delicate balance when applying AI to support the process of meditation. Tradition does not warn against distraction, and resistance to focus, without a reason. Tools are effective when they are adhered to rather than dictated by inner practice. The concentration starts with hard work, but gets relaxed as time progresses. Progress may be reflected in some machines, provided that self-study is the main point. Pairs of sensors with breathwork have already become available under some therapies, and depth can be provided by tech. The gadgets in question help even in chronic conditions, where they help provide guidance in an easy manner. It is important that a technique should never be placed above inner truth. Algorithms must, also, be submissive to silence. It is not data, but silent changes, familiar to the sitting only, which indicate progress.

In the event that brain data are gathered, privacy is a big issue. The federation techniques are useful because they leave EEG and HRV information in their place of origin. The risks involving meditation must be masked, in good faith under the international rules. Transparency manifests itself in terms of such tools as SHAP, which point toward the process of sorting the gamma patterns. Deep learning may deceive individuals, as dark results in radiographic images used to do. Ethical configurations are borrowed of ahimsa, which means no harm, particularly in monitoring body cues. Every VR session should be informed about what is being recorded before it starts. The evidence of access remains recorded in the course of the experiments with stressed learners. Open code will play a significant role in favor of all rather than a few groups. In such locations as India, equity implies the sharing of models widely in the wellness endeavors.

What would become the case with tech taking over too far? it is able to divide Dhyana out of its very essence. The alerts that are activated by touch can lead to dependence, and this disruption is incompatible with natural rhythm during the early stages of meditation. Practice games have the potential to evoke fidgety excitement, tranquil sanity at the edge of instability - which is opposite to the tenets of detachment found by Tripathi in 2025. When yoga is extended to clinical practices, something delicate is lost. Automated entries may run over the sophisticated consciousness of a teacher. Combining diverse methods introduces obsession with measurements without physical understanding as Basu-Ray and colleagues observed in 2022, followed by Biswas in 2025. How to respond? Expire set rules which gradually eliminate artificial aids. Weave the lines of ethical restraint of the ancient restraints of Patanjali. Such shields are used to maintain self-led growth, despite the spreading of intelligent machines in wellness areas (Sengar et al., 2024).

2.11. Research and Applied Domains

This macro perspective on previous research combines ancient yoga concepts with brain neuroscience, electrophysiology, and computer simulations, demonstrating that the AI-supported focus and meditation may open new directions in mind research. It transforms ancient practices of Patanjali into quantifiable indicators - such as frontal theta waves and P300 indications of focus, back area gamma bursts and vigilant control of the strong vagus nerve of deeper meditation - through machine learning tools, which also monitor their own uncertainty, establishing cautious protocols of long-term tests (Telles et al., 2012; Telles et al., 2016; Seoni et al., 2023).

Mental wellness Apps are increasing rapidly. As artificial intelligence drives care plans, certain tools today modify antique methods of focus to alleviate thoughts of anxiety in the face of years-long stress following an illness. The others are a combination of contemporary wisdom and ancient technique, which allow females to cope with sleepiness and stress in a more effective way. The studies on blood pressure and joint pain become sharper with the help of flexible body signals that help to change the treatment directions as time goes by. Study environments are opened up as well - virtual classrooms designed as small huts help the student to develop by exercising their brains on real-time. Emotional balance in courses in data science is also trained since it replicates the reaction of neurons to a load. These changes are subtle, but they transform the way schools are managing inner health without much ado.

A new fusion could combine brain scans and smart algorithms and could seek to follow the thoughts as they progress through time, particularly in mind-body connections associated with cancer treatment or diets. Others are based on old Indian activities, quantifying what alters the mind patterns, and artificial minds are experimented on artificial versions of mind. These tools are honestized by the ethical rules. The acts of introspection following trauma might be included in the organized experiments controlled by smart systems. Collectively, these trails outline a construct: ancient wisdom to the present encounter, creating a research that regards people as wholesome.

3. BIBLIOMETRIC ANALYSIS

This bibliometric review considers the academic situation regarding research topics of interest to AI-enhanced Dharana and Dhyana based on bibliographic information found in the Lens database. Lens was chosen because it is inclusive of interdisciplinary academic outputs, such as the publications in health sciences, neuroscience, yoga research, and computational approaches. The analysis uses a mixture of VOSviewer (Figures 1–4) to do the network-based visualizations of keyword co-occurrence and thematic density as well as Python-based scripts to analyze the trends of the data and visualize the frequency of keywords (Figures 5 and 6). The combination of these approaches can deliver a multi-dimensional perspective of thematic organization, development of research, and clustering of concepts in the field.

Figure 2 shows a map of key word co-occurrence networks created using the VOSviewer where nodes represent the key words and the edge will show the frequency of the key words appearing together in one and the same publication. The node size also shows the prominence of keywords, whereas the thickness of links shows how strong the co-occurrence relationships are.

In the visualization, it can be seen that there is a prevailing cluster around the word yoga which is closely related to hypertension, diabetes, lipid profile, health and memory. It means that modern yoga-related studies are highly rooted in cardiometabolic health outcomes and cognitive processes instead of unambiguous philosophic or spiritual aspects. The closeness of yoga to memory implies the growing attention to neurocognitive advantages that is immediately connected to Dharana and Dhyana as the practices based on attention and awareness.

Another, more concentrated cluster in the left part of the map contains keywords that are related to nutrition and metabolism, including obesity, 2′-fucosyllactose, amaranth, diet, and 024 months. The high level of internal cohesion and lower level of linkage of this cluster to the yoga node indicates that nutritional research is still an independent but more and more overlapping field especially in the field of preventive health and aging research.

Generally, the network suggests that yoga study can serve as a mediating variable between metabolical wellness, cognitive efficiency, and general wellbeing- developing empirical basis upon which AI-enhanced meditation studies can rely.

Figure 2. Keyword Co-occurrence Network Map Related to Yoga, Health, and Cognitive Outcomes (VOSviewer). (Data may vary slightly).

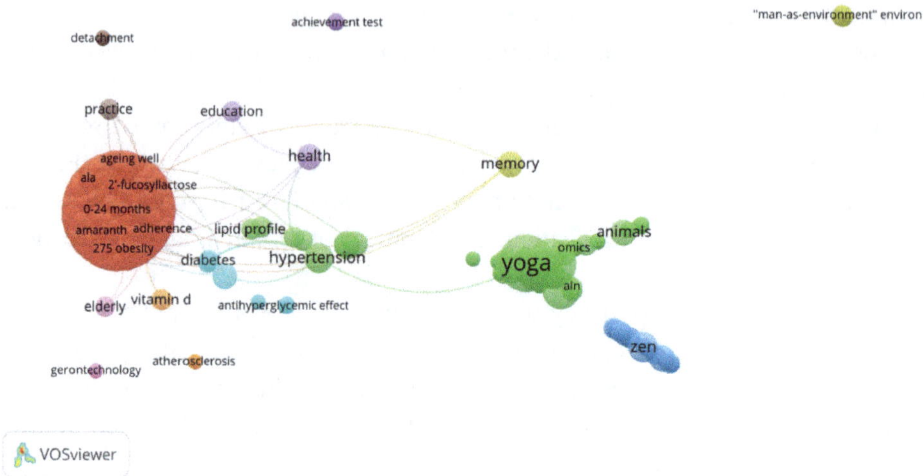

The co-occurrence analysis is further expanded in Figure 3 with a temporal overlay with node color corresponding to the mean publication year of each keyword. Colors that are colder (blue–purple) represent a time when the research has been conducted earlier whereas those that are warmer (green-yellow) represent more recent scholarly focus.

The overlay indicates that the use of the keywords like diabetes, hypertension, and health are linked to the previous years of publication, which is indicative of the very long-term interest in yoga as a form of intervention in the treatment of chronic illnesses. Conversely, the appearance of such terms as omics, animals, and memory are in warmer colours, which indicates the new research directions.

Interestingly yoga itself takes a central place and has had a rather modern look which means that the academic interest was continuous and increasing instead of diminishing. The paradigm shift in time between cognition-based and systems-level biological terms proposes a methodological change of shift, a clinical outcome study to a mechanistic, neurobiological and data-intensive one. The trend is especially applicable to the AI-enhanced Dharana and Dhyana research that is relying on the high-resolution data streams related to physiological and neural data.

Figure 3. Overlay Visualization of Keyword Co-occurrence by Publication Year (VOSviewer). (Data may vary slightly).

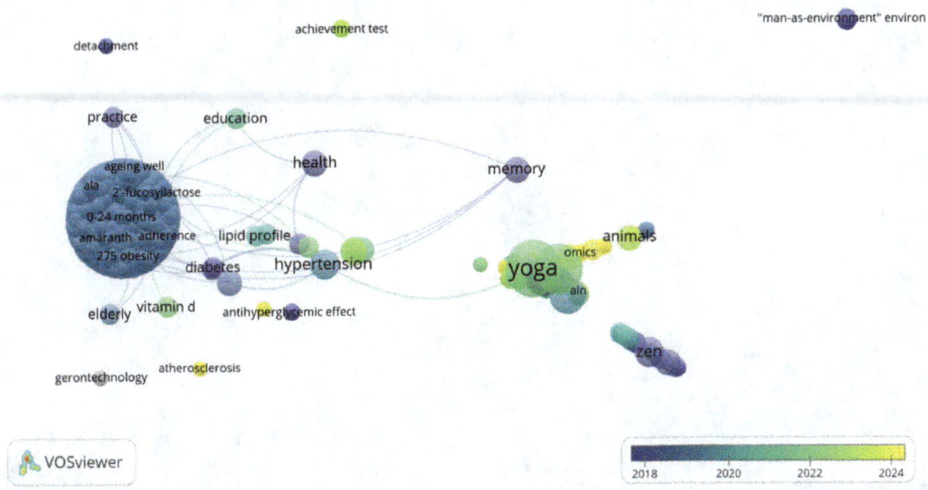

Figure 4 shows a mapping of key words density with color intensity being related to research activity concentration. The presence of yellow and green areas means a high density of the keywords, whereas the appearance of blue means lower intensity of research.

Two major hotspots of densities can be seen. The former, on the left, are related to nutrition- and metabolic-health topics, such as obesity, diet, and aging well. The second one, on the right, is focused on yoga and stretched towards memory, omics, and zen. This spacing confirms the fact that yoga research has a different yet becoming the integrative thematic territory.

Notably, the yoga-oriented hot spot also exhibits a tendency towards cognitive and reflective products, and this indicates that there is a gradual shift between peripheral health effects and those that are central to the mental functions of attention, memory and awareness. This distribution trend contributes to the thesis that Dharana and Dhyana which, as of tradition, have been underserved by empirical studies, are now becoming a part of the scientific mainstream, providing fertile soil to AI-based analysis schemes.

Figure 4. Keyword Density Visualization of Yoga-Related Research Themes (VOSviewer). (Data may vary slightly).

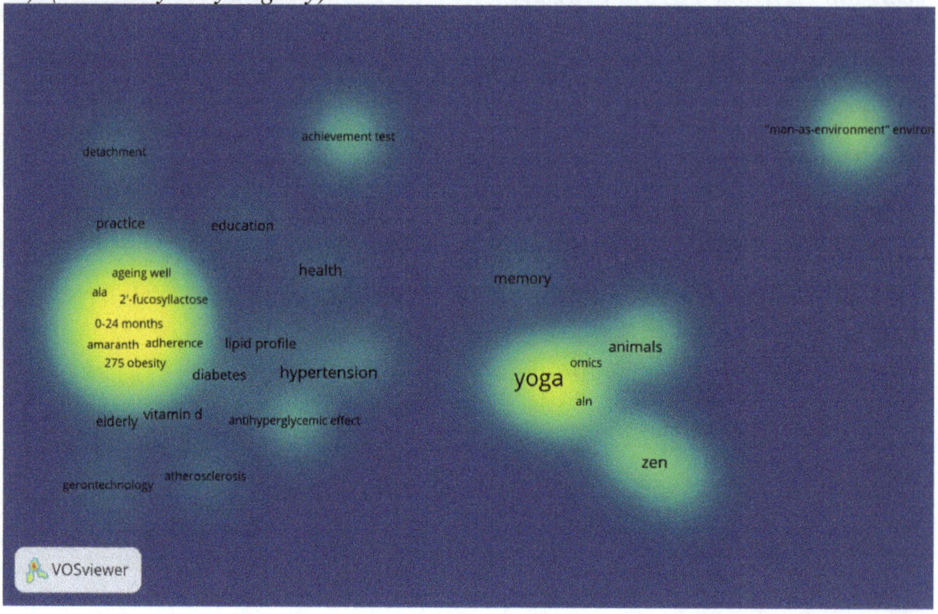

The temporal distribution of publications over time as shown in Figure 5 was created using the data visualization in Python. The trend displays three phases of the trend. The first stage, which can be described as the period between the late nineteenth and the mid-twentieth century, is marked by the scarcity and occasionality of publications, which indicates the lack of scientific interest toward the issues of yoga.

The second period of incremental development is evident in the second half of the twentieth century and it is accompanied by the rising interest in complementary and alternative medicine across the world. What is most interesting, though, is the sudden increase in the volume of publications since about 2010, which has a sharp peak in the first half of 2020s.

The given exponential increase is aligned with the development of neuroscience, wearable sensing technology, and machine learning that allow exploring meditative practices in a more rigorous manner. The trend supports the topicality of AI-augmented solutions to Dharana and Dhyana because the area has already entered a critical mass where data-driven methodologies are possible and even needed.

Figure 5. Publication Trend Over Time in Yoga- and Health-Related Research (Python-Based Analysis). (Data may vary slightly).

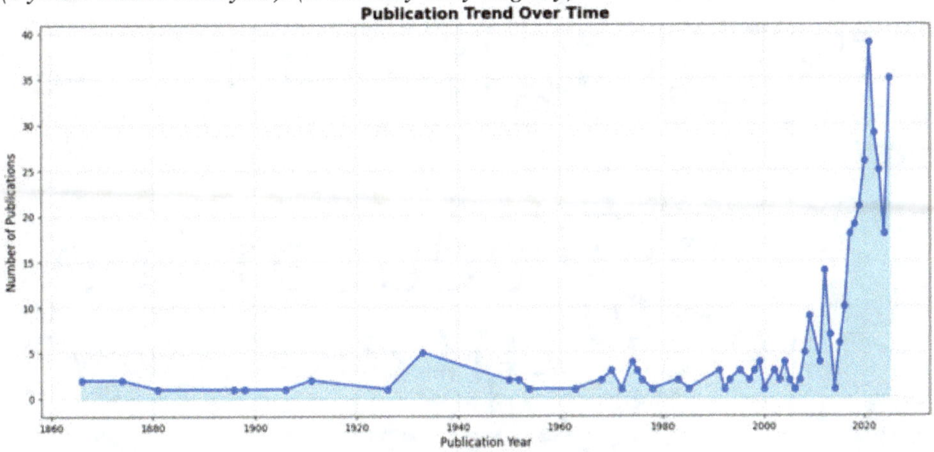

Figure 6 offers a word cloud of the most commonly used in the analyzed corpus keywords. The prevalence of the following terms like nutrition, diet, obesity, health, and children highlights the high level of public health orientation of up-to-date research. Meanwhile, the apparent focus on the mental and neural aspects can be seen through the more noticeable prominence of meditation, brain, cognitive, and function.

The combination of lifestyle, metabolic, and cognitive terminologies in the same visualization is indicative of the holistic framing that is becoming more common in yoga studies. Nonetheless, the conceptual gap is demonstrated in the relatively low levels of the exact meditative modes, like Dharana and Dhyana. This said divide supports the necessity of more sophisticated tools of analysis, like AI-based state detection and classification to surpass the generalized constructs of meditation in favor of more detailed and theoretically validated models.

Figure 6. Word Cloud of High-Frequency Keywords in the Dataset (Python-Based Analysis). (Data may vary slightly).

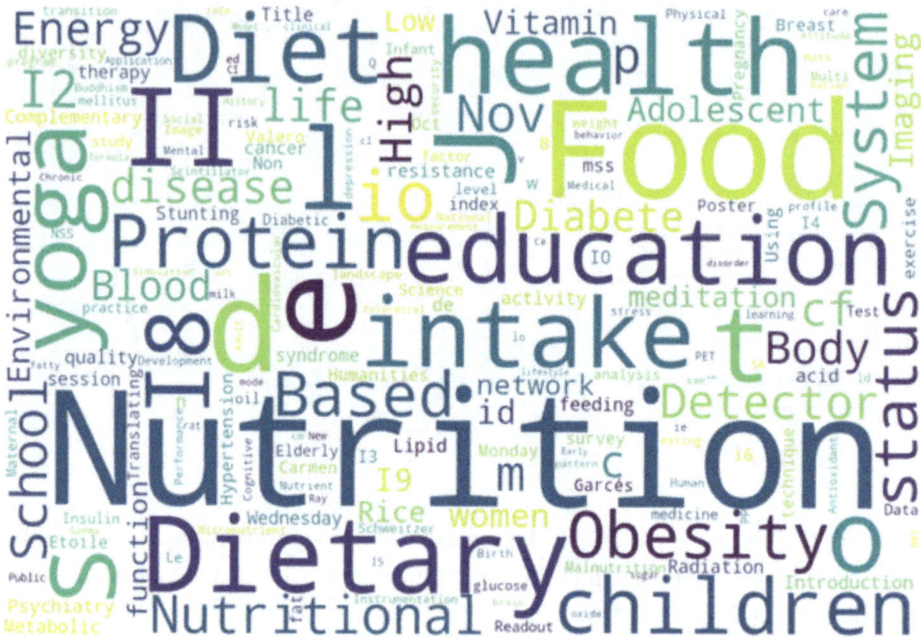

4. CONCLUSION

The purpose of this section was to dispel misunderstanding, introduce some order, and then revise the way we perceive Dharana and Dhyana - with the help of ancient yoga teachings as well as brain science and machine learning. Investigation of old source books, laboratory findings, and trends in literature reveal one concept reoccurring: these two practices are not of a similar nature of stillness. Rather, they entail various means through which the mind is attentive, perceives and is active within the body. One is based on intense concentration, coordinated by brain processes handling thinking processes, characterized by theta waves in the forefront, blanked-out distractions, and the constant control of heart rate. The other is smooth sailing, running like a silent brook bound to alpha-gamma rhythms in the dorsal parts, weaker chatter of the mind, stronger rest-and-digest, and an easy gradual fusion with whatever one is feeling.

Here we have an example of confusion in techniques and unequal outcomes in the study of meditation as an outcome of misunderstanding the sequence to be followed.

Surveys, general body cues and even brain scans loaded with labs, as opposed to down-cutting rapidly between trying hard and being caught up, lack clear timing and sharp concepts. Due to such gaps, the general thinking about meditation is not effective - more realistic models should be based on real mental stages associated with old teachings and real patterns of brain activity.

This is a new way of looking at things. Rather than intervening on the role of silent thinking, artificial intelligence appears as a handy assistant. Imagine it in the following way - computers combine brainwaves, breathing patterns, changes in heartbeat, as well as, how a person moves to think of all these simultaneously. That combination assists in distinguishing between two low key meditation phases as they occur even to demonstrate the degree of certainty of the guess. When intelligent algorithms come into play with intuitive reasoning techniques, it becomes far more precise to notice a shift in focus or profoundly relaxed. Issues that lingered over years - sharing practices, widespread results, adapting to people - begin to fade away. This time around the inner work can be explored further without the need to have an old-school mentor in place to bring it to fruition.

As it goes, the chapter continues to insist that ethics influence the use of tech. Developed on the principles of the yogic exercise, such values as inner control, doing no harm, personal freedom are considered as the first one, so artificial intelligence must support and not seize power, remain conscious of its functions, and retreat when necessary. Trust is increased when boundaries are respected, where data destination is open and shared and cultural context is treated. Progress implies the creation of tools that respect the goal as well as the form of yoga by means of attentive methods of learning and conscious designing.

The research trends further reinforce the primary concepts in this paper as it turns out that research on yoga has been rapidly increasing, with a change in the focus towards the brain science, complex biological networks, and one of the new methods of utilizing data. Yet, there is still a missing piece - despite the fact that yoga is given the appropriate attention, certain stages of meditation such as Dharana and Dhyana are almost never discussed as an independent study. Not having that is not only an issue, but it is an opening. As the theory is well coupled with the artificial intelligence tools, future research could be more successful at tracking the process of conscious training into a natural and fluid state of consciousness.

This chapter links old meditation practices with new concepts of computing to demonstrate that they do not lose their value. When these ways clash something useful can develop. It may be that science can better understand how people can be attentive, calm down, or come to pay attention. There might be new avenues in health and educational environments. The combination does not eliminate tradition - it gives it depth. Technologies may be altered, but it is the inside that matters.

REFERENCES

Basu-Ray, I., Metri, K., Khanra, D., Revankar, R., Chinnaiyan, K. M., Raghuram, N., Mishra, M. C., Patwardhan, B., Sharma, M., Basavaraddi, I. V., Anand, A., Reddy, S., Deepak, K. K., Levy, M., Theus, S., Levine, G. N., Cramer, H., Fricchione, G. L., & Hongasandra, N. R. (2022). A narrative review on yoga: A potential intervention for augmenting immunomodulation and mental health in COVID-19. *BMC Complementary Medicine and Therapies*, *22*(1), 191. DOI: 10.1186/s12906-022-03666-2 PMID: 35850685

Biswas, I., Kaur, J., Pearce, F., Lewis, S., & Chattopadhyay, K. (2025). E076 Key features of effective yoga interventions for treating rheumatoid arthritis: A systematic review and meta-analysis. *Rheumatology (Oxford, England)*, *64*(3, Supplement_3), keaf142.311. Advance online publication. DOI: 10.1093/rheumatology/keaf142.311

Demir, E., Uğurlu, B. N., Uğurlu, G. A., & Aydoğdu, G. (2025). Artificial intelligence in otorhinolaryngology: Current trends and application areas. *European Archives of Oto-Rhino-Laryngology : Official Journal of the European Federation of Oto-Rhino-Laryngological Societies (EUFOS) : Affiliated with the German Society for Oto-Rhino-Laryngology - Head and Neck Surgery*, *282*(5), 2697–2707. DOI: 10.1007/s00405-025-09272-5 PMID: 40019544

Hasan, M. K., Azad, M. K., & Hossain, M. S. (2025). 'Dharana' as the Gateway: Meditative Wit(H)Nessing and the transformation of trauma in Han Kang's The White Book. *INTERNATIONAL JOURNAL OF MULTIDISCIPLINARY RESEARCH AND ANALYSIS*, *8*(4). Advance online publication. DOI: 10.47191/ijmra/v8-i04-30

Nalbant, G., Hassanein, Z. M., Lewis, S., & Chattopadhyay, K. (2022). Content, Structure, and delivery Characteristics of Yoga Interventions for Managing Hypertension: A Systematic Review and Meta-Analysis of Randomized Controlled Trials. *Frontiers in Public Health*, *10*, 846231. Advance online publication. DOI: 10.3389/fpubh.2022.846231 PMID: 35419342

Rony, M. K. K., Parvin, M. R., & Ferdousi, S. (2023). Advancing nursing practice with artificial intelligence: Enhancing preparedness for the future. *Nursing Open*, *11*(1), nop2.2070. Advance online publication. DOI: 10.1002/nop2.2070 PMID: 38268252

Saeidnia, H. R., Firuzpour, F., Kozak, M., & Majd, H. S. (2025). Advancing cancer diagnosis and treatment: Integrating image analysis and AI algorithms for enhanced clinical practice. *Artificial Intelligence Review*, *58*(4), 105. Advance online publication. DOI: 10.1007/s10462-025-11117-w

Sak, J., & Suchodolska, M. (2021). Artificial Intelligence in Nutrients Science Research: A review. *Nutrients*, *13*(2), 322. DOI: 10.3390/nu13020322 PMID: 33499405

Sapci, A. H., & Sapci, H. A. (2020). Artificial Intelligence Education and Tools for Medical and Health Informatics Students: Systematic review. *JMIR Medical Education*, *6*(1), e19285. Advance online publication. DOI: 10.2196/19285 PMID: 32602844

Sengar, S. S., Hasan, A. B., Kumar, S., & Carroll, F. (2024). Generative artificial intelligence: A systematic review and applications. *Multimedia Tools and Applications*, *84*(21), 23661–23700. DOI: 10.1007/s11042-024-20016-1

Seoni, S., Jahmunah, V., Salvi, M., Barua, P. D., Molinari, F., & Acharya, U. R. (2023). Application of uncertainty quantification to artificial intelligence in healthcare: A review of last decade (2013–2023). *Computers in Biology and Medicine*, *165*, 107441. Advance online publication. DOI: 10.1016/j.compbiomed.2023.107441 PMID: 37683529

Telles, S., Raghavendra, B. R., Naveen, K. V., Manjunath, N. K., Kumar, S., & Subramanya, P. (2012). Changes in autonomic variables following two meditative states described in yoga texts. *Journal of Alternative and Complementary Medicine (New York, N.Y.)*, *19*(1), 35–42. DOI: 10.1089/acm.2011.0282 PMID: 22946453

Telles, S., Singh, N., Gupta, R. K., & Balkrishna, A. (2016). A selective review of dharana and dhyana in healthy participants. *Journal of Ayurveda and Integrative Medicine*, *7*(4), 255–260. DOI: 10.1016/j.jaim.2016.09.004 PMID: 27889426

Thakur, K. (2025). INDIAN KNOWLEDGE TRADITIONS: INTEGRATING MIND, BODY & SPIRIT FOR HOLISTIC WELLNESS. *International Journal of Research and Analytical Reviews*, *12*(2). Advance online publication. DOI: 10.56975/ijrar.v12i2.312734

Tripathi, R. L. (2025). AI Meets Mindfulness: Redefining spirituality and meditation in the Digital Age. *The Voice of Creative Research*, *7*(1), 17–26. DOI: 10.53032/tvcr/2025.v7n1.03

Tripathi, V., & Bharadwaj, P. (2021). Neuroscience of the yogic theory of consciousness. *Neuroscience of Consciousness*, *2021*(2), niab030. Advance online publication. DOI: 10.1093/nc/niab030 PMID: 34925910

Yadav, M., Sharma, A., & Sharma, I. (2025). The impact of Pragya Yoga and Savita Dhyana on stress levels and sleep quality of women. *Dev Sanskriti Interdisciplinary International Journal*, *26*, 01–06. https://doi.org/DOI: 10.36018/dsiij.26.376

KEY TERMS AND DEFINITIONS

Artificial Intelligence: Artificial Intelligence can be defined as the computational systems that can learn based on data, identify patterns and make decisions or predictions by involving minimum input by humans.

Awareness: Awareness is the ability to respond to, experience and be aware of internal and external phenomena in the current state.

Dharana: Dharana is the conscious effort to maintain a state of oneness of mind on one object, thought or sensation.

Dhyana: Dhyana refers to the effortless unbroken state of attention where the attention flows continuously and without conscious effort whatsoever.

fMRI: Functional magnetic resonance imaging (fMRI) is a neuroimaging process that indirectly measures the activity of the brain by assessing the change in blood oxygen levels that correspondingly relates to neural activity.

Focused Attention: Focused attention refers to the mental act of deliberately concentrating and keeping mental resources on a given target and eliminating distractions.

Meditation: Meditation refers to a methodical procedure of developing consciousness and awareness toward attaining mental clarity, emotional control and states of consciousness.

Yoga: Yoga is an old Indian philosophy that is a combination of physical exercises, breathing, moral values, and meditations to achieve mental and physiological equilibrium.

Chapter 8

A Comprehensive Review of AI and Machine Learning in Yoga:

From Pose Estimation to Personalized Training Systems

Kalpesh A. Popat
http://orcid.org/0000-0002-3818-3717
Marwadi University, India

Divyakant T. Meva
Marwadi University, India

ABSTRACT

Artificial Intelligence (AI) and Machine Learning (ML) transform physical wellness, with the yoga practice being one such area. The chapter is deep into development in the usage of AI and ML methods in yoga, recording the journey from simple pose recognizers to complex customized yoga trainers. The review highlights recent advances in Deep Learning and Computer Vision processes in pose estimation and classification on how to accurately detect and validate a yoga pose. One aspect of this is related to real-time feedback mechanisms and posture correction systems, leveraging AI to instantiate voice-guided or visual accuracy feedback for users. In addition, we investigate future applications, such as integrating ensemble learning for physiological tasks (e.g., EEG data) and building metaverse-based, customizable AI yoga coaches. The review critically evaluates datasets, algorithms, and performance metrics used from these studies, discusses the existing limitations in terms of generalization and diversity of data, and offers future research avenues.

DOI: 10.4018/979-8-3373-7625-7.ch008

1. INTRODUCTION: BRIDGING ANCIENT WISDOM AND MODERN TECHNOLOGY

Although many people now use yoga around the globe, there are still significant barriers to accessing high-quality teachers -- especially in rural or hard-to-reach areas or where cost, time, or disability may be an issue. Additionally, technological advancements in artificial intelligence and machine learning have greatly improved the delivery of health care, rehabilitation, sports science and digital fitness, and thus create a new question: can technology be used to enhance yoga practice while preserving the unique cultural and spiritual heritage that is at the heart of this ancient practice?

This fusion of traditional practice and modern technology necessitates thoughtful consideration. AI-enabled yoga platforms offer potential benefits including increased accessibility, customization, and objectivity; however, there exists a possibility of commercializing spiritual practice, continuing to appropriate culture, and diminishing yoga from a holistic practice into simply a form of physical activity.

The early forms of AI-based yoga platforms were limited to using computer vision to classify poses and treated yoga primarily as a pattern recognition problem. The latest forms of AI-based yoga platforms have begun to include real-time feedback, physiological monitoring and adaptable training; however, most of these systems focus on technical aspects and do not adequately address the experiential, cultural and ethical dimensions necessary for authentic yoga practice. In other words, how do we design AI-based yoga platforms that honor and preserve the rich and meaningful cultural and spiritual context of yoga?

1.1. Motivation: Toward Holistic Integration

This chapter comes from an understanding that much of the current work in this field has the potential to be more inclusive than it currently is. The majority of the research and reviews currently being published are focused solely on the technical aspects of the use of AI in yoga; such as, the accuracy of pose estimation, the metric used for the evaluation of classification algorithms, etc. There are no studies or reviews which address the cultural roots and/or philosophical basis of yoga, nor the experiential nature of the practice of yoga. While many researchers have developed very accurate and efficient systems (i.e., based upon their own technical standards), there may exist little if any, meaningful connection to the actual practice of yoga itself.

We argue for a model that is both technically innovative as well as culturally respectful, ethically responsible, and experientially authentic. Thus we are advocating for a review of not only what AI systems can do, but also what AI systems should do, how AI systems should be utilized, and what should remain as the exclusive domain of human instructional authority and individual experience.

1.2. Scope and Structure

The following is an overview of the six interdependent dimensions addressed by this comprehensive literature review:

Technical Foundations: A review of advances in both pose estimation and classification techniques (from convolutional neural networks to media pipe) as well as the abilities and limitations of these technologies.

Real-Time Systems: A description of architectures that allow for the practical implementation of real-time feedback mechanisms, personalization algorithms, and edge computing solutions.

Cultural and Philosophical Context: Investigating how Indian knowledge systems (such as concepts like prana and the subtle body) can be incorporated into the design of technology, and how the use of technology will influence the way in which traditional forms of yoga education are provided and learned.

Ethical and Social Dimensions: Reviewing a variety of issues that arise from the use of technology including: lack of diversity in datasets and the presence of biases within them; privacy concerns; potential for cultural appropriation; and the philosophic conflict between traditional practice and technological mediation of practice.

User Experience and Accessibility: A comparative analysis of user experience differences between the use of artificial intelligence and the use of human instructors; effectiveness of each instructional method with different populations; and design considerations for developing accessible systems.

Future Directions: Emerging application areas for AI in yoga include physiological monitoring; immersive environments; clinical rehabilitation; and human-AI collaborative models.

This comprehensive literature review will provide a reference model for researchers, practitioners, clinicians, and technologists who work at the intersection of AI and yoga by providing a synthesis of the technical, cultural, social/ethical, and experiential aspects of this field.

The interrelationship among these six dimensions is illustrated in Figure 1.

Figure 1. Conceptual framework illustrating the six interdependent dimensions of AI-enabled yoga systems

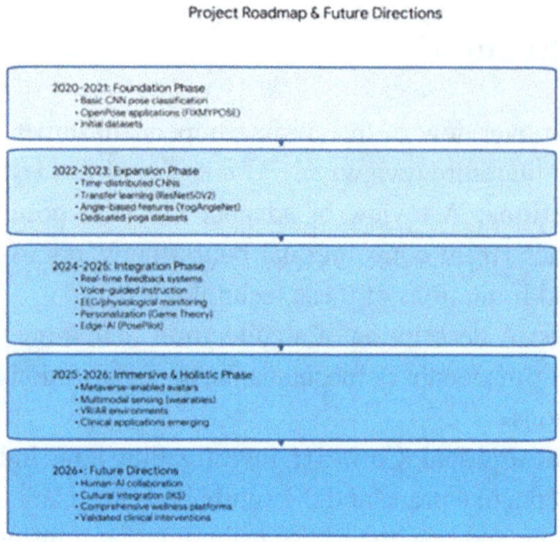

2. CULTURAL AND PHILOSOPHICAL FOUNDATIONS: YOGA BEYOND ASANA

Before looking at technology to support the application of yoga, it is helpful to know exactly what yoga is and how it differs from other forms of physical activity that promote development of the individual.

2.1. Yoga in Indian Knowledge Systems

The philosophical roots of yoga date back thousands of years and are described in many ancient Hindu texts such as the Vedas, Upanishads, Bhagavad Gita, and Yoga Sutras written by Patanjali (approximately 400 CE). In his writings, Patanjali outlines an eight-limbed path (Ashtanga Yoga), where he includes postures (asana) as only one of the components, in addition to ethics (yamas, niyamas), breath control (pranayama), removing distractions (pratyahara), focusing (dharana), meditation (dhyana), and ultimately achieving unity (samadhi).

Traditionally, yoga theory describes the "subtle body" in conjunction with the "physical body," outlining concepts not found in Western biomechanics:

Prana refers to the vital energy that exists throughout the body, different than the energy of breathing or metabolism. Pranayama practices are used to develop, direct and refine this subtle energy.

Nadis refer to the energetic pathways in which the prana flows, with traditional texts listing approximately 72,000 nadis, and identifying the three main nadis as ida (lunar/cooling), pingala (solar/heating), and sushumna (the central pathway associated with spiritual awakening).

Chakras refer to the energy centers or vortexes located along the spinal column of the body and are associated with various physiological, psychological and spiritual functions. There are seven major chakras that begin at the base of the spine (Muladhara) and end at the crown of the head (Sahasrara).

These concepts are central to the way yoga has been practiced historically and present unique problems for AI systems that will be limited to analyzing external physical positioning using computer vision. Will AI systems, when trained using only computer vision, be able to detect and measure the energetic dimensions reported by practitioners? If so, should these AI systems attempt to do so or does this create a category error — attempting to apply technological measurement tools to experiential domains that are inherently subjective?

2.2. Traditional Pedagogy and Experiential Learning

The guru-shishya (student-teacher) model of instructional yoga has historically been a highly relational experience where a student learns by being in an ongoing, close, and observational relationship with a teacher who is able to assist the student as they grow and develop over time. In addition to providing a student with the necessary information about how to perform postures and other aspects of yoga, a student's teacher is also responsible for guiding their student toward transformation — which includes:

Refining the student's observational skills: hrough observing a student's posture and movement, a teacher can see many small details about a student's alignment, compensation patterns, and energy quality that are often unseen in still images or even video recordings.

Providing individualized adjustments: When both parties are aware of the potential risks and benefits of using physical contact in teaching, teachers can use physical contact (such as hands on assists) to help students feel and learn how to correctly engage with their bodies.

Revealing new levels of awareness and knowledge to the student based on their ability to receive this new information: As a student develops a solid foundation of understanding about the basic principles of yoga, they will be prepared to receive additional information about advanced aspects of the practice.

Teaching the student about the whole of yoga, including the philosophical and ethical components of yoga as well as breathing practices and meditation: This allows the student to understand the role of the physical practice as part of a larger developmental process.

A key issue raised by this method of instructional yoga is whether it is possible for technology to replicate the relational, intuitive and energetic elements of instructional yoga. If so, what roles can technology fill as a complement, replacement, or something entirely new?

2.3. Implications for AI System Design

1. A holistic representation of quality of a pose is that a systems recognition of quality of a pose is not only physical alignment but also breath integration, mental focus, and subjective experience.
2. A culturally informed attribution of yoga materials, the materials should acknowledge the origins of yoga as well as avoid any presentation that divorces practice from its cultural context or claims innovation where traditional knowledge exists.
3. A transparent acknowledgment of limitations, clearly communicate to users that systems assess physical alignment and do not assess energetic dimensions, spiritual development, the full scope of yoga practice.
4. A complementary positioning of technology, technology should be framed as supporting rather than replacing human instruction particularly for deep learning and spiritual dimensions.

These considerations are largely absent in existing technical literature on AI in yoga domains and therefore need to become central to developing responsible AI in these domains.

3. EVOLUTION OF TECHNICAL APPROACHES: FROM STATIC CLASSIFICATION TO DYNAMIC ASSESSMENT

Having established cultural context, we now examine the technical evolution of AI in yoga, maintaining critical awareness of what these systems actually capture versus what they claim to assess.

3.1. Foundational Approaches: Image-Based Pose Classification

Researchers have applied early AI yoga systems using static image collection methods of practitioners in various asanas, labeling them by pose name, and then training Convolutional Neural Network (CNN) models on images to find recognizable patterns. In their study, Sharma et al. (2024), demonstrated that Deep Learning models were capable of predicting yoga poses with some level of success from asana images; similarly Duggal et al., (2025), and Battur et al. (2023) studied different Machine Learning (ML) techniques to classify yoga images. These foundational studies provided initial proof of concept; however they also identified several significant limitations for the use of static image analysis in this area.

In addition, most of these systems were primarily developed and tested using images of flexible, athletic people, all posed in a way that is aligned for what would be called "textbook" alignment; therefore, the systems created by these methods perform poorly when trying to generalize to those who are just beginning their practice, have a limitation, or come from a variety of body types.

3.2. Temporal Modeling: Incorporating Movement Dynamics

Static image-based methods were limited by their inability to model movement and sequence based on a single image; therefore, video-based methods have been proposed. Time Distributed CNN Architectures are designed to process each frame in a sequence as a separate input into the CNN architecture and therefore can analyze both the sequential pattern of a sequence of images, while also providing an opportunity to identify individual frames within that sequence.

The use of Time Distributed architectures has provided a means to detect and differentiate between movements that have the same static appearance but exhibit differences in their movement patterns, as well as the ability to track the transitions between different asanas (postures), identify when there is a decrease in stability or alignment during a posture and to assess the flow and continuity in dynamic practices.

However, one of the major drawbacks of using Temporal Modeling is the increased computational complexity which results in longer processing times. The processing time for a Static Image Analysis can be approximately 20-50 milliseconds, whereas the processing time for Video Sequence Analysis is typically 200-500 milliseconds. This could potentially degrade the quality of Real-Time Feedback.

3.3. Transfer Learning: Leveraging Pre-trained Networks

Transfer learning became a viable option because of limited availability of large-scale datasets for labeling yoga. A recent study (Chauhan et al., 2024), used a large-scale image dataset (ImageNet - millions of different images) to train ResNet50V2; then Chauhan et al. (2024) took the trained model and fine-tuned it specifically for yoga pose identification. The results showed that after fine-tuning ResNet50V2 achieved 92-97% accurate yoga pose identification in spite of having relatively small datasets for yoga pose training.

Transfer learning is based on the concept of utilizing early layers of a neural network to identify general characteristics such as edges, textures, etc. (without modifying those early layers) and using later layers to identify specific characteristics (such as those found in the yoga poses). Additionally, the last classification layer is replaced with a layer that includes categories for each type of yoga pose. This allows for the use of earlier layers that have already been trained on large amounts of images and significantly reduces the amount of images required to train the model and the time needed to train the model. Unfortunately, this method can inherit potential biases from the source datasets (e.g. the source datasets may not include enough images of people from all demographics, and may contain assumptions about what constitutes an ideal body type.)

The progression from static image classification to transfer learning-based adaptive models is summarized in Figure 2.

Figure 2. Evolution of technical approaches from static pose classification to transfer learning–based adaptive models.

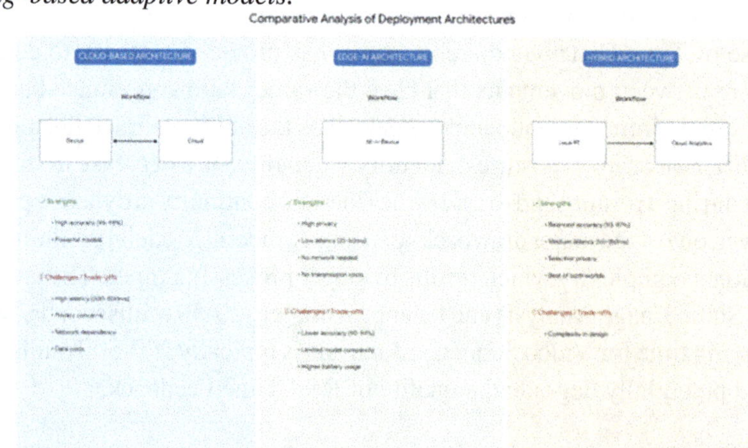

Table 1. Comparison of foundational technical approaches in AI-based yoga analysis.

Citation (First Author et al.)	Year	Primary Application Focus	Core Methodology/ Model	Key Contribution
Sharma et al.	2024	Pose Prediction/ Classification	Deep Learning	Approach for prediction of yoga posture using asana images
Meghana et al.	2025	Pose Detection/ Classification	ML Classifiers, Pose Estimation	Comprehensive analysis of ML classifiers for precise yoga pose classification
Talaat	2023	Pose Estimation	Novel Deep Learning Models	Development of new deep learning models for yoga pose estimation
Dhanyal & Nandyal	2023	Pose Classification	Time-Distributed CNN	Use of time-distributed CNN for yoga pose annotation and classification
Kumbhar et al.	2026	Pose Classification	OpenPose, PoseNet, MoveNet	Reviewing evolution and comparison of major deep learning pose estimation methods
Rajendran & Sethuraman	2025	Pose Classification	YogAngleNet (MediaPipe, Body Angles)	Classification using body angle features derived from MediaPipe
Duggal et al.	2025	Pose Classification	ML and Deep Learning	Exploration of AI techniques for yoga image classification
Battur et al.	2023	Pose Analysis	AI and ML Techniques	Analysis of yoga pose using general AI and ML techniques
Kim et al.	2021	Posture Correction	Pose Correctional Captioning	FIXMYPOSE system for generating corrective captions and retrieval
Ganesh & Ramudhin	2024	Posture Correction	Real-Time Application	Real-time posture correction to mitigate risks in yoga practice
Yenishettil et al.	2024	Posture Correction	AI Model, Virtual Teacher	Virtual Yoga Teacher for posture correction and health
Tripathi et al.	2025	Real-time Feedback	Real-time Pose Assessment	Voice-guided accuracy feedback for virtual yoga training
Saxena et al.	2025	Posture Feedback	Algorithmic and ML Approach	Methodologies for providing feedback on yoga asanas
Gadhvi et al.	2026	Posture Correction	Edge-AI Solution, PosePilot	Low-latency Edge-AI solution for posture correction

continued on following page

Table 1. Continued

Citation (First Author et al.)	Year	Primary Application Focus	Core Methodology/ Model	Key Contribution
Madhu et al.	2025	Physiological Monitoring	Ensemble Learning, EEG Classification	Investigating effects of yoga and meditation using EEG
Parab et al.	2023	Personalization	Game Theory, AI-Based Recommendation	Personalized AI-based yoga-pose recommendation system
Thushara & Abdul Jabbar	2026	Posture Assessment	PCA-Driven Feature Selection	Optimized posture similarity assessment using PCA
Wang et al.	2025	Immersive Training	Metaverse-Enabled Coach, Multimodal Sensing	Coach avatar in Metaverse using AI and insole sensing
Suryawanshi et al.	2023	Data Resource	Computer Vision	Introduction of dedicated Yoga dataset for computer vision analysis

4. POSE ESTIMATION FRAMEWORKS: TECHNICAL CAPABILITIES AND LIMITATIONS

Modern AI yoga systems are built upon pose estimation frameworks that use image or video to find skeletal keypoints, which need to be understood in terms of capability and limitation for developers as well as for evaluating what is measured by the systems.

4.1. OpenPose: High-Fidelity Multi-Person Detection

OpenPose, developed by the Perceptual Computing Lab at Carnegie Mellon University, is an important advancement in the field of pose estimation and has been evaluated by Kumbhar et al. (2026). OpenPose employed a novel "bottom-up" method where the system simultaneously identifies body parts (i.e., joints) and their association to create multi-person pose estimation without first detecting each person individually.

Technical Design: The architecture of OpenPose is a two-branch multistage CNN. The first branch produces confidence maps identifying the location of each joint while the second branch creates Part Affinity Fields (PAFs), which represent the orientation of limbs. Because PAFs can identify and describe the orientation of all limbs regardless of whether they are visible or partially occluded, this dual output architecture allows the system to detect people in a scene even if it is populated with multiple individuals or when there is partial occlusion of one or more of the subjects being detected.

Limitations for Yoga

- Requires high computational resources (typically GPUs for real-time processing)
- Performance degrades with occlusions common in many yoga poses (e.g., arms crossed behind back, seated twists)
- Designed for frontal/lateral views; unconventional camera angles reduce accuracy
- Captures external skeletal position but not muscle engagement, breath, or internal experience

4.2. Lightweight Models: PoseNet and MoveNet

To allow for deployment on consumer devices using general purpose hardware as opposed to specialized hardware, Google developed lighter weight versions of the algorithms that optimize the speed-accuracy trade-off.

PoseNet is based upon the MobileNet architecture and utilizes a depthwise separable convolutional layer to significantly reduce the number of model parameters and the amount of computation required. The PoseNet algorithm can detect 17 keypoints in approximately 30-50 ms of inference time on current generation smart phones; this enables real-time mobile applications. However, the accuracy (85-90%) of PoseNet is less than that of OpenPose and PoseNet only supports single person detection.

MoveNet further reduces computational requirements through the utilization of a feature pyramid network and center-based detection methods. MoveNet is available in two variants – Lightning (which prioritizes speed (inference time <20 ms)) and Thunder (which prioritizes accuracy (inference time 30-40 ms)). Both variants of MoveNet achieve 88-94% accuracy and are compatible with mobile applications.

The development of these lightweight models has helped to expand the scope of AI powered yoga instruction by enabling the development of web-based and mobile applications that operate locally on user devices, thus addressing both the issues of accessibility and privacy. However, because the lightweight models are attempting to address an accuracy-speed tradeoff, minor misalignments may be missed, and potentially lead to users developing unhealthy movement or practice habits unnoticed.

4.3. MediaPipe and Angle-Based Feature Engineering

MediaPipe Pose is a 3D pose detection system based on BlazePose, which recognizes 33 body landmark points in 3D space by way of x, y, and z coordinates, thus enabling differentiation of similar-looking poses that are viewed frontally versus those that differ in the sagittal plane, by virtue of its ability to capture depth.

Rajendran and Sethuraman (2025) designed a sophisticated example of feature extraction with MediaPipe, which they called YogAngleNet, and demonstrated how to apply MediaPipe's body landmark detection output to classify a set of biomechanically relevant joint angle values (e.g., knee flexion, hip extension, shoulder abduction) and/or body segment orientation values, rather than directly classifying raw body landmark coordinate values.

Advantages of Angle-Based Features

- **Scale and position invariance:** Angles remain constant regardless of distance to camera or position in frame
- **Biomechanical interpretability:** Angle features align with yoga instructional language (e.g., "maintain 90° at the knee in Warrior II")
- **Dimensionality reduction:** Converting 99 coordinate values (33 landmarks × 3) into 15-20 key angles simplifies models and reduces overfitting
- **Enhanced discrimination:** Poses with similar overall configurations but different joint angles become more distinguishable

Limitations: Angle based methods for assessing human movement assume that joints function as hinges which is a significant oversimplification of the complex dynamics of human movement. Angle-based methods are unable to represent qualities such as "grounding through the feet" or "lengthening the spine," which involve delicate muscle activation patterns as opposed to gross changes in angle.

Key characteristics of major pose-estimation frameworks are summarized in Table 2.

Table 2. Capabilities and limitations of major pose-estimation frameworks.

Framework	Developer	Keypoints	Inference Speed (Mobile)	Model Size	Accuracy	Best Use Case
OpenPose	CMU	25	150-300ms (requires GPU)	~200MB	95%+	Research, high-accuracy applications
PoseNet	Google	17	30-50ms	12-50MB	85-90%	Web applications, basic pose detection
MoveNet Lightning	Google	17	15-20ms	6MB	88-92%	Real-time mobile feedback
MoveNet Thunder	Google	17	30-40ms	12MB	90-94%	Mobile with balanced speed/accuracy
MediaPipe Pose	Google	33	20-30ms	8MB	90-93%	3D tracking, angle-based features
YOLOv8-Pose	Ultralytics	17	25-35ms	10-30MB	89-93%	Custom deployments, object detection integration

4.4. Critical Assessment: What Pose Estimation Actually Measures

Additionally, while highly sophisticated, current pose estimation systems can only measure the external skeletal positioning of an individual; thus, they provide only one necessary dimension of the complexity of yoga practice, but by no means sufficient to understand all dimensions of yoga. Pose estimation systems do not directly evaluate:

1.) Internal Experience: The sensations that arise during the performance of yoga movements, the flow of prana through the nadis, the mental focus required, the emotional states evoked.
2.) Muscle Activation Patterns: Which muscles activate, how the muscles engage, the level of subtle stabilization achieved.
3.) Breath Integration: Are the movements synchronized with breathing (i.e., inhale vs. exhale).
4.) Energetic Dimensions: The flow of prana through the nadis and the activation of the chakras as conceptualized in traditional yoga.
5.) Qualitative Aspects: How the body is engaged during movement i.e., whether it is a soft engagement or a gripping engagement, whether the body is opening or closing and whether the movements are performed easily or with strain.

The limitations of what these systems can measure and what yoga encompasses must be clearly articulated. The risk of relying too heavily on these types of systems is that it will reduce yoga to merely geometric representations, and the experiential and energetic dimensions of yoga will be lost, much like those experienced by traditional practitioners.

5. REAL-TIME FEEDBACK SYSTEMS: ARCHITECTURES AND USER EXPERIENCE

Transitioning from research prototype to deployable application, we are now dealing with a range of issues related to performance in real time, designing the user experience and the practical success of these tools for a wide variety of users.

5.1. Multimodal Sensing: Beyond Vision

At present, there is an overwhelming use of camera based systems to implement these technologies; however, assessments are increasing that incorporate a wide variety of other sensing modalities to evaluate the performance of each technology.

Primary reason for continued dominance by camera based systems is their non-invasive nature and the widespread availability of cameras on both smartphones and computer devices. To maximize accessibility Tripathi et al. (2025) implemented systems using everyday webcam or smartphone cameras. Field of view (full-body), robustness to light, optimal placement of the camera, minimum required frame rate (30fps), and the minimum required resolution (720p for reliable key point detection) are all critical design considerations when implementing camera based systems.

Three dimensional sensing systems (e.g., Microsoft Kinect, Intel RealSense) have the capability to measure the distance to body parts, rather than estimate this from monocular images. This has the advantage of being able to distinguish between poses that are very similar from the frontal view but significantly different along the z-axis. However, the requirement for special hardware and/or higher cost compared to cameras limits the ability for consumers to adopt depth cameras.

Emerging paradigms for wearable and embedded sensors were discussed by Wang et al. (2025). They proposed multimodal insole sensing systems that measured weight distribution, ground reaction forces, foot orientation and stability metrics derived from center-of-pressure measurements. These measurements capture aspects of gait and balance that are not visible through the use of cameras (for example, if weight is distributed properly between the ball and heel of the foot and whether subtle balance adjustments are indicative of instability).

Wearable and embedded sensors also allow for physiological sensor data collection to further expand the assessment process. Madhu et al. (2025) demonstrated ensemble learning based EEG classification to study the effects of combined yoga and Rajyog meditation, which showed how brain activity monitoring could be used to assess the efficacy of practice beyond body alignment. Additional examples of physiological sensor integration includes the integration of heart rate monitors, respiration sensors, and electromyography (EMG) for muscle activation patterns are at the forefront of assessing overall behavior and well-being.

A key aspect of using multimodal sensing is the added value of behavioral and wellness-related data provided by multimodal sensing can result in higher complexity of the system, higher costs and possibly higher user burdens. As a further example, when multiple sensors are attached to an individual, they may discourage users from experiencing the additional workload associated with casual use of the tool. Physiological sensor data may also pose a greater risk of violating an individual's right to privacy, thus appropriate ethical protocols should be developed to address this issue.

5.2. Feedback Modalities: Voice, Visual, and Haptic

Real-time feedback requires a practitioner to be able to translate technical data into easily understandable and actionable recommendations that he/she/they can act upon immediately during a practice session.

Voice-Guided Feedback: Tripathi et al. (2025) demonstrated how voice-based accuracy feedback could be used for real-time pose assessment. They recognized that a practitioner will rarely be able to continuously view their screen during a practice session. Therefore, any effective voice-based feedback system must consider the following factors:

Content Generation: The translation of numerical metrics into natural-language format requires the use of natural language generation (NLG), which generates natural language content from structured data. NLG also needs prioritization logic to identify the one most critical area of correction as well as context-aware phrasing to accommodate the flow of practice.

Timing and Frequency: Too much feedback can be distracting, while too little feedback does not give the practitioner the necessary guidance. Typically, an effective system allows 3-5 seconds of observation time prior to issuing corrections and limits the number of corrections to one every 10-15 seconds. An effective system also includes positive reinforcement when a practitioner holds a pose correctly. Finally, an effective system adjusts the frequency of corrections based on the skill-level of the practitioner.

Vocal Quality and Affect: As Yenishettil et al. (2024) have shown, the quality of a practitioner's voice affects the amount of feedback they receive. A practitioner who receives calming and encouraging feedback from a calm, supportive voice is more receptive than a practitioner receiving feedback delivered in a cold, clinical tone using a text-to-speech system.

Visual Feedback: Visual feedback provides practitioners with the ability to develop the proper alignment for the poses being practiced. Visual feedback is especially helpful in situations where the practitioner is holding a pose when it is possible to access a display device. There are several ways to provide visual feedback, including:

- Skeletal Overlay: Provides the practitioner with a visual representation of their detected skeletal structure by superimposing a color-coded representation of their detected skeleton over a video feed of themselves practicing the pose (correct joints are represented in green, minor errors are represented in yellow, and significant errors are represented in red).
- Reference Comparison: Provides the practitioner with a visual representation of what the correct pose looks like, either by showing the reference pose next to or overlapping the video feed of the practitioner attempting to replicate the pose.
- Angle Visualization: Provides the practitioner with a visual representation of specific joint angle measurements, such as knee angle (for example, "Knee: 102° (Target: 90°)") or other relevant joint angles.
- Progressive Indicators: Provide the practitioner with information about their overall performance, either through scores, progress bars, or percent correct measures (helps create a sense of competition or challenge for the practitioner while still providing them with feedback regarding their performance).
- Directional Cues: Provide the practitioner with arrows or graphic guides illustrating the direction in which the practitioner should move their body to make the corrections indicated by the feedback.

Saxena et al. (2025) noted that the method of feedback delivery should correspond to the type of learning environment — for example, voice feedback for flow sequences (where the practitioner has no way to visually reference a display device) and visual feedback for instructional mode (where the practitioner can visually reference a display device).

Limitations of Haptic Feedback Systems

Current haptic devices provide less sensory feedback compared to the physical corrections provided by human instructors. Controllers only provide vibration, do not provide directional pressure to guide the practitioner in placing their limbs, and do not provide sustained support to help the practitioner hold difficult poses or provide tactile feedback to confirm if the practitioner has engaged the appropriate muscles to perform the pose correctly. Although research is ongoing to develop more advanced haptic devices (pneumatic actuators, ultrasonic mid-air haptics, full-body haptic suits), the current high cost and low usability of these systems continue to limit their potential for widespread adoption.

The multimodal real-time feedback architecture integrating sensing, processing, and user interaction is depicted in Figure 3.

Figure 3. Multimodal real-time feedback architecture integrating sensing, processing, and user interaction.

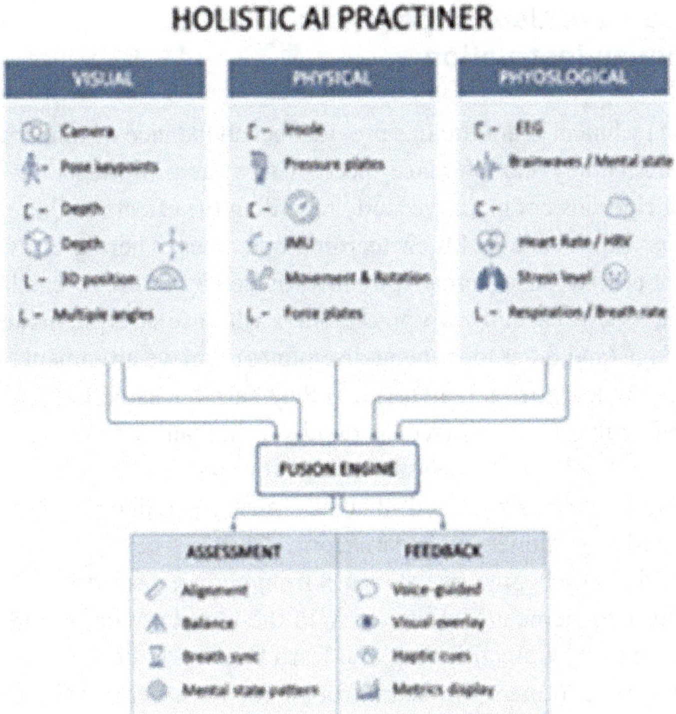

The principal real-time feedback modalities and their functional roles are outlined in Table 3.

Table 3. Real-time feedback modalities and usability characteristics.

System Type	Classification Accuracy	Correction Precision	Latency	Resource Requirements	Privacy Level
Cloud-based CNN	95-98%	85-90%	200-500ms	High server compute	Low (data transmitted)
Edge-AI Lightweight	90-94%	75-85%	25-50ms	Mobile device only	High (local processing)
Hybrid (Edge+Cloud)	93-97%	82-88%	50-150ms	Mobile + cloud	Medium (selective transmission)
Multi-modal (Vision+Sensors)	96-99%	88-95%	50-100ms	Sensors + compute	Variable

5.3. Comparative User Experience: AI Versus Human Instruction

While the technical literature has provided an abundance of information on the classification accuracy and inference speed of AI systems for teaching Yoga, there is a dearth of rigorous comparative study regarding the effects of these systems on both the users' experience and their learning outcomes. There are several critical questions that need to be systematically investigated by future researchers:

Effectiveness of Learning: Do practitioners who use AI systems to learn how to perform Yoga (and other movement disciplines) achieve alignment as rapidly as practitioners who learn from humans; will they have the same level of kinesthetic awareness and ability to self-correct as rapidly as human-instructed practitioners?

Prevention of Injury: Will AI systems help prevent many of the beginner injuries that occur when practicing Yoga and other movement disciplines? Will the number of injuries suffered by beginners who learn from AI systems be lower than the number of injuries suffered by beginners who learn from human instructors?

Long-Term Engagement/Motivation: Will the long-term engagement and motivation experienced by practitioners who learn from AI systems be similar to that experienced by practitioners who learn from human instructors? Which aspects of AI systems will lead to increased adherence and decreased dropout?

Developmental Progression of Skill: Will practitioners who learn from AI systems develop the skills to successfully move to intermediate/advanced poses, or will they "plateau" due to lacking certain subtle nuances that can only be taught by human instructors?

Perception of Support: How will practitioners perceive the support, understanding, and guidance provided by AI systems vs. human instructors? Will users feel that the technology-based experience is alienating or empowering?

Variation Based on Demographics: How will the perceptions of practitioners vary based on demographic factors such as age, body type, culture background, prior experience with technology, and prior experience with Yoga?

As important as it is to responsibly deploy AI systems into education, all of these questions remain largely unanswered. Therefore, it is essential for future researchers to conduct rigorous studies of the users' experience and learning outcomes of AI systems as well as their practical effectiveness, safety, and experiential quality across various demographics.

6. PERSONALIZATION AND ADAPTIVE SYSTEMS: BEYOND ONE-SIZE-FITS-ALL

Recognizing that individuals differ dramatically in flexibility, strength, experience, body structure, and wellness goals, advanced systems incorporate personalization mechanisms.

6.1. Game-Theoretic Pose Recommendation

In their 2023 study, Parab et al. applied game theory for developing individualized, AI-based systems that recommend yoga poses based on a multi-criteria decision-making framework in which each objective is represented by a player with opposing goals:

- Skill appropriateness (no recommendations for poses that are either too easy or too hard).
- Focus on target body part (recommendation of specific body parts such as back, hip etc.)
- Variety of practice (reducing monotony due to repetitive practices).
- Quality of sequence (smooth transition from one pose to another).
- Timing (limitations imposed by time constraints of the practice).

The system identifies sequences of poses that simultaneously achieve a Nash Equilibrium or Pareto Optimality with respect to these competing objectives. User capability models are continually updated based on the success of the user's practice of the recommended poses; thus providing continuous improvement in recommendations.

This methodology exceeds both the limitations of content-based filtering (i.e., recommending poses with similarities to poses previously taken) and collaborative filtering (i.e., recommending poses that were preferred by other users with similar characteristics). Thus, this methodology achieves true multi-objective optimization while considering all constraints and pedagogically relevant considerations.

6.2. PCA-Driven Feature Selection for Personalized Assessment

Thushara and Abdul Jabbar (2026) suggested an approach to evaluating the similarity of optimal yoga postures by determining the most relevant characteristics through principal component analysis-based feature selection. The authors acknowledge that not all characteristics of a given yoga pose will be equally important in the evaluation of each posture. In addition, the physical capabilities of individuals vary greatly requiring customized assessments.

Principal Component Analysis is used to identify the variables of greatest variability which can distinguish the correct from incorrect execution of a specific yoga posture. For example, when executing Tree Pose (Vrksasana), Principal Component Analysis may determine that the angle of the hip of the standing leg and the lateral alignment of the spine are the primary variables which distinguish expertly executed poses from those executed incorrectly. Conversely, the position of the arms can have high variability even among experts in this posture. Thus, the assessment system can focus on the critical characteristics of a pose and allow for flexibility in assessing other dimensions where the position does not impact the overall quality of the posture.

In addition to focusing on critical characteristics of a posture, the personalized assessment process takes into account the unique body type and baseline flexibility of the individual being assessed. Calibration measurements are established based on these factors to adjust criteria accordingly. Improvement is measured against an individual's baseline, and not against absolute standards, and areas of asymmetry or limitations are identified and addressed with targeted instruction.

Existing personalization strategies and their constraints are synthesized in Table 4.

Table 4. Personalization strategies and adaptive assessment mechanisms.

Dataset	Number of Poses	Subjects	Images/ Videos	Body Type Diversity	Skill Levels	Annotations
Yoga-82	82	50+	28,000 images	Limited	Mostly advanced	Pose labels
YogaSet	50	30	15,000 images	Moderate	Mixed	Pose + keypoints
Custom (Suryawanshi et al.)	107	40+	23,000+ images	Moderate	Advanced	Multi-label

continued on following page

Table 4. Continued

Dataset	Number of Poses	Subjects	Images/ Videos	Body Type Diversity	Skill Levels	Annotations
Typical Research Dataset	20-50	10-20	5,000-10,000	Very limited	Advanced	Pose labels only
Ideal Future Dataset	100+	500+	100,000+	High diversity	All levels	Pose + keypoints + corrections + metadata

6.3. Limitations of Current Personalization

The first point is that although there has been a lot of progress in the area of personalization, it is still somewhat limited by what is being done today:

There are coarse categories that most people use as their primary way of describing someone's skill level, as opposed to creating a detailed picture of a person's skills and limitations.

Most people do not take into consideration the vast number of things that can affect how well they are able to perform such as an injury within the last week or two, the phase of their menstrual cycle (which affects both their flexibility and energy), whether they are stressed out right now or at what time of day they are practicing, etc.

Very few systems track how well someone is doing from month-to-month or year-to-year, therefore they are not able to adapt to someone who is developing capabilities at a slower pace over time, or regressing because of life events.

Homogeneous optimization objectives: Systems generally try to optimize for "alignment," but recognize that the practice goals of different individuals can be vastly different (for example, some may want to develop their flexibility, while others may want to build strength, recover from therapy, reduce stress, etc., or deepen their spirituality).

7. ETHICAL, CULTURAL, AND SOCIAL DIMENSIONS: CRITICAL CONSIDERATIONS

Beyond technical sophistication, responsible AI yoga systems must address profound ethical, cultural, and social considerations largely neglected in existing literature.

7.1. Dataset Diversity and Algorithmic Bias

The main limitation of current AI yoga systems is their lack of a large, representative dataset that would allow them to generalize well and avoid being biased by their training data.

Lack of Body Types: The majority of all the current training datasets contain mostly individuals who are thin, flexible and strong; are relatively young (young adult) to middle aged; are primarily white/Caucasian and have an athletic/lean body type. Because of this limited representation of body types, systems will perform poorly when trying to evaluate individuals who are bigger, older, injured/disabled, new to yoga and inflexible, or ethnically/racially diverse and have different body proportions.

There are several ways that under-representation of body types affects the performance of AI yoga systems. First, algorithms for estimating pose based upon images of "typical" athletes/individuals may be unable to detect key points on larger bodies since these landmarks may be visually indistinct. Second, classification systems may not identify valid pose variations associated with physical limitations. Finally, assessment systems may require practitioners to assume poses that they cannot attain because their bodies do not fit the criteria established in a traditional studio setting; such unrealistic expectations may lead to discouragement or unsafe attempts to make their bodies conform to an unnatural configuration.

Limited Environmental Representation: Training data is usually generated in a studio environment using professional lighting, neutral backgrounds, idealized camera angles and high quality video capture equipment. Practitioners conduct their yoga in a variety of home environments including cluttered rooms, outdoors in changing light, and from a variety of vantage points using cameras and/or cell phones with varying quality. Since most systems are trained on data generated in a studio environment, they are not equipped to handle a variety of backgrounds, varying light sources, or atypical camera positions.

Lack of Cultural and Style Diversity: Different yoga traditions place emphasis on the alignment of the body for poses which share the same name. Thus, if one tradition places greater importance on precise alignment with the use of props, while another does not, then it is possible that a system trained on the first tradition's data may misclassify a valid pose from the second tradition as an error. For instance, Iyengar yoga has a focus on precise alignment using a variety of props. Ashtanga yoga involves a very specific sequence of postures with dynamic movement between each posture. Restorative yoga makes heavy use of props to support the practitioner in each posture. Power yoga, on the other hand, is characterized by fast flowing movements and athletic poses.

Responsible Development: Creating datasets that represent a wide range of body types, ages, abilities and ethnicities and include a number of skills levels (from novice to expert), and represent a number of different environmental and recording conditions, and represent a number of different yoga traditions and styles. These datasets should be subjected to fairness testing with regard to demographic groupings and the results of these tests should be reported in a transparent manner and include a discussion of the limitations of the systems.

7.2. Cultural Appropriation and Respectful Representation

In the context of a yoga practice, there are some important things to be aware of when working with an AI system. First, many Westernized versions of yoga, which have been commercialized, reduce the complexity of the practice and the underlying philosophy to simply the physical movements themselves, fail to honor the source community, and do not fairly compensate those who share their knowledge. Therefore, it is possible for an AI to further amplify this issue by promoting the use of yoga as a form of technology that has no connection to its historical, cultural, and spiritual roots; failing to provide the user with a complete understanding of the historical context of the practice, including the philosophical and spiritual aspects; discounting traditional forms of pedagogy in favor of what may be perceived as innovative; and misrepresenting the work of others as new when in fact it is rooted in centuries-old traditions.

Therefore, there are certain respectful integration principles that you can follow to avoid potential pitfalls:

1.) Cultural Attribution: In order to respect the culture from which yoga originates, an AI system should clearly indicate that yoga originated in India and that it has a deep philosophical foundation. The system should also provide the user with information about how traditional yoga is practiced, as opposed to just presenting itself as the originator of a new type of technology.
2.) Traditional Consultation: When developing an AI system related to yoga, it would be best to consult with individuals who are well-versed in both the philosophy and the pedagogy of traditional yoga, as opposed to consulting with primarily computer scientists and/or fitness professionals.
3.) Holistic Representation: An AI system that addresses only physical alignment, and does so without acknowledging that such a representation is limited to only one aspect of yoga, will likely not adequately represent the full range of what yoga encompasses. Therefore, it is essential that an AI system acknowledge that there is more to yoga than just the physical aspects, and to represent the entire

practice of yoga, which includes breath control, meditation, ethics, and spiritual development.

4.) Terminology Respect: Finally, an AI system should demonstrate respect for the language associated with yoga, particularly with regard to the use of Sanskrit terminology. It is therefore recommended that an AI system provide users with access to accurate pronunciations of Sanskrit terms, and refrain from using reduced or culturally insensitive terms to refer to yoga practices or philosophies.
5.) Ethical Frameworks: A final principle that should guide the development of AI systems related to yoga is the inclusion of the ethical frameworks that exist within the practice. These include the yamas and niyamas, and as such, an AI system should not be designed solely around the mechanical execution of poses, but should also promote the ethical and moral dimensions of the practice.

7.3. Privacy and Data Security in Wellness Applications

There are serious privacy implications associated with collecting a person's private video recordings of their body, and/or their health information and other performance metrics by an artificial intelligence "yoga" system.

Data minimization: Ethical systems can only collect the data that they need to function. This represents a "privacy by design" approach; as edge-AI approaches process video locally, thus transmitting nothing and representing privacy by design. The system should clearly explain what data is being collected and why; default to a "privacy favoring setting" (i.e., local processing, no transmission); allow the user to control how long data will be retained in the system, and allow the user to delete data from the system; and, if any data is used for improving the system, it should be anonymous.

Informed consent: Users should be aware of how their data is going to be used prior to providing their consent to the collection of said data. As such, the system's use of the data must be explained within a clear, plain language, non-legalistic privacy policy. In addition, the system must obtain specific, affirmative consent for the use of sensitive data (e.g., when such data is shared with third-party entities, or when the data is used for marketing purposes). Furthermore, the system should offer the user a choice of whether they wish to grant consent for each type of data collection/use separately. Finally, once a user has granted consent for the collection and use of their data, the user should have the ability to revoke that consent at any time, and have the data deleted from the system.

START_TEXT Protection of personal information: All of the data sent needs to be encrypted so others can't intercept it. The data also has to be stored in a secure manner with proper access control, auditing capabilities and the ability for users to verify their identity. Regularly assessing the security of the overall system as well as each component, and having a plan in place to respond to an incident when a breach occurs are two other ways to help protect the user's information.

Specific considerations: Body capture videos are very sensitive, and therefore, they can only be shared/transmitted with the user's direct knowledge and consent. In addition, because of this sensitivity, retention of the data should be limited and video captured by local devices should be processed locally.

Ethical and socio-cultural considerations for responsible AI-enabled yoga systems are summarized in Table 5.

Table 5. Ethical, cultural, and privacy considerations in AI-enabled yoga systems.

Challenge Area	Current State	Research Gaps	Proposed Solutions	Expected Timeline
Dataset Diversity	Limited body types, studio environments	Underrepresentation of diverse populations	Community data collection efforts, synthetic data generation	2-3 years
Subtle Error Detection	Gross misalignments detected well	Micro-adjustments, muscle engagement invisible	Multi-modal sensing, advanced biomechanical modeling	3-5 years
Personalization	Basic difficulty adjustment	Limited individual adaptation	Longitudinal learning, constitutional modeling	2-4 years
Contextual Assessment	Fixed standards	Goal-dependent, therapeutic modifications	Expert system integration, contextual AI	3-5 years
Physiological Integration	Emerging EEG studies	Limited multi-sensor fusion	Standardized protocols, integrated platforms	4-6 years
VR/Metaverse	Conceptual prototypes	Haptics, tracking, comfort limitations	Hardware advances, algorithm optimization	3-7 years
Ethical Frameworks	Minimal guidance	Privacy, bias, cultural appropriation concerns	Interdisciplinary guidelines, community input	Ongoing
User Experience Research	Very limited	Learning effectiveness, safety outcomes	Rigorous comparative studies, longitudinal tracking	1-3 years
Clinical Validation	Lacking	Safety/efficacy for clinical populations	RCTs for rehabilitation, chronic disease, mental health	3-5 years
Cultural Integration	Absent	IKS perspectives, philosophical context	Collaboration with traditional practitioners, curriculum integration	2-4 years

7.4. The Philosophical Tension: Technology Versus Traditional Practice

Yoga, which is traditionally a holistic and experiential method of promoting personal growth, has historically relied upon the teacher/student relationship, the development of internal awareness and ultimately, spiritual development. The introduction of technology into this space raises a number of philosophical questions:

1. Disconnection From Human Experience: Can Artificial Intelligence (AI) replicate the intuitive adjustments made by a human teacher, the physical presence and energy of a human teacher, the relationships formed between a student and teacher and the transmission of spirit from one human being to another that occurs when two human beings interact?

If AI can make some of these adjustments then what will be lost in the transition from a shared experience in a community, to the interaction with an individualized technology, versus a group learning environment in which the participants learn together within the context of a shared culture and tradition?

2. Focus On The External Versus Internal: The focus of traditional practices is on an individual's internal awareness (breathing, proprioception, mind), whereas technology-based practices may move the focus of attention away from the internal awareness of the practitioner toward the collection and analysis of external quantitative data (heart rate variability, body temperature, etc.).

This could result in a reduction of the internal awareness that practitioners have come to rely upon for their understanding of the practice.

3. Commodification Paradox: On the one hand, technology offers individuals the ability to connect with qualified instructors and thereby gain access to yoga instruction that was previously unavailable to them; however, technology also has the potential to transform a deeply spiritual practice into a commodified form of yoga, where convenience replaces depth, and yoga is reduced to a consumable product rather than a transformative discipline.
4. Alternative Practice Goals: Traditional Yoga (Hatha Yoga, Raja Yoga, etc.) aims to facilitate Self-Realization (Atma Samadhi), Liberation (Moksha), and Spiritual Development (Sadhana); whereas many technology-directed systems aim to provide Physical Fitness, Stress Reduction, or Measurable Results -- all of which are valuable, but incomplete expressions of what yoga entails.

5. Moving Toward An Integrated Equilibrium: Instead of viewing technology and tradition as mutually exclusive, I suggest combining them in a manner that enables students to develop the fundamental skills of yoga via technology, while utilizing human teachers to attain Deep Learning. Design systems that promote an individual's internal awareness rather than simply recording an individual's performance, and include the philosophical teachings of yoga in conjunction with the instructional components of the physical practice of yoga. Furthermore, consider technology as a supportive tool for your practice rather than a replacement for the practice itself. Finally, honor the origins of yoga while incorporating modifications to support contemporary cultural contexts.

In Rajput et al.'s (2024) study of Chakra software applications, they were able to demonstrate the possibility of accessing the spiritual dimensions of the chakras via software applications. However, they identified the need for culturally sensitive approaches to the subtle energy systems, as well as acknowledging the variety of beliefs related to these systems.

8. CLINICAL APPLICATIONS AND THERAPEUTIC POTENTIAL

Beyond general wellness, AI yoga systems show promise for clinical rehabilitation, chronic disease management, and mental health support—applications requiring rigorous validation and specialized design.

8.1. Rehabilitation and Physical Therapy

The benefits of using an AI-assisted yoga program to aid in recovery after an injury, recovery from surgery, or to manage chronic pain include:

Accessibility: Because many patients face barriers to traveling to visit a physical therapist due to mobility or transportation issues or because of scheduling conflicts, these patients can practice yoga at home and receive real-time, automated feedback about their form and positioning during every session.

Consistent Instruction: Through the use of automated feedback, patients receive the same instructions throughout every session, regardless of whether or not a physical therapist is available to provide them.

Quantifiable Data: By using measurable data (e.g., range of motion, percentage of accurate alignment, degree of stability), clinicians are provided with quantifiable evidence to support their clinical decision-making and quantify a patient's progress.

Automated Injury Detection: Although an automated system will never be able to prevent injuries from occurring entirely, it can potentially identify when a patient performs an unsafe movement and alert the patient to correct their movement, which could reduce the risk of the patient suffering a repeat injury.

Therapeutic Applications: For therapeutic application of AI-based yoga programs, the following requirements will need to be met:

1. AI-assisted yoga programs should be integrated into clinical protocols that were developed by certified physical therapists.
2. The programs must ensure contraindications are managed so that patients do not attempt to perform exercises that may exacerbate a particular condition.
3. The programs must establish emergency response procedures if a client experiences an adverse reaction to a movement or exercise.
4. Clinical oversight will be required as opposed to allowing clients to utilize the system independently as part of their overall treatment plan.
5. A rigorous study will be required to validate the safety and effectiveness of the system prior to implementation.
6. Depending upon the type of assistance being provided by the system it may also require regulatory approval (i.e., FDA approval).

8.2. Chronic Disease Management

The use of AI in yoga provides some evidence for the treatment of chronic health conditions such as high blood pressure, diabetes, chronic pain syndromes, arthritis, and breathing problems. Using a combination of AI technology, a user can have an automated system that will provide a personalized yoga routine tailored to their condition(s) and physical limitations (e.g., modify poses to make them easier/difficult to do). The use of sensors in a yoga program can also track the physiological responses of the user (e.g., heart rate, blood pressure), which can trigger alerts if they exceed certain limits, allowing the user to take action to prevent further harm. In addition, an AI-based yoga program can track long term trends, and correlate the user's yoga practice patterns with improvements in managing symptoms, providing data to help guide better treatments/interventions.

Limitations: Although there is potential to use AI in yoga programs for the treatment of chronic conditions, the amount of evidence supporting its use is limited. The majority of the current AI-based yoga programs were developed and evaluated using healthy young adults rather than individuals who are at risk for developing chronic conditions or those already experiencing chronic conditions. Therefore, it is critical that more rigorous randomized controlled trials be conducted to evaluate the safety, effectiveness and cost-benefit of using AI-based yoga for the treatment of chronic conditions prior to large scale clinical implementation.

8.3. Mental Health Support

Yoga studies have shown that yoga is effective in reducing anxiety, depression, post-traumatic stress disorder (PTSD) symptoms, and overall stress levels. AI systems can:

Increase the number of people who receive evidence-based treatments as there are many areas where people do not have access to these services.

Provide continuous support to an individual between therapy appointments so that the individual can continue practicing the same techniques learned during therapy while continuing to work on issues with a trained mental health professional.

Allow for customization based on how someone is feeling at the time of use and adjust practice accordingly based on self-reported feelings/moods and physiological indicators of stress (e.g., heart rate variability).

Include biofeedback capabilities using devices such as heart rate monitors or electroencephalograms (EEGs), allowing individuals to become more aware of their body's physiological responses to different stimuli and develop skills to better manage their nervous systems.

Important Factors To Consider: The AI will be unable to provide sufficient help to an individual who is experiencing severe psychological distress; as such, the developers and marketers of this application should clearly state what this application can and cannot do, and advise users that they must seek help from a licensed practitioner if needed. Provide users with access to emergency services and crisis lines; avoid stating that this application will diagnose any mental health condition, or provide a "cure" for any condition; and work with experienced practitioners in the field of mental health to develop this application so that it utilizes established practices and methods.

9. EMERGING TRENDS: PHYSIOLOGICAL INTEGRATION AND IMMERSIVE ENVIRONMENTS

The frontier of AI yoga systems extends beyond pose correction toward comprehensive wellness assessment, immersive training, and integration with broader health ecosystems.

9.1. EEG and Neurological Assessment

Madhu et al. (2025) conducted an investigation into the neurological and cognitive effects of yoga and Rajyog meditation by developing an ensemble learning-based method for EEG classification that represented a shift in paradigms from evaluating physical performance to determining how these practices affect one's nervous system and cognitive abilities.

Electroencephalography (EEG): EEG is a non-invasive way of collecting signals of the brain's electrical activity via electrodes placed on the scalp. The signals produced are associated with various frequency bands corresponding to different mental states. There are five types of frequency bands; delta waves (0.5 – 4 Hz) correspond to deep sleep, unconsciousness and other similar processes; theta waves (4 – 8 Hz) correspond to meditation and the creative process; alpha waves (8 – 13 Hz) correspond to relaxation, awareness and being in a meditative state; beta waves (13 – 30 Hz) represent focused thought; and gamma waves (30+ Hz) represent intense concentration and integration.

Both yoga and meditation can influence these patterns of brain activity. Many regular practitioners of both practices tend to have higher levels of alpha wave activity while practicing (relaxed focus), higher levels of theta wave activity during deep meditation, better synchronized gamma waves (more aware), and lower levels of high-beta wave activity (less stressed/anxious).

Ensemble Methods for Multi-Class Classification of Meditation States Based on EEG Signals: Ensemble methods involve training multiple classifiers using different subsets of features to predict more than two classes of meditation states, which is what Madhu et al. did in their study. Their approach included preprocessing the EEG signals to remove artifacts, extracting features from the frequency bands using wavelet transforms and power spectral density, training multiple classifiers on the extracted features and then combining the predictions of the classifiers using either voting or stacking, resulting in accuracy rates of 87 – 92% in classifying meditation states.

Future Integration: Future applications could integrate EEG monitoring with pose estimation to evaluate the relationship between the quality of one's physical postures and their mental states, to determine which physical postures best induce desired mental states in specific individuals, to provide practitioners with biofeedback so they may more easily access meditative states, to monitor and document long term improvement in both physical and mental practice dimensions, and to recognize when physical discomfort or poor alignment prevents a practitioner from focusing mentally.

Ethics: EEG monitoring raises significant ethical concerns related to privacy. Brain activity data is some of the most private data possible regarding an individual. Any use of this data must be secured with the highest level of security protocols, each participant must sign an informed consent form prior to the collection of any neurological data, all participants must be provided with full disclosure as to how their collected data will be used, and no participant's data should ever be shared or sold without their explicit approval.

9.2. Cardiovascular and Respiratory Monitoring

Using a combination of heart rate variability (HRV), a measure of the autonomic nervous system's status and the level of stress, and integrating it into a yoga program helps verify that restorative poses have been effective in reducing sympathetic activity, identify poses that are being completed at a level of intensity that is too high for the cardiovascular system, provide biofeedback to assist practitioners in improving their HRV through breathing practices, and monitor for cardiovascular issues in practitioners who have them.

Breathing Analysis: The analysis of how an individual is using his/her breathing to practice yoga, through the use of wearable technology such as heart rate monitors and blood oxygen sensors, or video based technologies which measure the motion of the chest and abdomen, will allow a practitioner to determine if he/she has achieved a consistent breathing pattern while performing a difficult pose; alert him/her to breath holding, a common occurrence among beginners when they are struggling with a difficult pose; provide real time feedback to assist the practitioner in performing pranayama (breath control); and correlate the breathing patterns used by a practitioner with the quality and stability of the poses they perform.

9.3. Muscle Activation Assessment

Surface electromyography (EMG) allows systems to identify patterns of muscle activation allowing a distinction between proper muscle recruitment and the activation of muscles that are being used as substitutes for proper muscles. The use of EMG will provide a more accurate indication of which muscles are being engaged by the user in order to facilitate correction when the user is using incorrect or compensating muscle(s).

However, EMG requires electrodes to be placed on the individual muscles, thus requiring additional setup time prior to each training session, possibly increasing the amount of user friction; reducing the likelihood of casual practice and therefore limiting its potential usage as a training tool in a home environment or other environments where training occurs outside of a clinical or serious training context.

9.4. Metaverse and Virtual Reality Yoga

Virtual Reality and Augmented Reality are increasing in popularity and are being used in a wide range of ways; the medical field is one area where VR and AR are becoming more prominent. Research has focused on developing Virtual Reality (VR) systems to aid individuals learning to perform surgery. One example is the "Simulation-Based Training Program," which was developed at the University of

California San Francisco (UCSF). The purpose of the Simulation-Based Training Program was to train surgeons to perform complicated surgical procedures and increase their comfort levels when performing these complicated procedures.

There are two types of simulation technologies that are the basis for the Simulation-Based Training Program. The first is known as the "Robotic Surgery Simulator." This is an interactive computer-based system that teaches surgeons to perform robotic surgeries. It utilizes a combination of virtual reality and robotics to enable the surgeon to practice a procedure prior to performing it in a real operating room. By practicing a procedure using a robotic surgery simulator, the surgeon gains familiarity with a variety of different robotic instruments and techniques prior to performing a real surgery.

The second type of simulation technology used in the Simulation-Based Training Program is known as the "Virtual Patient Simulator." Similar to a robotic surgery simulator, a virtual patient simulator is an interactive computer-based system. However, a virtual patient simulator does not include robotics and instead simulates the experience of performing a surgical procedure on a live patient. This includes simulating the sounds, sights and sensations experienced during a procedure. The virtual patient simulator enables the surgeon to practice various scenarios and test his/her decision-making skills in a controlled environment.

The Simulation-Based Training Program also contains components that assist surgeons in preparing for emergencies that may occur during a surgery. The program simulates emergency events such as fires, explosions and equipment failure. This allows the surgeon to develop the necessary skills and confidence to rapidly and effectively respond to emergencies that may occur during surgery.

Studies have demonstrated the Simulation-Based Training Program to be very successful. Studies have indicated that surgeons participating in the program are able to complete surgical procedures faster and with fewer complications than surgeons who did not participate in the program. Additionally, the program has increased the confidence of surgeons in their ability to perform complex surgical procedures.

One of the greatest advantages of this program is that it minimizes the risk of complications occurring during surgery. Complications arising from surgery may result in serious health consequences and potentially death. The Simulation-Based Training Program can assist in minimizing the occurrence of complications by providing surgeons with the opportunity to practice surgical procedures prior to performing them in a real operating room.

A further advantage of the program is that it increases patient safety. When surgeons are confident in their abilities to perform a procedure, there is less likelihood of error. Additionally, the program assists in enhancing communication between surgeons and other team members involved in the surgical process. Enhanced communication may also minimize the potential for errors occurring during a surgical procedure.

Overall, the Simulation-Based Training Program provides surgeons with a valuable resource for developing their skills and increasing their confidence in their ability to perform complex surgical procedures. It is particularly beneficial for surgeons who are transitioning into a new area of specialization or technique. The program is also beneficial for surgeons who are returning to work after a prolonged period of time away from surgery to develop their skills and confidence again.

In summary, the Simulation-Based Training Program is an excellent method for surgeons to develop their skills and increase their confidence in their ability to perform complex surgical procedures. It is a valuable resource for decreasing complications and increasing patient safety. Surgeons who take part in the program will be able to perform their duties more confidently and efficiently.

The only drawback to this program is the cost and time associated with it. A surgeon must be capable of accessing high end simulation tools and personnel and have the time to practice in the simulator. Some surgeons could find the program to be to stressful and/or to overwhelming to handle. Surgical procedures are already an extremely stressful event.

The added stress of knowing someone is watching and judging your every move, through the simulator, could be to much for some surgeons to handle. Overall however, this Simulation-Based Training Program is a wonderful resource for surgeons to increase their skill levels and build their confidence. This program can greatly improve patient outcomes and ultimately save lives.

Finally, Virtual Reality has grown so much since its beginning in the early 80's and is now more advanced than ever. Besides the medical industry, Virtual Reality is also being used in the education industry, the entertainment industry and the advertising industry. Education, Virtual Reality is creating new ways of teaching students. Using Virtual Labs and Classrooms, Virtual Lectures and Virtual Discussions with other students. Entertainment, Virtual Reality is changing how people watch movies and play video games.

Virtual Reality Headsets allow users to enter a completely virtual world and get immersed in the action. Advertising, Virtual Reality allows companies to create advertisements that people will remember. Creating a first hand look at products, services and experiences for customers. As stated earlier, Virtual Reality has the potential to greatly improve the quality of life of people across the globe. Virtual Reality has the ability to transform Medicine, Education, Entertainment and Advertising. However, there are several obstacles that must be conquered before Virtual Reality becomes a common form of entertainment. One of the largest problems facing the growth of Virtual Reality is the cost.

Currently, most Virtual Reality devices are very expensive and most consumers cannot afford them. Therefore, they are unable to benefit from the many advantages of Virtual Reality. Another problem facing Virtual Reality is the technology itself.

Even though Virtual Reality technology has improved dramatically in the last few years, it is still very rudimentary.

Most current Virtual Reality devices are cumbersome and tend to make the user dizzy and nauseous due to the lag in the graphics and the heavy weight of the headset. Despite the challenges, Virtual Reality is here to stay and will continue to evolve in the years to come. As the technology improves and the price of the devices decrease, we will begin to see more and more people use Virtual Reality as a form of entertainment.

Overall, Virtual Reality has the potential to significantly affect society and improve the quality of life of people worldwide. Virtual Reality is a revolutionary technology that has the potential to revolutionize Medicine, Education, Entertainment and Advertising. Therefore, I believe Virtual Reality will continue to grow and eventually be a huge part of our lives in the future.

10. HUMAN-AI COLLABORATION: HYBRID TEACHING MODELS

Rather than positioning AI as human teacher replacement, emerging models explore complementary human-AI collaboration leveraging respective strengths.

10.1. Complementary Strength Profiles

AI Strengths:

- Measurement consistency and objectivity on alignment metrics
- Persistent availability for training at any time
- Broad accessibility with a large population with no local instruction options available
- Timing-based quantitative tracking of individual progress
- Lack of subjective personal bias and judgment

Human Teacher Strengths:

- Sensitivity to subtle qualities that are invisible to the sensors
- The relational and energetic aspects of training
- Metaphysical and philosophical perspectives for training
- Creativity in response to emerging training needs
- Empathy and motivation in providing emotional support to students
- Transmission of cultural and historical practices

10.2. Hybrid Model Architectures

Tiered Learning: AI is used by beginners for a baseline for pose learning and to help them be consistent with their home practice, which will create a foundation for alignment and build confidence.

As they develop further they will have an opportunity to review their development with human instructors, and receive refinement on the subtleties of practice, philosophical understanding, and direction on how to advance; meanwhile, they will continue to use AI to maintain their home practice as they wait for their next session with a human instructor.

Augmented Human Teaching: Teachers use the analytical capabilities of AI to monitor student development through all of their home practice sessions, and identify patterns and difficulties that will inform in-class teaching.

While AI can provide objective data to support teacher's instinctive thinking; it cannot replace teacher's ability to guide students in energetic ways, provide spiritual context to practice, and establish relationships with students; this is what allows students to connect with their teachers, and ultimately receive wisdom from their teachers.

The use of AI for tracking of student development, frees up teacher time to focus on developing the whole student — both physically and spiritually.

Remote Teaching Enhancement: AI technology allows teachers to teach students who are geographically far away from the teacher, and allow teachers to give students daily feedback, while teachers offer occasional remote sessions for more in-depth guidance.

This type of remote teaching also increases access to quality instruction for those students living in under-served communities, while allowing students to maintain their relationship with their teacher, and ultimately receive wisdom from their teacher.

Specialized Applications: AI is being used in specialized clinical or therapeutic applications where consistent monitoring of a patient's condition is required (rehabilitation protocol, chronic disease management); while human teachers focus on developing the whole student — both physically and spiritually — as well as the creation of community.

The proposed hybrid human–AI instructional ecosystem is illustrated in Figure 4.

Figure 4. Hybrid human–AI instructional ecosystem for collaborative yoga learning and guidance.

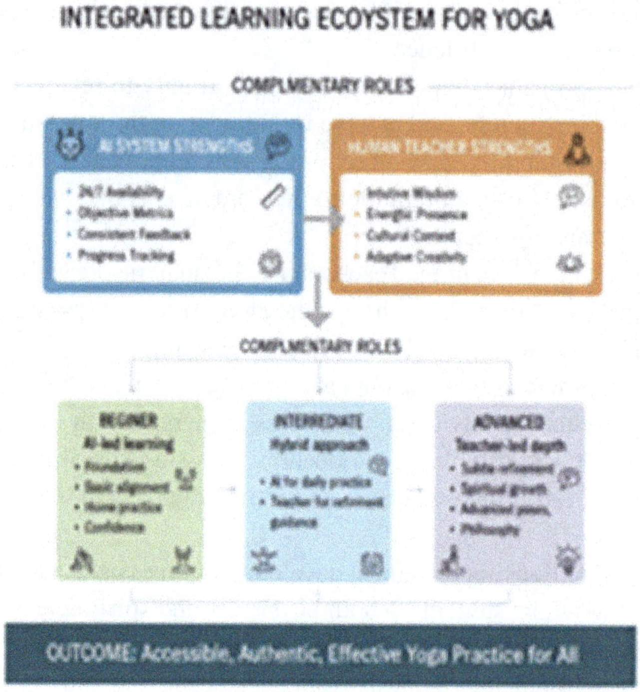

10.3. Design Principles for Hybrid Systems

The following are necessary for effective human-AI collaboration:

Clearly Defining Roles & Responsibilities: Clearly communicating the physical alignment assessments made by an AI and those aspects that remain within a human's role (the energetic qualities, spiritual guidance, relationship).

Empowering Teachers: Systems designed to support teachers rather than replace them; systems provide the tools that can assist with enhancing the effectiveness of a teacher's role as opposed to potentially threatening their employment.

Student Autonomy: Students retain choices and control over whether they want to utilize an AI-based assessment tool versus utilizing a human as a guide; students will choose to use the tools at times when it is beneficial to do so based upon their own needs and preferences.

Human Teacher-Driven Improvements: As human teachers gather insight from the use of the AI system, these insights will help improve the AI system; conversely, the AI will provide additional information to human teachers regarding the learning needs of each individual student.

Ethically/Grounded Developmentally: The AI system is developed under the auspices of ethical considerations and grounded principles of traditional yoga philosophy; this means the AI system will be developed to meet specific criteria other than optimizing the technology itself or meeting commercially driven objectives.

11. DATASET DEVELOPMENT AND STANDARDIZATION: A RESEARCH PRIORITY

Addressing the fundamental limitations of current AI yoga systems requires community-wide efforts to create comprehensive, diverse, standardized datasets.

11.1. Current Dataset Limitations

Suryawanshi et al. (2023) introduced a dedicated yoga dataset for computer vision analysis, yet even dedicated datasets remain limited. Typical characteristics include 20-50 poses, 10-20 subjects, 5,000-10,000 images, very limited body type diversity, predominantly advanced practitioners, and pose labels only without detailed annotations.

11.2. Ideal Dataset Characteristics

Comprehensive datasets should include:

Scale and Diversity

- 100+ poses representing various traditions and styles
- 500+ diverse subjects across ages, body types, abilities, ethnicities
- 100,000+ images/videos capturing varied conditions
- Multiple skill levels from absolute beginner to advanced
- Different yoga traditions (Iyengar, Ashtanga, Vinyasa, Restorative, etc.)

Rich Annotations

- Pose labels with standard Sanskrit and English names
- Skeletal keypoint annotations (33-point or richer)

- Joint angle measurements
- Correctness assessments with common error patterns
- Metadata (practitioner demographics, experience level, props used, camera specifications, lighting conditions)
- Expert commentary on subtle qualities beyond alignment

Environmental Diversity

- Studio, home, and outdoor settings
- Varied lighting conditions (natural, artificial, mixed)
- Complex backgrounds (cluttered, simple, variable)
- Multiple camera angles and distances
- Different recording equipment quality

Standardization

- Consistent keypoint definitions enabling cross-dataset compatibility
- Standardized pose taxonomy with clear inclusion/exclusion criteria
- Quality criteria defining correctness and acceptable variation ranges
- Metadata schemas enabling systematic querying and analysis
- Open access or reasonable licensing supporting research

11.3. Ethical Data Collection

Dataset development must address:

Informed Consent: Participants are entitled to know exactly how their images/videos will be used, by whom and where; participants must also give specific informed consent in order to allow the researcher to use their image/video(s) for the intended purpose(s).

Compensation: Practitioners who contribute images have a right to be fairly compensated for their contributions to commercially valuable systems.

Cultural Sensitivity: The recruitment process should include an emphasis on diversity and representation, so as not to continue to perpetuate homogeneous representation.

Privacy Protection: Faces should be either blurred or removed from images/videos unless absolutely necessary for research purposes, and identifying information should be minimized to protect privacy.

Licensing: Clearly defined, transparently stated licensing agreements that specify permitted uses, requirement for attribution, etc., and any restrictions.

12. FUTURE RESEARCH DIRECTIONS: A SYSTEMATIC ROADMAP

Based on identified gaps, we propose a systematic research agenda organized by timescale and priority.

12.1. Near-Term Priorities (1-2 Years)

Dataset Creation: A community effort that develops multiple diverse, large scale annotated yoga datasets; datasets will be created to reflect diverse demographics and varying environmental conditions.

User Study Research: Comprehensive comparative research is conducted to compare the relative effects of AI versus human instructional methods on learning, injury rates, user engagement and overall user satisfaction across a variety of population types.

Bias Evaluation: Systematically evaluating how well an AI Yoga System performs in comparison to other population types or demographics; transparency about limitations and development of methods to mitigate bias.

Development of Standardized Practices: Community standardization of common key point definition terms, pose taxonomy terminology, quality standards, metadata schema, and evaluation methodologies for AI Yoga Systems.

Development of Ethical Guidelines: Interdisciplinary collaboration to develop ethical guidelines and standards for the creation of AI Yoga Systems including but not limited to: cultural sensitivity, privacy issues, potential for bias, and proper use of AI Yoga Systems.

12.2. Medium-Term Goals (3-5 Years)

Multimodal Sensing: Developing real-world, multi-sensory systems that combine sensory inputs from multiple modalities including Vision, Depth, Force and Physiological Sensors, in order to provide a complete assessment.

Studies of Clinical Validity: Systematic, randomized, controlled studies examining the safety and efficacy of the system with various clinical populations (rehabilitation, chronic illness, mental health).

AI in Context: The integration of contextual information (goal of user, physical constraints, emotional state, historical practices) in systems in order to provide a completely personalized assessment and direction.

Detection of Subtle Errors: Techniques that capture micro-movements, patterns of muscle engagement, and qualitative characteristics of the movement that are not visible to current systems.

Hybrid Human-AI Teaching Models: Practical demonstrations of the implementation of hybrid models for teaching, the study of their effectiveness, and refinements made as a result of feedback from both teachers and students.

Systems Incorporating Cultural Content: Systems that include philosophical content, pranayama guidance, meditative content and ethically sound content in addition to physical content.

12.3. Long-Term Vision (5+ Years)

Holistic Wellness Platforms: Systems that combine a full range of wellness through the practice of yoga as well as health monitoring and providing personalized wellness recommendations, and integrating into the healthcare system.

The Development of Immersive Virtual Reality: Haptic feedback and tracking are both being improved, VR is becoming increasingly comfortable and can be used for extended periods of time; Social-emotional AI avatars will allow for the development of engaging virtual instructors.

Energetic and Experiential Dimensions: Research as to whether or how technology could potentially interact with our understanding of subtle energy (prana, chakra), in a manner that is culturally respectful and empirically supported.

Democratizing Access: Systems that are affordable and available to enable high quality instruction to be delivered to those who have historically been underserved throughout the world, while at the same time support rather than replace traditional teachers.

Tradition Preservation and Evolutionary Adaptation: Technology which enables the passing down of tradition knowledge from one generation to another, while enabling evolution and adaptation of the information to fit the context of the current day.

A consolidated roadmap of future research priorities is presented in Table 6.

Table 6. Future research roadmap across temporal horizons.

Dimension	AI Systems	Human Teachers	Research Priority	Status
Alignment Accuracy	Objective, quantifiable	Subjective, experienced-based	Comparative accuracy studies	Needed
Injury Prevention	Rule-based safety checks	Intuitive risk assessment	Injury rate comparisons	Critical
Learning Effectiveness	Standardized feedback	Adaptive, personalized	Skill development trajectories	Urgent
Engagement	Gamification, metrics	Relationship, community	Long-term adherence studies	Needed

continued on following page

Table 6. Continued

Dimension	AI Systems	Human Teachers	Research Priority	Status
Subtle Refinement	Limited to external alignment	Internal awareness, energetic	Progression to advanced poses	Needed
Cultural Transmission	Information delivery	Tradition, context, values	Cultural authenticity assessment	Critical
Cost/Accessibility	Low cost, high access	Variable cost, limited access	Cost-effectiveness analysis	Needed
Flexibility Accommodation	Standardized modifications	Individualized adaptations	Body type performance studies	Urgent

13. CONCLUSIONS: TOWARD INTEGRATIVE, ETHICAL AI YOGA SYSTEMS

This review has taken a holistic look at the current state of use of AI and ML in yoga; technical (from basic pose classification to advanced real-time feedback), cultural, ethical, and experiential. A great deal of technical advancement has occurred in terms of yoga applications for AI and ML. However, there is much work to do to address the cultural and philosophical bases of yoga, as well as its experiential nature.

13.1. Key Insights

Technical achievements have been made possible by new open-source frameworks that allow real-time, accurate pose estimation of humans using skeletal keypoints; this has allowed for an increased amount of mobile processing of these estimations. Techniques such as transfer learning, feature extraction based upon angles and temporal models have been able to improve the ability to classify and assess poses to 90-95% on controlled datasets.

Current limitations of current technologies include, they only measure the external physical alignment of the body and are unable to capture the internal experience of the practitioner, energetic dimensions of movement, breathing integration into the practice, muscle engagement during movement and the qualitative aspects of traditional yoga. Homogenized datasets limit the applicability of current systems to be generalized across a wide range of body types, age ranges, abilities and styles of yoga. The user experience of current systems is also not well researched which leaves fundamental questions about the learning effectiveness, safety and long term outcomes of current systems unanswered.

Most of the development of current systems has occurred in isolation from the deep philosophical roots of yoga, traditional methods of teaching yoga and the energetic framework of yoga (prana, nadis and chakras) resulting in a lack of engagement with the cultural and ethical implications of developing technology that utilizes and potentially appropriates the yoga tradition. There are many privacy concerns regarding collecting video and physiological data of users that need to be addressed through more stringent protocols.

The use of multimodal sensing devices and physiological sensors, personalized algorithms, and immersive virtual reality (VR) environments all provide promise to provide a more complete picture of the practitioner's overall wellness. Models of collaborative work between humans and AI provide potential pathways to leverage the unique strengths of each entity. In addition, clinical applications of technology that utilizes pose estimation may prove beneficial in rehabilitation and chronic disease management but will likely require careful validation.

13.2. Recommendations for Responsible Development

Address the technical base of yoga using a cultural lens: Any system developed should incorporate individuals knowledgeable of both the philosophy and traditional teaching practices of yoga; i.e., practitioners-not just computer scientists. In addition, any system that utilizes yoga should be cognizant of the Indian roots of yoga; the system should utilize a philosophical base; and the system should provide technology as a means to enhance the traditional transmission of yoga-not as a replacement for it.

Create data sets that are representative of diversity: Community wide initiatives to create data sets that are representative of a wide variety of body types, ages, abilities, ethnicities, skills, environmental settings, and Yoga styles is required. Developing standards for annotation, taxonomy, and evaluation methods will allow for systematic progress and reproducible research.

Put the user experience and safety at the center: Comparative studies must evaluate the learning efficacy, injury prevention, engagement, and outcomes for different populations, using both AI and human instructors. The safety of the users must always be considered above the performance of the system.

Develop an ethical framework for the development of systems: Collaborative work by interdisciplinary teams should develop comprehensive frameworks for the ethics of developing systems including issues such as privacy, cultural appropriation, informed consent, limits of the system, and transparency.

Promote the integration of humans and machines: Instead of replacing teachers with machines, develop hybrid models that leverage the benefits of AI for consistent measurement and access, while allowing the human teachers to continue to fulfill their role as the source of intuitive, relational, and spiritual guidance for students.

Include holistic dimensions: Expand the focus of systems from just providing corrective feedback on poses, to providing systems that can also support breath awareness, meditation, philosophical education, and the incorporation of ethical principles into Yoga. When exploring energetic concepts (e.g., prana, chakras), be culturally sensitive and recognize that these are subjective and experiential concepts.

Empower and support the continued success of traditional teachers: Design systems that empower, instead of replace teachers; extend their reach, enhance their effectiveness, and provide a means to earn a living, rather than threaten their livelihoods.

13.3. Final Reflections

Both tremendous opportunity and enormous risk are associated with the integration of AI with yoga. With the help of technology it may become possible to make yoga accessible to a larger number of people as it provides an objective means for providing feedback, allows for personalized coaching, and supports the development of clinical applications – all of which could result in millions of individuals having access to yoga's benefits that currently do not have access to qualified instruction. At the same time technology has the potential to reduce a profoundly spiritual practice into a commodity, continue to appropriate from other cultures, reduce a comprehensive, holistic practice into simply physical movement and diminish the importance of human interaction and the transfer of traditional wisdom.

To move forward in this area will require more than just technological advancements; it will also require cultural humility, an ethic of commitment, and the acknowledgment that yoga involves much more than what any algorithm can quantify. Even the most advanced AI systems cannot replicate the transformative nature of long-term practice under the direction of a knowledgeable teacher; the AI systems cannot convey the subtle energetic and spiritual aspects of the experience that many practitioners report; and AI systems cannot assist in developing the awareness of self and ability to observe one's inner experience that are fundamental to the ultimate goals of yoga.

Technological developments in AI must ultimately serve yoga and not the other way around. When AI systems are developed with an appreciation for the culture from which yoga originates, a sense of responsibility, the highest level of technical expertise, and a clear understanding of its capabilities and limitations, then these systems can become valuable tools for both practitioners and instructors. Conversely, when AI systems are developed without consideration for the culture from which yoga originated (i.e., with a focus on achieving a high level of technical achievement or generating profit), then there is the possibility of creating actual harm to this ancient and sacred tradition.

The blending of technology (AI) into the practice of yoga allows us to incorporate ancient principles with modern innovations, to honor where we have come from while contributing to the wellness of those who will follow us; as we continue along this journey, may we also celebrate the tradition of yoga by expressing it in new and innovative ways; may we quantify when we can but appreciate when we cannot; and ultimately may we remember that true success in yoga lies in integrating all aspects of ourselves and in liberating the total human being to flourish.

REFERENCES

Battur, R.; Kunchur, P.; Bangarashetti, S.; Managuli, M.; Kulkarni, G.L. (2023). Artificial Intelligence and Machine Learning Techniques for Analysis of Yoga Pose. *Lecture Notes in Electrical Engineering*, 1007 LNEE, 457–466.

Chauhan, S., Chetwani, P. S., & Mahajan, S. (2024). Yoga Pose Recognition through Fine-Tuned ResNet50V2 Model with Projection Head. In: *IC3TES* (Conference paper). DOI: 10.1109/IC3TES62412.2024.10877545

Dhanyal, S. S., & Nandyal, S. S. (2023). Yoga pose annotation and classification by using time-distributed convolutional neural network. *Indonesian Journal of Electrical Engineering and Computer Science*, *32*(3), 1639–1647. DOI: 10.11591/ijeecs.v32.i3.pp1639-1647

Duggal, A., Kumar, S., & Tripathi, P. (2025). Exploring AI Techniques for Yoga Image Classification: A Focus on Machine Learning and Deep Learning. In: *ICISCN* (Conference paper). DOI: 10.1109/ICISCN64258.2025.10934197

Gadhvi, R., & Desai, P. Siddharth (2026). PosePilot: An Edge-AI Solution for Posture Correction in Physical Exercises. *Lecture Notes in Computer Science*, 15938 LNCS, 208–219.

Ganesh, K., & Ramudhin, A. (2024). Leveraging AI to Mitigate Risks in Yoga Practice: A Real-Time Posture Correction Application. *International Conference on Sport Sciences Research and Technology Support, icSPORTS - Proceedings*, 241–250. DOI: 10.5220/0013063300003828

Kim, H., Zala, A., Burri, G., & Bansal, M. (2021).. . *FIXMYPOSE: Pose Correctional Captioning and Retrieval. AAAI, 14B*, 13161–13170.

Madhu, S., Kumar, P., & Chandra, S. (2025). Ensemble Learning based EEG Classification – Investigating the Effects of Combined Yoga and Rajyog Meditation. *Journal of Scientific and Industrial Research*, *84*(1), 36–47.

Meghana, J. H., Chethan, H. K., Santhosh Kumar, K. S., & Shiva Prakash, S. P. S. (2025). Comprehensive Analysis of Pose Estimation and Machine Learning Classifiers for Precise Yoga Pose Detection and Classification. *Procedia Computer Science*, *258*, 3345–3356. DOI: 10.1016/j.procs.2025.04.592

Parab, N. P., Rampurawala, A. A., Khade, S. S., & Mahato, M. (2023). Personalised AI Based Yoga-Pose Recommendation System Using Game Theory. In: *ICACTA* (Conference paper). DOI: 10.1109/ICACTA58201.2023.10393658

. Patanjali (circa 400 CE). *Yoga Sutras of Patanjali*. (Classical text - multiple modern translations available, e.g., Bryant, E.F. (2009). *The Yoga Sutras of Patañjali: A New Edition, Translation, and Commentary*. New York: North Point Press.)

Rajendran, A. K., & Sethuraman, S. C. (2025). YogAngleNet: Body angle-based yogic posture classification approach using MediaPipe from single-person images. *Turkish Journal of Electrical Engineering and Computer Sciences*, *33*(5), 613–630. DOI: 10.55730/1300-0632.4147

Rajput, G. S., Khan, M. A., Jain, T., Khandelwal, T., & Sharma, U. (2024). Exploring Chakra Balancing Practices in Software Applications. In: *ACROSET* (Conference paper). DOI: 10.1109/ACROSET62108.2024.10743620

Saxena, P., Sharma, V., Yadav, A., Singh, R. P., & Laiphrakpam, L. D. (2025). An Algorithmic and Machine Learning Approach for Yoga Asanas Feedback. In: *ISACC* (Conference paper), 7–12. DOI: 10.1109/ISACC65211.2025.10969307

Sharma, H. K., Choudhury, T., Mahapatra, S., Satish Kumar, G. A. E. S., & Maganti, S. B. (2024). Deep Learning based approach for Prediction of Yoga Posture using Yoga Asana Images. *AIP Conference Proceedings*, *2942*(1), 20006. DOI: 10.1063/5.0197215

Suryawanshi, Y., Gunjal, N., Kanorewala, B., & Patil, K. (2023). Yoga dataset: A resource for computer vision-based analysis of Yoga asanas. *Data in Brief*, *48*, 109257. DOI: 10.1016/j.dib.2023.109257 PMID: 37383745

Talaat, A. S. (2023). Novel deep learning models for yoga pose estimator. *SN Applied Sciences*, *5*(12), 341. DOI: 10.1007/s42452-023-05581-8

. Thushara, L.; Abdul Jabbar, P. (2026). Beyond the General Pose: An Optimized Yoga Posture Similarity Assessment Method With PCA-Driven Feature Selection. *Communications in Computer and Information Science*, 2475 CCIS, 323–337.

Tripathi, A., Tyagi, A., Dubey, A., Vijh, S., & Verma, P. (2025). Enhancing Virtual Yoga Training: Real-time Pose Assessment with Voice-guided Accuracy Feedback. In: *ICETM* (Conference paper).

Wang, H. (2021). Neural Network-Oriented Big Data Model for Yoga Movement Recognition. *Computational Intelligence and Neuroscience*, *2021*(1), 4334024. DOI: 10.1155/2021/4334024 PMID: 34751226

Wang, L., Guo, X., Zhang, Z., & Lee, C. (2025). Metaverse-Enabled Yoga Coach Avatar Using AI-Enhanced Multimodal Insole Sensing System. *Advanced Functional Materials*.

Yenishettil, S., Karajkhede, G., & Panat, L. (2024). Virtual Yoga Teacher with AI Model for Yoga Posture Correction for Good Health. In: *ITUK* (Conference paper). Indian Knowledge Systems (IKS) and Philosophical Foundations DOI: 10.23919/ITUK62727.2024.10772930

Chapter 9

Complementary Management of PCOD (Polycystic Ovarian Disorder) Among Women Through an Integrative Approach of Yoga and Artificial Intelligence (AI)

Ayushi Singh
http://orcid.org/0009-0002-0411-0605
Banasthali Vidyapith, India

Sakshi Chaturvedi
http://orcid.org/0000-0002-4979-3430
Banasthali Vidyapith, India

Murlidhar Mishra
Banasthali Vidyapith, India

ABSTRACT

Polycystic ovarian disorder (PCOD) is a complex and prevalent endocrine disorder affecting women of reproductive age. It is characterized by hormonal imbalance, irregular menstruation, hyperandrogenic symptoms, and polycystic ovarian morphology. Sedentary lifestyle, unhealthy dietary habits, stress, and obesity are the primary factors that contributes to PCOD among women's. In recent years, Yoga

DOI: 10.4018/979-8-3373-7625-7.ch009

therapy has emerged as a promising integrative modality in the management of PCOD. Yoga therapy targets the root cause of PCOD and it is a safe, cost-effective, with minimal side effect. It is a holistic approach that improves quality of life. By Combining Artificial intelligence with Yoga is helpful in real-time monitoring, personalized sessions, facilitates self-paced learnings, facilitates instant support for clearing doubts in a healthcare. This chapter explores the efficacy of yoga as a complementary therapeutic approach in women for Polycystic Ovarian Disorder (PCOD) management

INTRODUCTION

Polycystic ovarian disorder (PCOD) is hyper androgenism (male hormones) with chronic anovulation in women without specific underlying adrenal or pituitary gland disease. PCOD is a hormonal and lifestyle disorder that affects women's of reproductive age (Chithra et al., 2024). In this disorder Insulin, Follicular stimulating hormone, Testosterone, Luteinizing hormone and Adrenal hormones are affected (Chithra et al., 2024). The primary symptoms of PCOD are hyperandrogenism, infertility, irregular menstruation and additional symptoms includes hirsutism, acne, pelvic pain, diabetes, obesity etc. (Chithra et al., 2024).

Following are the signs and symptoms of Polycystic Ovarian Disorder:

1. **Hyperandrogenism**: Hyperandrogenism is a medical condition characterized by an excess of androgen hormones (like testosterone) in the body, most commonly affecting women.
2. **Infertility**: Infertility is a disease of the reproductive system where a person or couple cannot achieve pregnancy after one year of regular, unprotected intercourse
3. **Irregular menstruation**: The most common irregular menstruation includes following-
    - Amenorrhea – Amenorrhea is a condition of absent menstrual periods.
    - Oligomenorrhea – Oligomenorrhea is a condition of infrequent menstrual periods.
    - Menorrhagia – Menorrhagia is condition of excessive bleeding.
    - Prolonged menstrual bleeding - Prolonged menstrual bleeding is condition when bleeding exceeds 8 days.
    - Dysmenorrhea – Dysmenorrhea is condition of severe menstrual cramps and painful periods.
4. **Hirsutism**: Hirsutism is the excessive growth of dark, coarse hair on the face, chest, back, or other areas in a male-like pattern, most often in women. It is a

symptom of an underlying issue, frequently caused by an excess of male hormones (androgens).

5. **Alopecia (hair loss)**: Alopecia is a general term for hair loss that can be temporary or permanent and affect any part of the body
6. **Obstructive sleep apnea**: Obstructive sleep apnea (OSA) is a common sleep disorder where breathing repeatedly stops and starts due to the upper airway becoming partially or completely blocked during sleep

This disorder adversely impacts women's fertility and reproductive health due to its nature (Chahar et al., 2023). According to international surveys, between 4 and 10% of women who are of reproductive age struggle with PCOD (Chahar et al., 2023). About 5–10% of people around the world and 20% of Indian women are affected by a disease (Dilip & Prashant, 2023)(Uma, 2024). It has an adverse impact on mental health, including depression, anxiety, and low self-esteem . The possibility of PCOD in urban women is higher as compared to rural women (Chahar et al., 2023). Polycystic Ovarian Disease (PCOD) is an emerging lifestyle-related disorder among women that contributes to infertility and increases the risk of developing cardiovascular diseases, type 2 diabetes, and endometrial cancer.

Pharmacological treatments provide symptomatic relief; however, they are often associated with side effects and a higher risk of recurrence once the medication is discontinued. Therefore, it is essential to explore the effectiveness of non-pharmacological interventions including yoga, naturopathy, ayurveda to manage such disorders, as these approaches have minimal side effects and a lower likelihood of recurrence.

Yoga has been practiced for thousands of years as a holistic discipline promoting physical, mental, and spiritual well-being. In recent years, it has emerged as an effective complementary and alternative therapy in managing various women's health concerns, including menopause, Polycystic Ovarian Disease (PCOD), Polycystic Ovarian Syndrome (PCOS), leucorrhoea or abnormal vaginal discharge, breast cancer, cardiovascular diseases, osteoporosis, and cervical cancer.

There are limited scientific evidence demonstrating the effectiveness of yoga as a complementary and alternative therapy for the management Polycystic Ovarian Disease (PCOD) among women. The primary aim of this chapter is to explore the effectiveness of yoga as a complementary and alternative therapy in the management of Polycystic Ovarian Disease (PCOD). Because of rapid technological development and continuous innovation, the integration of Artificial Intelligence (AI) into yoga therapy represents a promising approach in applying traditional practices within modern healthcare systems. The incorporation of AI in yoga therapy substantially enhances accessibility, efficiency, and personalisation while also advancing holistic health management (Sinha & Sinha, 2024).

PCOD vs PCOS:

Table 1. PCOD and PCOS appears to be similar but there are minor differences that exists between PCOD and PCOS. PCOD is a Disorder whereas PCOS is a Syndrome.

PCOD	PCOS
PCOD refers to Polycystic Ovarian Disorder.	PCOS refers to Polycystic Ovarian Syndrome.
PCOD is a disorder in which ovaries produces immature eggs, which transforms into cysts.	PCOS is a syndrome and a severe condition, in which ovaries produces high level of male hormones which results in formation of large number of cysts.
Usually, PCOD has less severe health complications.	PCOS leads to severe irreversible health complications including Type-2 diabetes, High blood pressure, Cardiovascular issues, and endometrial cancer etc.
PCOD is a lifestyle disorder hence it can be reversed naturally with a balanced diet, and complementary therapy.	PCOS is hard to reverse but lifestyle changes and medicines are helpful in controlling symptoms.
PCOD affects fertility but with medication it is possible to conceive.	PCOS affects fertility in females, it is hard to conceive and there is high risk of miscarriage, premature child birth.
In PCOD severity is mild to moderate.	In PCOS severity is high and complex.
In PCOD hormonal imbalance is mild.	In PCOS hormonal imbalance is highly notable.
In PCOD male hormones are slightly elevated	In PCOS male hormones are markedly elevated.

EVIDENCE BASED LITERATURE REVIEW

After thorough comprehensive and detailed literature review indicates that a considerable number of studies have examined the effectiveness of yoga on Polycystic Ovary Syndrome (PCOS) (Nidhi, Padmalatha, Nagarathna, & Ram, 2012) (Nidhi, Padmalatha, Nagarathna, & Amritanshu, 2012) (Mohseni et al., 2021) (Selvaraj et al., 2020), whereas limited studies have specifically focused on its effectiveness in Polycystic Ovarian Disorder (PCOD).

Devi & Rani, 2022 has conducted a study on "Exploring on the Comparative merit of Allopathy Medicine and Yoga Therapy for PCOD Condition". The result of the study demonstrated the effectiveness of both yoga intervention and allopathy treatment in PCOD management. There was significant improvement in psychological and hormonal factors. There is risk of side effects and repetition of PCOD when medication is stopped in allopathic treatment, whereas Yoga intervention is helpful in reducing hormonal imbalance, and anxiety level without any side effects (Devi & Rani, 2022). Mathur, 2023 has conducted a case study on "Managing Polycystic

Ovarian Disorder through Yoga". The findings of the study indicates that yoga is helpful in managing PCOD and it symptoms. Yoga is a holistic approach that improves psychological, physiological, emotional health and wellbeing of women (Mathur, 2023).

Challenges in Conventional treatment: Several pharmacological treatments are available such as hormonal therapy and insulin therapy, but it provides short term relief, they may have side-effects too. These treatments do management of symptoms but don't address the root cause of the disorder. Conventional treatments are standardized treatment which lacks personalization and patients' satisfaction. There may be many side effects of these treatments including mood swings, weight gain, nausea, and issues related to metabolism. Pharmacological treatments often show inadequate focus on psychological well-being including stress, anxiety, depression, and emotional instability. There are some long-term complications too such as type-2 diabetes, infertility, cardiovascular disease, and also reduces quality of life of PCOD women. These limitation of the convention treatment highlights the importance and need of complementary treatment.

Women's health condition

The World Health Organization (WHO) defines women's health as "a state of complete physical, mental, and social well-being, and not merely the absence of disease or infirmity, in all matters relating to the female reproductive system." Women plays an essential role in the progress and stability of society, they are serving as the strongest pillar in the development of society and nation. They plays a crucial role in strengthening and empowering the nation. Therefore, it is extremely essential to give utmost priority to women's health, including physical, mental, emotional, intellectual, and social well-being. There are several factors as mentioned in (Figure 1), that affect women's health, including biological, psychological, lifestyle, environmental, and socio-economic factors. These factors negatively affects all the aspects of health and well-being of women's. Hence, it is necessary to focus on their health and wellness.

Figure 1. Factors affecting women's health

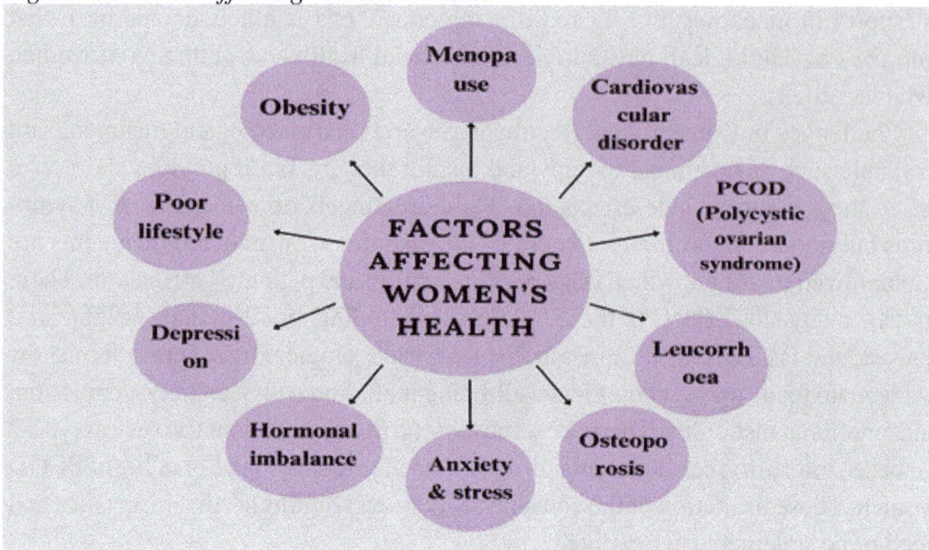

Life stages of women: The life stage of women are given below and are mentioned in (Figure 2)

A. Childhood
B. Adolescence
C. Reproductive years
D. Pregnancy and Postpartum stage
E. Perimenopausal stage
F. Menopausal stage
G. Postmenopausal or Elderly stage

Childhood: Childhood age is from birth to 10-12 years. It is an age of rapid physical growth, development of emotions and skills motor including motor, cognitive, and social.

Adolescence: Adolescence age is from 10-19 years. This age is transition between the childhood and adulthood. During this age there are development of emotional sensitivity, changes in hormones, beginning of puberty and secondary sexual characteristics.

Reproductive years: Reproductive age is from approximately 20-40/45 years. This age is an epitome of fertility, stability in hormones, regularity in menstrual cycle and phase of huge responsibilities.

Pregnancy and Postpartum stage: Pregnancy and Postpartum age is from pregnancy and up to one year after child birth. During this age there are huge physiological and psychological changes, weight gain, high risk of anxiety and postpartum depression.

Perimenopausal stage: Perimenopausal stage is usually between 40-50 years. During this stage there is gradual decrease in ovarian functioning, hormonal fluctuation, irregularities in menstrual cycle, mood swings, sleeping problem.

Menopausal stage: Menopausal stage occurs between the age of 45-55 years. During this phase there is permanent cessation of menstruation, sudden decline in level of oestrogen, increase in risk of osteoporosis, metabolic, and cardiovascular health issues.

Postmenopausal or Elderly stage: Postmenopausal or Elderly stage occurs at the age of 55 years and above. During this phase there is low level of oestrogen, high risk of depression, feeling of loneliness, loss of muscle density and muscle mass, changes in metabolism.

Figure 2. Flow chart of stages of women

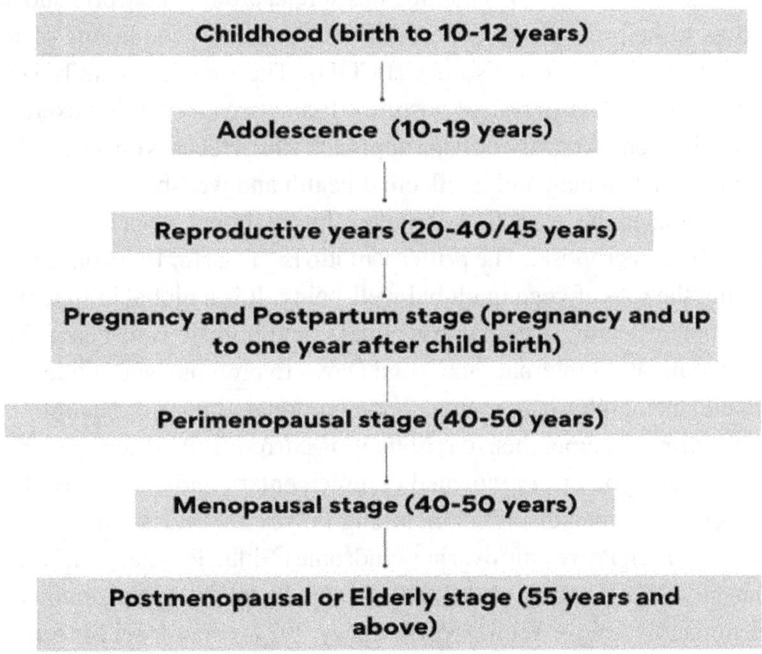

ROLE OF YOGA AS A COMPLEMENTARY THERAPY IN PCOD

Yoga is derived from the Sanskrit root 'yuj', which means 'to join or unite', mind; body; and soul. According to World Health Organization (WHO, 2019) "Yoga is a group of physical, mental, and spiritual practices or disciplines which aim to improve health and well-being." According to Maharishi Patanjali 'Yoga' is defined as "yogah citta vrtti nirodhah" which means "the cessation of the fluctuations of the mind". It is a combination of eight limbs Yama; Niyama; Asana; Pranayama; Pratyahara; Dharana; Dhayana; Samadhi.

According to Swami Satyananda Saraswati "Yoga is not an ancient myth buried in oblivion. It is the most valuable inheritance of the present. It is the essential need of today and the culture of tomorrow." There are many branches of yoga including Raja yoga; Hatha yoga; Jnana yoga, Karma yoga; Bhakti yoga; Mantra yoga; Kundalini yoga and Laya yoga. In twentieth century hath yoga is most famous and is widely practiced worldwide. Hath yoga commonly includes asana; pranayama; mudra; and bandh.

Since the last few years, Yoga therapy has spread around the world and has been studied so as to help people to cope with various health conditions of women's including Polycystic Ovarian disorder (PCOD). The most commonly performed yoga practices are Asana (physical posture); Pranayama (breathing exercise); and Dhayana (meditation). Yoga is a holistic approach which focuses on physical, mental, spiritual, emotional, social; and intellectual health and well-being.

United Nations in the year 2014, initiated 'International Yoga Day' on 21st June by following India's proposal. The primary motto is "Yoga for Harmony and Peace," for promoting the role of yoga in global well-being. It is a global initiate by United Nations for better health, sustainable wellness, and holistic well-being. The main aim of commemorating International Yoga Day is to promote worldwide awareness of yoga in enhancing physical, mental, and emotional aspects of health.

After a thorough comprehensive review of current scientific literature, it has been observed that yoga is a renowned complementary and alternative therapy in managing several women disorders including Polycystic ovarian disorder (PCOD) (Devi & Rani, 2022); Polycystic ovarian syndrome (Nidhi, Padmalatha, Nagarathna, & Amritanshu, 2012) (Selvaraj et al., 2020) (Nidhi, Padmalatha, Nagarathna, & Ram, 2012); Menopause (Abiç & Yilmaz Vefikuluçay, 2024) (Elavsky & McAuley, 2007) (Jorge et al., 2016); leucorrhoea (Mittal et al., 2025), breast cancer (Chakrabarty et al., 2015). Yoga has been shown to enhance quality of life by reducing stress, alleviating symptoms of depression, and promoting overall psychological well-being.

Role of Asana in PCOD: Asana plays an important role in the management of PCOD physiological and psychological symptoms and improves quality of life. Regular Yogasana practice enhances blood circulation in pelvic region, helpful in weight management, reduces visceral fat, regulates hypothalamic–pituitary–ovarian function, strengthens pelvic muscles and abdominal muscles. It improves the functioning of ovaries, reproductive system, and endocrine system. Asana reduces somatic stress and provides deep physical relaxation. Asana has been classifying into 3 categories namely meditative asana, cultural asana, and relaxative asana, that promotes mental stability, physical functioning, and stress reduction respectively.

- Meditative asana: Meditative asana are comfortable and stable sitting postures especially performed for prolonged pranayama and dhyana. It promotes steadiness, calms nervous system and improves concentration. Such asanas include Padmasana, Siddhasana, Sukhasana, Swastikasana, Simhasana.
- Cultural asana: Cultural asana are dynamic physical postures, it improves flexibility, strength, balance and coordination in the body. It enhances muscular health, metabolism and blood circulation. Such asanas include Bhujangasana, Trikonasana, Dhanurasana, Pawanmuktasana
- Relaxative asana: Relaxative asana are performed for physical and mental relaxation. It reduces fatigue and stress, balances parasympathetic system, provides mental calmness and restore energy. Such asanas include Shavasana, Makrasana, Balasana.

Role of Pranayama in PCOD: Pranayama plays a significant role in the regulation of autonomic nervous system, reduction of stress and anxiety among women diagnosed with PCOD. It is helpful in kundalini activation, lowering cortisol level in the body, balances sympathetic and parasympathetic system activities, increases oxygenation in the body, improves metabolic system functioning, enhance insulin resistance, better sleep cycle, promotes psychological calmness and emotional stability, balances endocrine system, support harmony, and regulates hormones. Therefore, regular practice of pranayama improves overall psychological and physiological well-being in women with PCOD. According to Hatha Yoga Pradipika Pranayama is classified into eights types namely Suryabhedi pranayama, Ujjayi pranayama, Shitali pranayama, Seetkari pranayama, Bhramari pranayama, Bhastrika pranayama, Murcha pranayama, and Plavini pranayama. Pranayama is an alternative and complementary medicine in the holistic management of PCOD.

- Suryabhedi pranayama: Suryabhedi pranayama involves inhalation from right nostril and exhalation from left nostril. It is helpful in activating Agni (digestive fire), stimulates metabolic and endocrine system, weight management, activates sympathetic nervous system, improves blood circulation, and balances hormones.

- Ujjayi pranayama: Ujjayi pranayama involves slow, deep breathing with gentle pressure on throat, producing soft sound. This pranayama promotes calmness, increases oxygenation, regulates stress level, balances autonomic system functioning, improves concentration and emotional instability, enhances hypothalamic–pituitary–ovarian functioning.
- Shitali pranayama: Shitali pranayama involve inhalation with rolled tongue and exhalation through both nostrils. It provides cooling effect to both mind and body, regulates inflammation, excessive heat, and irritability, balances hormones, reduces anxiety and stress, improves sleep quality, lowers body temperature and blood pressure.
- Seetkari pranayama: Seetkari pranayama involves inhalation with clenched teeth and exhalation with both nostrils. It provides cooling and calming effect to mind and body, helps in reducing stress, anxiety, mood disturbance and emotional fluctuation, provides relaxation, and stabilizes hormones.
- Bhramari pranayama: Bhramari pranayama involves inhalation with a followed exhalation with a humming sound. It helps in calming nervous system, reduces stress and anxiety, supports parasympathetics nervous system, regulates hormones, and emotional well-being.
- Bhastrika pranayama: Bhastrika pranayama involves rapid and forceful inhalation and exhalation. Regular practice improves lungs capacity and insulin sensitivity, alleviates metabolism and detoxification, and energizes the body.
- Murcha pranayama: Murcha pranayama involves prolonged inhalation with retention. It promotes deep relaxation, provides mental calmness, reduces psychological stress, fatigue, and emotional instability, balances neuroendocrine system and helps in withdrawal of the senses.
- Plavini pranayama: Plavini pranayama involves deep inhalation that creates a feeling of lightness in the body. It promotes digestive system functioning, and balances mind-body. It is traditionally associated with floating and should be practiced under expert supervision.

Role of Dhayana in PCOD: Dhayan plays a crucial role in maintaining psychological and neurological health in women with PCOD. It improves mental self-awareness, emotional regulation, reduces stress and anxiety, calms internal mental fluctuations, regulates menstrual cycle and alleviates sleep pattern. Regular dhyana practice promotes hypothalamic–pituitary–adrenal system functioning and activates brain waves. There are five types of brain waves Beta waves, Alpha waves, Theta waves, Delta waves, and Gamma waves.

- Beta waves (13-30 Hz): Dhayana gradually reduces excessive beta waves, calms mind and brain activity, and reduces stress and anxiety.

- Alpha waves (8-13 Hz): Dhayana enhances theta waves, which helps in improving calmness, stabilizing mood, and provides mental relaxation. Regular practice of Deep yogic breathing, Ujjayi pranayama and Nadi shodhan pranayama can activate alpha waves.
- Theta waves (4-8 Hz): Dhayana increases theta waves, helps in stress reduction, and emotional stability. It is a state of deep meditation and awareness. Yoga Nidra and Bhramari pranayama, are helpful in the activation of theta waves.
- Delta waves (0.5-4 Hz): Delta wave is a state of deep sound and dreamless sleep. It promotes physical relaxation and healing. Yoga Nidra and Shavasana provides deep relaxation and activate delta waves
- Gamma waves (30-100 Hz): Regular dhyana practice increases gamma waves, it help in regulating emotions, promotes awareness, and provides mental clarity.

The combination of asana (physical posture), pranayama (breathing technique), and dhayana (meditation) addresses physiological health, psychological health, and metabolic dimensions for holistic and sustainable treatment.

History of yoga:

Yoga has its existence in India and world for more than ten thousand years ago. During archaeological excavations several statues resembling lord shiva and mata Parvati were found from Indus Valley at Harappa and Mohenjo-Daro performing asanas and meditation. According to mythology, and it is also mentioned in the Yoga Granth namely "Yoga Beej" in which Shiva is considered as the founder of yoga and Parvati, was his first disciple. Lately yoga was slowly promoted by various sages and yogis across the world. In ancient time yoga sadhana were kept secret and were never written or never exposed to public. It was passed from guru or teacher to disciple verbally. There is mention of yoga in Vedas, Upanishads, hathyoga Granth. The history of Yoga is categories into 6 parts on the basis of historical periods:

1. Pre-Vedic Period (Before 3000 BCE)
2. Vedic Period (1500-500 BCE)
3. Upanishadic Period (800-200 BCE)
4. Classical Period (200 BCE-500 CE)
5. Post-Classical Period (500–1700 CE)
6. Modern Period (19th Century–Present)

Pre-Vedic Period (Before 3000 BCE): During Indus Valley Civilization traces of yoga were found. Seals of meditative postures were excavated during Pre-Vedic Period. The yoga was performed for spiritual awareness.

Vedic Period (1500-500 BCE): There is mention of yoga in Vedas especially in 'Rigveda'. During Vedic period the primary focus of yoga was on rituals, discipline, and meditation. Yoga was defined as spiritual knowledge and self-control.

Upanishadic Period (800-200 BCE): During Upanishadic Period concept of atman (self) and Brahman (universal unity) were introduced. Yoga was more philosophical and introspective. In Upanishads yoga was defined as path of meditation, breathing technique, and self-realization.

Classical Period (200 BCE-500 CE): During Classical Period Maharishi Patanjali assembled eight components of yoga known as 'Ashtanga Yoga' under four chapters known as 'Paad' in his book namely 'Patanajal Yoga Sutra'. Ashtanga Yoga (eight-fold path) were introduced including Yama, Niyama, Asana, Pranayama, Pratyahara, Dharana, Dhyana, Samadhi. The Paads are Samadhi Paad, Sadhana Paad, Vibhuti Paad, and Kaivalya Paad. Yoga was defined as 'control of mental fluctuations.

Post-Classical Period (500–1700 CE): During Post-Classical Period focus was shifted to Hatha Yoga. Text like Hatha Yoga Pradipika by Swami Swatmaram, Ghera a Samhita by Maharishi Ghera a, Gorakhsh Samhita by Guru Gorakhnath, and Yoga Beej were introduced. Hatha Yoga primarily focuses on physical postures (asanas), purification (Shatkarma), and energy control. The main objective of yoga was to achieve spiritual growth.

Modern Period (19th Century–Present): During modern Period the primary objective of practicing yoga is physiological health, psychological well-being, and management of diseases such as PCOD (polycystic ovarian disorder), menopause, hypertension, diabetes, cancer. Several yoga gurus spread importance of yoga globally including Swami Vivekananda, Sri Aurobindo, Swami Sivananda, B.K.S. Iyengar, T. Krishnamacharya, Pattabhi Jois, Swami Satyananda Saraswati.

Relevance of yoga in present time:

The present scenario is an era of modernization, technological advancement and stress dominant lifestyle, which result in physical inactivity, mental stress, emotional imbalance, unhealthy diet, and psychosocial issues. Yoga is emerged as an effective alternative and complementary therapy in stimulating physical, mental, emotional, social health, and overall-wellbeing. It is cost-effective and holistic approach that promote mind and body harmony. Regular yoga practice increases flexibility, regulates hormones, reduces stress, improves reproductive health, boost immunity, alleviates emotional imbalance, and enhances immunity. In present time yoga is helpful in addressing following challenges which are mentioned below:

- Physical Health
- Mental Health
- Stress Management
- Lifestyle disorder

- Preventive and complementary therapy
- Social and Emotional well-being
- Global Acceptance

Physical Health: Yoga maintains physiological health by improving flexibility, postures, balance, and strength. It helps in prevention and management of lifestyle disorders including obesity, PCOD (polycystic ovarian disorder), hypertension, diabetes.

Mental Health: Yoga is helpful in reducing anxiety, stress, and depression, by providing calmness and improving emotional stability. Pranayama and meditation improve clarity, memory and concentration.

Stress Management: Regular yoga practice activates nervous system functioning reduces level of cortisol, and provides relaxation. It is helpful in maintaining work stress, academic pressure and any emotional instability.

Lifestyle disorder: Yoga manages lifestyle disorders generates due to stress, diet, sleep disturbance and physical inactivity. It is helpful in the management of hormonal imbalance, and metabolic dysfunction cause because of unhealthy lifestyle.

Preventive and complementary therapy: Yoga is an effective alternative, preventive, and complementary therapy along with pharmacological medicines. It improves healing capacity of body and boost immunity.

Social and Emotional well-being: Yoga promotes social harmony and emotional well-being by enhancing self-discipline, inner peace, ethical values.

Global Acceptance: Yoga is now globally accepted as a complementary therapy. Every year on 21st June 'International Yoga Day' is celebrated worldwide for better holistic health.

Components of yoga:

'Maharishi Patanjali' in his text 'Patanjali Yoga Sutra' mentioned eight fundamental components of yoga collectively known as "Ashtanga Yoga". These components include Yama; Niyama; Asana; Pranayama; Pratyahara; Dharana: Dhayana; Samadhi. These are classified in two categorized: Bahayah sadhana (Yama; Niyama; Asana; Pranayama; Pratyahara) and Antaranga sadhana (Dharana: Dhayana; Samadhi).

A. Yama: Yama refers to social disciple. It includes ahimsa (non-violence), satya (truthfulness), asteya (non-stealing), brahmacarya (continence), and aparigraha (non-possessiveness). Maharishi Patanjali defines Yama as "ahi sā-satyāsteya-brahmacaryāparigrahā yamā ."
B. Niyama: Niyama refers to self-discipline and inner purification. It includes sauca (purity), samtosa (contentment), tapas (austerity), svadhyaya (scriptural

study), and isvarapranidhana (surrender to God). Maharishi Patanjali defines Niyama as "śauca-sa to a-tapa -svādhyāyeśvara-pra idhānani niyamā ."

C. Asana: Asana refers to physical posture to enhance physical strength, and flexibility. Maharishi Patanjali defines Asana as "Sthira-sukham-āsanam", which means asana should be steady and comfortable.

D. Pranayama: Pranayama refers to breathing technique, to regulate the flow of vital energy (prana). It is helpful in strengthen respiratory system and improving its functioning, calming the mind, and stimulate nervous system. Maharishi Patanjali defines Pranayama as "tasmin satiśvāsa praśvāsayo gativiccheda prā āyāma ".

E. Pratyahara: Pratyahara refers to withdraw of senses, to reduce external distractions. It is helpful in promoting inner peace and mental awareness. Maharishi Patanjali defines Pratyahara as "svavi aya asa prayoge cittasya svarūpāanukāra iva indriyā ā pratyāhāra ."

F. Dharana: Dharana refers to concentration. It is helpful in stimulating mental stability. Maharishi Patanjali defines Dharana as "deśa bandha cittasya dhāra ā", which means attention on a single object, and it helps to prepare practitioner for mediation.

G. Dhyana: Dhyana refers to meditation. It is a state of continuous and uninterrupted flow of awareness on an object. It promotes mental clarity, inner awareness and emotional stability. Maharishi Patanjali defines Dhyana as "tatra pratyaya ekatānatā dhyānam".

H. Samadhi: Samadhi refers to continuous and effortless attention to an object, force, or person. Maharishi Patanjali defines Samadhi as "tadeva arthamātranirbhāsa svarūpaśūnyam iva samādhi ". It is the highest state of yoga.

Table 2. Yogic intervention recommended for PCOD:

A. Shuddhi kriya/ Shatkarma	**Kapalbhati (Dilip & Prashant, 2023); Jal neti, Basti**
B. Asana	Paschimottanasana (Chithra et al., 2024); Bhujangasana (Chithra et al., 2024); Sarvangasana (Chithra et al., 2024); Matsyasana (Chithra et al., 2024); Setubandhasana (Chithra et al., 2024); Vajrasana (Chithra et al., 2024); Surya Namaskara (Dilip & Prashant, 2023); Malasana; Pawanmuktasana; Shavasana; Tadasana; Baddha konasana; Mandukasana; Padhastasana; Sarpasana; Janu sirasana; Naukasana (Dilip & Prashant, 2023); Shalbhasana; Tiryak tadasana; Marjariasana; Bitilasana; Ardha chakrasana; Chakki chalanasana (Dilip & Prashant, 2023); Nauka chalanasana; Mayurasana; Dhanurasana (Dilip & Prashant, 2023); Halasana (Dilip & Prashant, 2023) Suptabandhkonasana (Dilip & Prashant, 2023)
C. Pranayama	Ujjayi pranayama; Suryabhedhan pranayama; Seetkari pranayama; Shitali pranayama; Bhramari pranayama (Dilip & Prashant, 2023); Nadi shodhana (Dilip & Prashant, 2023); Deep yogic breathing
D. Mudra	Yoni mudra; Vipreetkarni mudra; Ashwini mudra
E. Bandha	Jalandhara bandha (Chithra et al., 2024); Mool bandha (Chithra et al., 2024); Uddiyana bandha (Chithra et al., 2024)
F. Dhyana	Om Chanting (Chithra et al., 2024)

S. No.	**Yoga intervention**	**Benefits of an intervention**
1.	Kapalbhati	Kapalbhati is shuddhi kriya that enhances ovarian functioning, improves digestion; metabolism; and detoxification, alleviates abdominal organs functioning, controls hormonal imbalance.
2.	Jal neti	Jal neti balances hormones, activates parasympathetic functioning, reduces stress level, improves respiratory system functioning.
3.	Basti	Basti is also known as yogic enema. It helps in improving digestion; gut health and detoxification, regulates hormonal functioning, enhances metabolism, relieves in constipation.
4.	Paschimottanasana	Paschimottanasana stimulates and improves blood flow in ovaries, uterus and pelvic organs, reduces stress; anxiety; depression, regulates cortisol, relieves menstrual irregularities and abdominal discomfort.
5.	Bhujangasana	Bhujangasana improve blood flow in uterus, strengthens reproductive organs and enhances its functioning, reduces central abdominal fat and improves body postures.
6.	Sarvangasana	Sarvangasana regulates metabolism; menstrual cycle and thyroid function, improves endocrine and hormonal functioning, alleviates menstrual irregularities.
7.	Matsyasana	Matsyasana practice reduces stress and balances hormones; improves respiratory functioning by increasing breathing capacity, enhances blood flow in reproductive organs, stimulates functioning of thyroid and parathyroid glands.
8.	Setubandhasana	Setubandhasana regulation thyroid glands and reproductive organs functioning, improves blood flow in pelvic region, reduces stress; anxiety and abdominal fat.

continued on following page

Table 2. Continued

S. No.	Yoga intervention	Benefits of an intervention
9.	Vajrasana	Vajrasana improves digestion, reduces bloating and gastric issues which is very common in PCOD, reduces stress and anxiety, improves blood flow in pelvic region.
10.	Surya Namaskara	Surya Namaskara is helpful in reducing weight, improves cardiovascular; metabolic and reproductive system functioning, enhances circulatory system functioning, reduces stress and regulates hormones.
11.	Malasana	Malasana improves blood circulation in pelvic region, ovaries; and uterus, regulates menstrual cycles, improves digestion and reduces constipation.
12.	Pawanmuktasana	Pawanmuktasana reduces constipation; bloating; and abdominal issues, improves blood flow in pelvic region, enhances reproductive organs functioning, reduces stress; anxiety, useful in impotence; sterility; and menstrual issues.
13.	Shavasana	Shavasana is helpful in improving sleep quality, reduces stress; anxiety, and cortisol level, activates parasympathetic system, relaxes psycho-physiological system.
14.	Tadasana	Tadasana improves blood circulation; and body postures, reduces muscular stress and anxiety, regulates breathing and endocrine system functioning.
15.	Baddha konasana	Baddha konasana improves blood circulation in hips, ovaries, uterus and pelvic region, enhances reproductive functioning, alleviates menstrual discomfort.
16.	Mandukasana	Mandukasana improves digestion, reduces abdominal fat, balances hormones, regulates pancreas and reproductive system functioning.
17.	Padhastasana	Padhastasana reduces stress and anxiety, regulates hormones, improves blood flow in abdominal and pelvic region, enhances flexibility and strengthens core.
18.	Sarpasana	Sarpasana reduces abdominal fat, improves reproductive system and adrenal system functioning, reduces stress; anxiety; and fatigue.
19.	Janu sirasana	Janu sirasana increases blood flow in pelvic region; uterus and ovaries, regulates menstrual cycle, improves pelvic flexibility, reduces stress; anxiety; and cortisol level, provides relaxation.
20.	Naukasana	Naukasana regulates uterine and ovarian functioning, reduces abdominal fat, strengthens abdominal muscles, improves metabolic functioning, stimulates functioning of muscular, digestive, circulatory, nervous and hormonal systems.
21.	Shalbhasana	Shalbhasana improves blood circulation in pelvic and reproductive organs, strengthens lower back muscles, regulates hormones, reduces stress.
22.	Tiryak tadasana	Tiryak tadasana improves digestion, regulates hormonal imbalance, enhance flexibility and circulation,
23.	Marjariasana	Marjariasana improves blood circulation in reproductive organs and pelvic region, reduces stress and menstrual discomfort, enhances adrenal glands functioning.
24.	Bitilasana	Bitilasana reduces cortisol levels, regulates hormones, improves reproductive organs functioning and abdominal muscles flexibility.

continued on following page

Table 2. Continued

S. No.	Yoga intervention	Benefits of an intervention
25.	Ardha chakrasana	Ardha chakrasana regulates function of thyroid glands, improves blood circulation to uterus and ovaries, reduces central abdominal fat.
26.	Chakki chalanasana	Chakki chalanasana improves reproductive and ovarian system functioning, alleviates digestion, regulates menstrual cycle, reduces abdominal fat.
27.	Nauka chalanasana	Nauka chalanasana improves blood circulation of reproductive organs, reduces abdominal fat, strengthens abdominal and pelvic muscles, regulates menstrual cycle.
28.	Mayurasana	Mayurasana enhances digestive fire, alleviates obesity, strengthens core muscles, improves metabolism functioning, eliminates toxins from the body.
29.	Dhanurasana	Dhanurasana stimulates pelvic and abdominal organs, alleviates menstrual irregularities, enhance ovarian functioning, reduces stress, improves spinal flexibility.
30.	Halasana	Halasana practice regulates thyroid glands; reproductive organs; and metabolism functioning, reduces abdominal fat, improves blood circulation.
31.	Suptabandhkonasana	Suptabandhkonasana provides deep relaxation, stimulates pelvic region and reproductive organs, reduces stress and anxiety, regulates hormonal balance, relieves menstrual discomfort.
32.	Ujjayi pranayama	Ujjayi pranayama activates parasympathetic system functioning, reduces stress, improves sleep quality, enhances thyroid and metabolic functioning.
33.	Suryabhedhan pranayama	Suryabhedhan pranayama activates sympathetic system functioning, improves digestion and boost metabolism, reduces insulin resistance, helpful in managing lethargy which I s common in PCOD.
34.	Seetkari pranayama	Seetkari pranayama calms nervous system and cools the body, reduces body inflammation, manages and reduces stress.
35.	Shitali pranayama	Shitali pranayama calms nervous system, reduces inflammation and body heat, balances cortisol levels, improve digestion and provides mental clarity, balances hormones.
36.	Bhramari pranayama	Bhramari pranayama reduces stress, anxiety and sympathetic overactivity significantly, improves pituitary gland functioning, regulates menstrual cycle, alleviates sleep quality; insomnia; and overall emotional well-being.
37.	Nadi shodhana	Nadi shodhana balances autonomic nervous system, reduces stress and fatigues, regulates endocrine system functioning, increases oxygen level, provides mental clarity and emotional stability.
38.	Deep yogic breathing	Deep yogic breathing reduces stress; anxiety and cortisol levels, provides deep relaxation, enhances lungs capacity and bodily oxygen level, regulates hormones.
39.	Jalandhara bandha	Jalandhara bandha regulates menstrual irregularities, stimulates thyroid and parathyroid glands, calms mind and body.
40.	Mool bandha	Mool bandha strengthens pelvic floor muscles, improves ovarian functioning, regulates menstrual cycle.

continued on following page

Table 2. Continued

S. No.	Yoga intervention	Benefits of an intervention
41.	Uddiyana bandha	Uddiyana bandha massages reproductive and abdominal organs, improves digestive and metabolic system functioning, improves insulin resistance, strengthens core muscles.
42.	Om Chanting	Om Chanting provides deep relaxation to mind and body, reduces stress; and anxiety, promotes emotional well-being, improves mind-body connection, and balances hormones.

ROLE OF ARTIFICIAL INTELLIGENCE IN MANAGEMENT OF PCOD

Artificial Intelligence (AI) is emerged as a substantial transformation and innovation in the global health sector, contributing noticeably to prediction of disease, its early diagnosis, prevention, personalized treatment planning, clinical decision-making, and management of patient. It is a substantial revolution in the advancement of women's healthcare. Artificial intelligence can be used in tracking menstrual cycle; pregnancy monitoring; hormonal health monitoring; mood tracking; virtual counselling; sleep monitoring; stress monitoring; irregular cycle prediction.

Artificial intelligence in health is a considerable revolution in women healthcare, by making healthcare more safe, personalized, smarter and holistic. In recent years, numerous Artificial intelligence (AI)-enabled devices have become available that facilitate real-time monitoring and management of health parameters, include smart-watches, fitness bands, and wearable sensors. These AI-based devices continuously monitor various physiological health parameters, including heart rate, stress levels, sleep patterns, physical activity, and blood pressure.

What is an Artificial Intelligence?

Artificial intelligence is an emulator of human knowledge and intelligence in a machines which is design to think, analyse, learn, and make decisions. AI is able to perform several tasks including analysis of data, predictions, recognitions of any patterns, critical problem solving, reasoning, language understanding, perception, and learning from previous experiences by using algorithms, machine learnings, and deep learning methodology. AI is a modern and latest technology unlike old traditional computer programs, AI uses existing data and improves its performance by continuous learning of large database. AI is a branch of computer science and is based on an advanced computation models. It is capable of performing tasks that usually requires human intelligence. The core components of Artificial Intelligence are as following:

- Machine learning (ML)
- Deep learning (DL)
- Natural Language Processing (NLP)
- Computer vision
- Wearable and sensor based AI

Machine learning (ML): Machine learning uses and studies previous data and recognizes pattern and on the basis of it makes and provides decisions. No other explicit programme is being used in machine learning.

- Prediction of improvement in PCOD symptoms on the basis of yoga intervention.
- Identification of participants response towards yoga protocol.

Deep learning (DL): Deep learning is an advance version of machine learning that utilizes artificial network and works like human brain. It studies complex patterns from large database.

- MRI and ultrasound analysis.
- Identification of hormonal, physiological, neurological changes through a medical scans.

Natural Language Processing (NLP): Natural Language Processing enhances the capability of computer to understand and analyse human language. It is helpful in reading, interpreting and summarizing the text or speech.

- Analysis feedback of patients.
- Summarized yoga practitioners feedback and experiences.
- Abstracts symptoms from patients medical records or reports.

Computer vision: Computer vision helps computer in seeing and interpreting images and videos. It allows computers to understand visual information just like human do.

- Examines yoga asana and body alignment.
- Analysis facial expression related to pain and fatigue.
- Reads medical records including CT scans, MRI, sonography.

Wearable and sensor based AI: Wearable and sensor based AI utilizes data obtains from smart devices and sensors. They are helpful in tracking health signals and monitoring body in real-time.

- Monitoring of blood pressure, heart rate, sleep, and stress during yoga intervention.
- Tracking physiological activity.
- Analysing lifestyle patterns.
- Providing real-time feedback to PCOD patients.

Types of Artificial Intelligence: There are majorly three types of Artificial intelligence which are as following-

- Narrow or Weak AI
- General AI
- Reactive and Adaptive AI Systems

Narrow or Weak AI: Narrow or Weak Artificial intelligence is use to perform specific task including posture corrections, health tracking, and vocal guidance. Most health care and complementary therapy based AI applications falls under this category.

General AI: General AI is also termed as theoretical AI, and is used to perform intellectual task just like human do.

Reactive and Adaptive AI Systems: Reactive and Adaptive AI Systems gives immediate response and are based on behaviour, progress, and outputs of an users.

Levels of Intelligence in Artificial intelligence systems: Levels of Intelligence in Artificial intelligence systems are as the following-

- Perceptual intelligence
- Cognitive intelligence
- Predictive intelligence
- Adaptive intelligence

Perceptual intelligence: Perceptual intelligence uses images, videos, sound, audio and physiological signals as an inputs. In yoga therapy it is useful in recognising posture, detecting breathing patterns, and analysing facial expression.

Cognitive intelligence: Cognitive intelligence levels is use for reasoning, problem solving, and decision making. In a yoga therapy this intelligence is use to design personalized yoga interventions including asanas, pranayama, and dhayana.

Predictive intelligence: Predictive intelligence is generally use for future predictions based on real-time database including progression of symptoms, personalised yoga intervention, symptoms improvement, risk predictions.

Adaptive intelligence: Adaptive intelligence provides modified suggestions, recommendations and guidance based on behaviour, progress, participants feedback. It will be helpful in long-term engagement.

What is the Relevance of an Artificial Intelligence in Health care?

Artificial Intelligence has a great relevance and transformation in health care sector due to its ability to improve efficiency, accuracy, personalization, and accessibility in health sector. Relevance of an Artificial Intelligence in Health care are as following:

1. AI is helpful in the analysis of clinical database, early detection and diagnosis of signs or symptoms of disease, laboratory data results, and patients health history.
2. AI can provide personalised yoga intervention and treatment based on patients history, lifestyle, psychological and physiological parameters, and genetics. It will enhance the effectiveness of treatment and minimize any side-effects
3. AI provides clinical decision support by providing facilities including recommendations based on evidence, assessment and predictions of risk.
4. AI is capable to perform routine task such as data entry, scheduling and generation of reports automatically, which increases the efficiency of healthcare providers, reduces there burdens, and enhances focus on patients health.
5. AI based wearable devices and health application continuously monitor patients, which is helpful in managing chronic illness, reduces unnecessary hospital visits, and provides immediate virtual assistant in remote areas.
6. AI is cost-effective and provides quality care by reducing unnecessary tests, hospital visits, and hospital admissions.
7. AI based healthcare is efficient as it increases accessibility in remote and undeserved areas.
8. AI provides health assistance enhances patients engagement and adherence by including chatbots, routines, reminders, chatbots, and virtual assistance.
9. AI intensifies healthcare research as it is able to access and evaluate large database.
10. AI is helpful in complementary therapies including yoga, naturopathy, ayurveda, and chakra healing.

What is the Relevance of an Artificial Intelligence in yogic science?

Artificial intelligence is emerged as an encouraging and transformative technology in yogic science as it enhances the accessibility, assessment, delivery, and monitoring of yoga as a complementary and alternative therapy. Yoga is a traditional and ancient holistic practice which is deeply rooted. Artificial intelligence without replacing its traditional foundation strengthens it by improving its scientific, therapeutic, and educational dimensions.

1. AI based platforms for yoga practice ensures detailed step-by-step instructions, virtual guidance, clear prompt, and accurate sequencing of asanas, pranayama, and dhyana (meditation technique). It is helpful in providing correct and consistent support especially to beginners and remote practitioners.
2. AI analyses body movement and posture during yoga practice. This ensures safety, posture correction, correct body alignment, error reduction, minimal risk of injury, and improves quality of life.
3. AI provides personalized yoga intervention based on characteristics of an individuals including age, gender, medical history, stress level, physical ability, and health condition. Personalised yoga intervention enhances the effectiveness and adherence.
4. AI based yoga platforms continuously monitors practice parameters including frequence, duration, accuracy, and physiological changes. The primary objective is to determine progress and outcome.
5. AI is helpful in tracking health parameters and symptoms changes, hence by integrating it with yoga therapy it strengthens the role of therapeutic yoga as a complementary and alternative medicine in the treatment of lifestyle-based psychological and physiological disorders.
6. AI provides virtual platforms for online and home-based yoga practice, therefore it expands the accessibility of quality yoga in remote and backward areas populations beyond geographical limitations.
7. AI supports research in yogic science as it enables large-scale data collection and its analysis, pattern identification, and outcome evaluation based on psychological, physiological, and behavioural responses.
8. AI provides virtual support, tracks progress, and reminders which enhances adherence to yoga practice. For long term benefits continuous motivation and engagement is necessary.
9. AI integrates asana, pranayama (breathing technique) and dhyana (meditation technique) and provides personalized structured yoga programs to practitioners and responses to feedback.
10. AI is helpful for yoga instructor or teachers as it serve as an assistance tool by monitoring symptoms, provides personalized guidance, and records feedback. In this way AI complements traditional yoga techniques.

Evidences for AI effectiveness in yogic science?

Several studies have demonstrated the effectiveness and relevance of Artificial Intelligence in yogic science. Presently AI focuses especially on yoga posture recognition, alignment correction, virtual assistance, feedback, and enhances practice. It is a digital and personalised transformation that incorporates traditional yoga wisdom with modern technology. The primary aim of this integration is to promote accessibility, effectiveness and customization of the yoga interventions. AI based systems are proficient to correct and classify postures in real-time, and provides feedback. Along with the postures correction this AI based system also encourages practitioners for better health and fitness, and improves their overall holistic health including physical, mental, emotional, spiritual, and social.

1. Numerous studies have shown that Artificial Intelligence based deep learning (DL) and machine learning (ML) enhances the accuracy of correct yoga postures in real-time. By integration of AI in yoga practice substantially increases health benefits, transforms healthcare sector, and reduces burden of diseases. Utilizing deep learning (DL) and machine learning (ML) models in yogic science improves asanas alignment in real-time in healthy persons. Incorporating AI in yoga programs is safest and effective technique in home-based yoga learning (Özsezer & Mermer, 2025).
2. A research study demonstrated the effectiveness of applying Artificial Intelligence for analysing and supporting yoga practice in real time. AI is helpful in recognising accuracy of yoga posture in real time, correcting postures, proving instant feedback, identifying wrong body alignment, enhancing safety, enhancing accessibility of yoga intervention, minimizing injury during yoga practice, reducing dependency on in-person yoga session, providing learning at your pace and time. AI is a complement for yoga trainers or instructor but cannot replace them (Pawar & Kulkarni, 2025).
3. Several studies have identified the effectiveness of integrating deep learning and machine learning in yoga practice estimation. These studies have shown significant results for both researchers and practitioners. The primary aim was to effective utilize technology in enhancing performance of the practitioners. AI based platforms provides real-times postures correction and instant feedback, this helps in improving practice, creating user-friendly environment, and evaluating long term benefits (Raj et al., 2025).
4. Research studies have demonstrated that AI based yoga program provides real-time inference. It shows 98.43% accuracy, 98.30% sensitivity, 99.88% specificity, and 0.9831 of Matthews correlation coefficient in yoga postures recognition. Through AI it is possible to capture movement during yoga intervention, in real time. It provides a guidance for selected yoga asanas and avoids incorrect

postures. After covid-19 the demand for AI based yoga program has increased for better home training (Long et al., 2022).

5. Studies have identified that AI-driven technologies including wearable devices, machine learning, and computer vision are useful in tracking patients progress, provides individual feedback to practitioners, presents precise and standardized outcomes. AI-based computer vision algorithms monitors safety and correctness of yoga postures. Artificial Intelligence enhances the advantages of yoga by incorporating modern technology with tradition therapy (Sapna, 2025).
6. Numerous studies have demonstrated that the integration of Artificial Intelligence (AI) with a traditional Yoga therapy is a transformation in a holistic healthcare system. It offers personalization, efficacy and accessibility and enhances effectiveness and scalability of yoga as therapeutic interventions. Incorporation of AI a modern computer based technology with a yoga a complementary and non-conventional therapy is a great revolution in medical science for better health, and improving quality of life. AI is highly capable in analysing large database and recognising patterns which significantly impacts health care system. Integration is helpful in the transformation, management, diagnosis, and treatment of diseases (Sinha & Sinha, 2024).

Therefore, Artificial Intelligence based platforms for yoga intervention uses techniques including deep learning, machine learning, computer vision, and pose estimation models that effectively recognizes and corrects yoga asanas, provides real-time feedback, enhances engagement of practitioners, improves body alignment, reduction in injury, provides better safety and increases home based yoga practice.

Benefits of artificial intelligence in PCOD management: The benefits of integrating an artificial intelligence in the management of Polycystic Ovarian Disorder (PCOD) are as following (Sinha & Sinha, 2024):

A. Advanced data analytics
B. Personalised interventions
C. Remote monitoring and guidance
D. Scalability and accessibility
E. Enhanced research and development
F. Real time monitoring and feedback
G. Virtual assistants and telehealth platform
H. Remote and telehealth services
I. Health promotion and prevention
J. Operational and cost efficiency

Advanced data analytics: Artificial intelligence enables analysis of large and complex database including hormonal profile, clinical history, vital signs, and lifestyle factors. It facilitates the early detection of risk, prediction of progression of disease, customised clinical treatment.

Personalised interventions: Artificial intelligence is helpful in developing personalised interventions based on individual lifestyle, dietary habits, clinical, and hormonal factors. These personalised interventions including diet, yoga intervention, and stress management are effective in improving overall health and wellbeing.

Remote monitoring and guidance: Wearable devices and mobiles promotes physical health and provides continuous and uninterrupted health monitoring of menstrual pattern, blood pressure, heart rate, oxygen level, metabolic parameters, and physical activity. Through this it is possible to provide timely management and guidance of PCOD.

Scalability and accessibility: Artificial intelligence provides a platform through which it is easy to reach large populations in limited time. Through it the accessibility of healthcare to remote and undeserved areas is possible.

Enhanced research and development: Artificial intelligence intensify research by identifying outcome over large database of the population. It accelerate research by providing scientific evidence and also evaluates the effectiveness of complementary and alternative therapy including yoga and diet in management of PCOD.

Real time monitoring and feedback: Through Artificial intelligence it is easy to monitor symptoms and progression of PCOD in real-time and provide feedback. Instant and immediate feedback reduces risk and improves symptoms.

Virtual assistants and telehealth platform: Artificial intelligence provides virtual assistants, health educations, answer patients queries, and send reminders. It provides an uninterrupted and continuous virtual interaction between patients and healthcare workers.

Remote and telehealth services: Artificial intelligence promotes remote consultations, virtual assessment, and digital follow-up care to patients. Hence remote and telehealth services are beneficial as they provide long term consultations and management of PCOD, which is necessary for better outcome.

Health promotion and prevention: Through Artificial intelligence promotion and prevention of health is easily possible. As it is helpful in identifying high risk and management of symptoms of PCOD. It provides sustainable monitoring and continuous support to the patients diagnosed with PCOD.

Operational and cost efficiency: Artificial intelligence is beneficial as it provides cost-effective healthcare facilities. It improves diagnostic accuracy, reduces unnecessary clinical visits, and provides timely management of any chronic conditions. Through this functioning of health care system will get better in remote and backward areas.

How Artificial Intelligence Assists Yoga Trainers Without Replacing Them?

Artificial Intelligence based Yoga intervention are design to assist, support, and reduce workload of yoga trainer and primarily to enhance their work, not to replace them from their professional role. Yoga trainers have human presence, empathy, personal connection, emotional intelligence, motivation, feeling, and cultural & tradition values, which Artificial intelligence based technology cannot replace.

1. Artificial intelligence is a supportive technology for the yoga trainers but they can't be a substitute of them. They can help yoga trainer in monitoring and managing intervention efficiently but cannot replace their intelligence, expertise, intuition, and decision making.
2. AI tools can assess posture accuracy, breathing technique, heart rate, blood pressure through sensors which helps trainers in tracking progress, but final interpretation and assessment is always remain a responsibility of the trainers.
3. AI can help trainers in analysis of data and personalization of yoga intervention on the basis of participants medical history, and health data but final decision-maker will always be trainers.
4. AI helps in maintaining discipline and practice continuity when yoga trainer is not physically available for session by providing reminders and recorded sessions, this is helpful for yoga trainers but it cannot replace trainers' personal guidance.
5. Yoga is a tradition complementary therapy and deeply rooted in human connection, guidance, and mindfulness, whereas AI lacks emotional intelligence, empathy, moral counselling, and human understanding. Therefore AI-based tools can support, serve as an adjunct and complement yoga trainers rather replacement of them.

INTEGRATION OF YOGA AND ARTIFICIAL INTELLIGENCE IN PCOD

When Artificial intelligence is combined with Yoga therapy, it can serve as a boon for women's healthcare, especially in the prevention and management of numerous disorders. This integration is a significant breakthrough in healthcare as it provides an innovation, personalization, comprehension, and holistic approach for the management of diseases, reducing their symptoms, and promoting the overall health and well-being of women. Artificial Intelligence (AI) is a valuable evolution in health sector which propound, personalized and continuous monitoring of health, analysis of psychological and physiological health data, and continuous tracking of physiological parameters including blood pressure, heart rate, respiratory rate, sleep quality, stress and anxiety level, menstrual cycle, and irregularities.

Yoga is a traditional, non-pharmacological and holistic therapy that has been determined to be effective in improving all the aspects of health, including physiological, psychological, emotional, spiritual, and social well-being. Therefore, incorporating Artificial Intelligence into yoga research and practice may enhance all aspects of health and contribute to the overall well-being of women.

Artificial Intelligence can assist in correcting posture and body movements, designing personalized yoga sessions based on the specific disease and its severity, and detecting physiological irregularities that may indicate potential health problems. This AI integration have the potential to completely transform the diagnosis, treatment, and management of diseases (Sinha & Sinha, 2024).

Artificial Intelligence (AI) is playing a crucial and transformative role in healthcare, as it can identify abnormalities in the body in real time. AI, which is widely recognised for its capacity to analyse enormous datasets, identify trends, and generate predictions based upon data, has started to have significant impacts on healthcare (Sinha & Sinha, 2024). Nowadays, real-time physiological parameter monitoring during yoga practice is now possible by wearable technology and sensors, allowing for customised interventions (Sinha & Sinha, 2024).

It is a new emerging era of online yoga sessions that facilitate worldwide awareness and accessibility of yoga. By integrating yoga with artificial intelligence, online yoga delivery becomes more efficient, personalized, and user-friendly, thereby enhancing global participation and engagement. There are some applications that integrates AI in yoga practices including YogMudra; YOGI; TrueYogi; AsanaAI; YogaPose AI; Yoga: Ai Personal Trainer.

Challenges for Yoga trainer during online session:

A. It is difficult for trainer to monitor every participant's posture, body alignment and body movement closely.
B. Sometimes during an online session direct communication and real-time feedback is not possible between trainer and practitioner's
C. Trainer is not able to identify any discomfort, improper posture, and risk of injury during an online session.
D. In an online session trainer is not able to consistently monitor and observe multi participants at a time.
E. There is huge administrative burden on trainer including attendance, management of session schedule, and it is time consuming too.
F. It is difficult to assess all the participants simultaneously especially during an online session.

G. In an online session as they are practice in home-based environment there will be several difficulties including interruptions, limited space, and background noise which will impact participants performance and result in lack of focus.
H. An online session is completely based on continuous verbal instructions, and screen monitoring, which can leads to mental fatigue.
I. During an online yoga session it is difficult for the yoga trainer to demonstrate asanas, monitor and observe them simultaneously.
J. Online session requires addition time due to which there will be time management issues because of login, troubleshooting, camera placement.
K. In an online yoga sessions professional accountability becomes complex.
L. Without a standardized online assessment tool it is difficult to do assessment of participant progress, consistency and long-term outcome during an online sessions.
M. Sometime it is difficult for yoga trainer to receive real-time verbal or non-verbal immediate feedback regarding the discomfort, and fatigue of the participants.

How integrating Artificial intelligence will help in overcoming these challenges:

A. There will be more accuracy in assessment of yoga postures during session, as AI based motion tracker is able to capture the body alignments, and movement quality. Hence it will be easy for yoga trainer to identify error.
B. AI can generate personalized report of every participant which will help them in analysing their flexibility, mobility and progress.
C. AI algorithm is design in a way that it can detect micro-movement, improper posture which can help trainer in corrections.
D. By analysing movement pattens AI is able to highlight any potential injury and unsafe posture
E. AI is helpful in consistently monitor postures, movements and giving progress report based on performance of participants.
F. AI can automatically perform administrative tasks including reminders, class scheduling, and management which is helpful for trainer to focus only on teaching yoga.
G. AI based yoga sessions provides personalized on screen intervention, reminders, and guided prompts which will help participants in maintaining attention even with environmental distractions.
H. AI based yoga sessions provides noise-filtering algorithms and recorded sessions.
I. AI driven yoga session provides pre-recorded asanas, and pranayama demonstrations session which will help participants to view correct techniques, and trainer will focus only on monitoring, observation, and guidance during live virtual sessions.

J. AI works on automate session management which reduces setup time.
K. Ai minimizes cognitive load and mental fatigue during online virtual session because of automate instructions, ai-assisted voice prompts, and trainer can provide real-time feedback too.

CHALLENGES OF INTEGRATING ARTIFICIAL INTELLIGENCE IN YOGA SESSIONS

There are following challenges of integrating Artificial intelligence in a Yoga session for Yoga Trainers:

A. By integrating Artificial intelligence in health dependency on technology increases which is highly challenging .
B. Digital awareness is extremely important for attending yoga session, therefore it is mandatory for trainer and practitioners' both to have familiarity with technology.
C. Maintenance and development of an Artificial Intelligence based yoga session is costly.
D. The dependency on Artificial intelligence increases which sometimes results in lack of interpersonal interaction between participants and trainers.
E. There will be risk of disruption in yoga session because of system errors, tracking failure, or software glitch, which results in session interruption and misleading instructions.
F. There will be risk related to practitioner's consent, confidentiality and data security, as Artificial intelligence uses practitioner's biometric data and tracks there motions.
G. Artificial intelligence lacks emotional sensitivity.
H. By amalgamation of Artificial intelligence with yoga therapy there may be a risk of commercialization of yoga and dilution of its essence.
I. In rural, economically backward and financially disadvantaged populations there is restriction on use of Artificial intelligence based platforms for yoga sessions because of no or limited access of smartphones, poor internet connectivity, and lack of digital education and literacy.
J. The dependence on Artificial intelligence based yoga sessions increases dependency on technology which will contradicts the svadhyaya (self-discipline) which is a yogic principle and it is termed as 'Niyama'.
K. Yoga is an ancient therapy based on Indian philosophy and is deeply rooted with values including self-awareness, calmness, discipline. By integration of yoga

with artificial intelligence there may an inadequate philosophical, ethical, and experimental component of yoga, and turns yoga purely into a physical exercise.

L. Artificial intelligence based yoga sessions may face difficulties in monitoring accuracy of complex asana, posture detection, alignment and level of flexibility. Due to incorrect feedbacks the risks of injury may increase.

M. Yoga is a tradition therapy and is purely based on guru-shishya Parampara. But due AI based Yoga intervention lacks this aspect.

N. AI based yoga intervention rely only on virtual or sensor-based data, hence it is difficult to monitor the rhythm, depth, internal retention (kumbhaka) of the pranayama.

O. It is difficult to monitor and do assessment of meditation and mindfulness as it is subjective and based on individual inner experience which may lack in AI based yoga intervention.

FUTURE DIRECTIONS

Currently, there is only a single randomized controlled trial titled "Exploring the Comparative Merit of Allopathy Medicine and Yoga Therapy for PCOD Condition", which demonstrated the effectiveness of yoga as a complementary therapy. The study highlighted that yoga is a safe, cost-effective intervention with minimal chances of recurrence. Therefore, further research involving larger sample sizes, longer intervention duration, standardized yoga protocols, diverse populations and Artificial intelligence (AI) integration is needed to establish the efficacy of yoga as a complementary therapy for PCOD and to ensure generalizability of the outcomes. As yoga is a multidimensional practice that enhances physical, mental, emotional, spiritual, and social well-being, more longitudinal, multicentric studies, and along with artificial intelligence (AI) incorporation are essential to provide vigorous scientific evidence supporting its role as a complementary and alternative therapy in the management of PCOD. Exploring the benefits of yoga in managing PCOD as a non-conventional treatment can contribute to the development of holistic and sustainable management strategies.

CONCLUSION

The amalgamation of Yoga, a traditional, and holistic therapeutic curative system, along with an Artificial Intelligence (AI), a modern and advanced technological approach, has the potential to revolutionize women's healthcare and is helpful as a complementary therapy in managing Polycystic Ovarian Disorder. Artificial Intelligence (AI) is helpful in accurately tracking both physiological and psychological parameters of health.

REFERENCES

Abiç, A., & Yilmaz Vefikuluçay, D. (2024). The Effect of Yoga on Menopause Symptoms: A Randomized Controlled Trial. *Holistic Nursing Practice*, *38*(3), 138–147. DOI: 10.1097/HNP.0000000000000646 PMID: 38709129

Chahar, K., Sharma, Y., Kumar, M., Kumari, L., Mishra, L., Patel, P., & Kurmi, B. D. (2023). A recapitulation of the polycystic ovarian disorder in adult women and the risk of disease associated with the polycystic ovarian disorder. *Health Sciences Review (Oxford, England)*, *8*, 100110. DOI: 10.1016/j.hsr.2023.100110

Chakrabarty, J., Vidyasagar, M., Fernandes, D., Joisa, G., Varghese, P., & Mayya, S. (2015). Effectiveness of pranayama on cancer-related fatigue in breast cancer patients undergoing radiation therapy: A randomized controlled trial. *International Journal of Yoga*, *8*(1), 47–53. DOI: 10.4103/0973-6131.146062 PMID: 25558133

Chithra, S., Sriram, S., Rajalakshmi, P., & Brindha, P. (2024). Yoga theraphy in the management of polycystic ovarian disease –. *RE:view*, *9*(4).

Devi, C. R., & Rani, N. J. (2022). Exploring on the Comparative Merit of Allopathy Medicine and Yoga Therapy for PCOD Condition. *International Journal of Health Sciences (Qassim)*, *III*, 308–324. DOI: 10.53730/ijhs.v6nS3.5187

Dilip, D. K. A., & Prashant, D. D. (2023). *IMPORTANCE OFAAHAR VIHAR IN PCOD. 12*(13).

Elavsky, S., & McAuley, E. (2007). Physical activity and mental health outcomes during menopause: A randomized controlled trial. *Annals of Behavioral Medicine : A Publication of the Society of Behavioral Medicine*, *33*(2), 132–142. DOI: 10.1007/BF02879894 PMID: 17447865

Jorge, M. P., Santaella, D. F., Pontes, I. M. O., Shiramizu, V. K. M., Nascimento, E. B., Cabral, A., Lemos, T. M. A. M., Silva, R. H., & Ribeiro, A. M. (2016). Hatha Yoga practice decreases menopause symptoms and improves quality of life: A randomized controlled trial. *Complementary Therapies in Medicine*, *26*, 128–135. DOI: 10.1016/j.ctim.2016.03.014 PMID: 27261993

Long, C., Jo, E., & Nam, Y. (2022). Development of a yoga posture coaching system using an interactive display based on transfer learning. *The Journal of Supercomputing*, *78*(4), 5269–5284. DOI: 10.1007/s11227-021-04076-w PMID: 34566258

Mathur, D. A. (2023). *Endowing to good Health: A Case Study on Managing PCOD through Yoga. 10*(6).

Mittal, A., Krishna, N. R., Singh, D., & Kavuri, V. (2025). Study Protocol for a Yoga-Based Lifestyle Modification Program for Leucorrhea Disorders. *Cureus*. Advance online publication. DOI: 10.7759/cureus.78294 PMID: 40027048

Mohseni, M., Eghbali, M., Bahrami, H., Dastaran, F., & Amini, L. (2021). Yoga Effects on Anthropometric Indices and Polycystic Ovary Syndrome Symptoms in Women Undergoing Infertility Treatment: A Randomized Controlled Clinical Trial. *Evidence-Based Complementary and Alternative Medicine : eCAM*, *5564824*, 1–9. Advance online publication. DOI: 10.1155/2021/5564824 PMID: 34221076

Nidhi, R., Padmalatha, V., Nagarathna, R., & Amritanshu, R. (2012). Effect of holistic yoga program on anxiety symptoms in adolescent girls with polycystic ovarian syndrome: A randomized control trial. *International Journal of Yoga*, *5*(2), 112–117. DOI: 10.4103/0973-6131.98223 PMID: 22869994

Nidhi, R., Padmalatha, V., Nagarathna, R., & Ram, A. (2012). Effect of a yoga program on glucose metabolism and blood lipid levels in adolescent girls with polycystic ovary syndrome. *International Journal of Gynaecology and Obstetrics : The Official Organ of the International Federation of Gynaecology and Obstetrics*, *118*(1), 37–41. DOI: 10.1016/j.ijgo.2012.01.027 PMID: 22507264

Özsezer, G., & Mermer, G. (2025). Real-Time Prediction of Correct Yoga Asanas in Healthy Individuals With Artificial Intelligence Techniques: A Systematic Review for Nursing. *Nursing Open*, *12*(8), e70278. DOI: 10.1002/nop2.70278 PMID: 40768382

Pawar, M. P. U., & Kulkarni, M. H. H. (2025). Real Time Yoga Pose Detection Using AI. *International Journal of Latest Technology in Engineering Management & Applied Science*, *14*(10), 151–155. DOI: 10.51583/IJLTEMAS.2025.1410000020

Raj, gokul, Ramakrishnan, R., Parasuraman, T., Ganesh, R., & Natesamurthy, V. (2025). *Pose Estimation in Yoga: A Bibliometric Exploration of Technological Advancements in Sports Sciences | Journal of Neonatal Surgery*. https://www.jneonatalsurg.com/index.php/jns/article/view/1689?utm_source=chatgpt.com

Sapna, D. (2025). Yoga and Artificial Intelligence: A Review of The Potential Applications of AI in Yoga Research and Practice for Neurological Disorders. *Indian Journal of Ayurveda & Alternative Medicines*, *2*(1), 8–14.

Selvaraj, V., Vanitha, J., Dhanaraj, F. M., Sekar, P., & Babu, A. R. (2020). Impact of yoga and exercises on polycystic ovarian syndrome risk among adolescent schoolgirls in South India. *Health Science Reports*, *3*(4), e212. DOI: 10.1002/hsr2.212 PMID: 33305014

Sinha, N., & Sinha, R. K. (2024). Harnessing the Potential of Artificial Intelligence in Yoga Therapy. *International Journal of Yoga*, *17*(3), 242–245. DOI: 10.4103/ijoy.ijoy_124_24 PMID: 39959510

Uma, G. (2024). *An Analytical Study about Awareness and Knowledge on PCOD among Coimbatore People. 1043.*

Compilation of References

Abiç, A., & Yilmaz Vefikuluçay, D. (2024). The Effect of Yoga on Menopause Symptoms: A Randomized Controlled Trial. *Holistic Nursing Practice*, *38*(3), 138–147. DOI: 10.1097/HNP.0000000000000646 PMID: 38709129

Abràmoff, M. D., Tarver, M. E., Loyo-Berrios, N., Trujillo, S., Char, D., Obermeyer, Z., Eydelman, M. B., & Maisel, W. H. (2023). Considerations for addressing bias in artificial intelligence for health equity. *NPJ Digital Medicine*, *6*(1), 170. DOI: 10.1038/s41746-023-00913-9 PMID: 37700029

Adamson, A. S., & Smith, A. (2018). Machine learning and health care disparities in dermatology. *JAMA Dermatology*, *154*(11), 1247–1248. DOI: 10.1001/jamadermatol.2018.2348 PMID: 30073260

Adebisi, E., Balogun, S. T., Oguntuase, S. B., & Olajide, F. O. (2025). Leveraging artificial intelligence (ai) for stress management in peak athletic performance: An integrative review. *Scientific journal of engineering and technology., 2* (2), 94-106. DOI: 10.69739/sjet.v2i2.999

Agarwal, V., Sharma, K., & Rajpoot, A. K. (2022). AI based Yoga Trainer - Simplifying home yoga using mediapipe and video streaming. *2022 3rd International Conference for Emerging Technology, INCET 2022*. DOI: 10.1109/INCET54531.2022.9824332

Aguilera, A., Hernandez-Ramos, R., Haro-Ramos, A. Y., Thapa-Chhetry, B., & Figueroa, C. A. (2024). A machine learning approach for personalized autonomous digital mental health interventions in underrepresented populations. *Journal of Medical Internet Research*, *26*, e59673. DOI: 10.2196/59673

Anand Thoutam, V., Srivastava, A., Badal, T., Kumar Mishra, V., Sinha, G. R., Sakalle, A., Bhardwaj, H., & Raj, M. (2022). Yoga Pose Estimation and Feedback Generation Using Deep Learning. *Computational Intelligence and Neuroscience*, *2022*, 1–12. Advance online publication. DOI: 10.1155/2022/4311350 PMID: 35371230

Anuradha, T., Krishnamoorthy, N., Kumar, C. S. P., Prasad, L. V. N., Chunduru, A., & Moorthy, U. (2024). A Method for Specifying Yoga Poses Based on Deep Learning, Utilizing OpenCV and Media Pipe Technologies. *Scalable Computing: Practice and Experience*, *25*(2), 739–750. Advance online publication. DOI: 10.12694/scpe.v25i2.2590

Applied Sciences. (2023). Machine learning for respiratory behavior classification. *Applied Sciences*, 13(11), 6489. DOI: 10.3390/app13116489

Attar, E. T., Balasubramanian, V., Subasi, E., & Kaya, M. (2021). Stress Analysis Based on Simultaneous Heart Rate Variability and EEG Monitoring. *IEEE Journal of Translational Engineering in Health and Medicine*, *9*, 1–7. DOI: 10.1109/JTEHM.2021.3106803 PMID: 34513342

Aydın, V. A. (2024). Comparison of CNN-based methods for yoga pose classification. *Turkish Journal of Engineering*, *8*(1), 65–75. Advance online publication. DOI: 10.31127/tuje.1275826

Ayub, F., Gul-E-Sehar, Javed, M. M., & Iqbal, H. H. (2025). Mindfulness and focus in AI based learning platforms: A cognitive behavioral analysis. *The critical review of social sciences studies, 3* (3), 778-796. DOI: 10.59075/zpy09450

Bansal, R., Sharma, R., Jain, P., Arora, R., Pal, S., & Vishal, . (2024). DeepYoga: Enhancing Practice with a Real-Time Yoga Pose Recognition System. *Engineering. Technology and Applied Science Research*, *14*(6), 17704–17710. Advance online publication. DOI: 10.48084/etasr.8643

Barton, A. C., Do, M., Sheen, J., & Byrne, L. K. (2024). The restorative and state enhancing potential of abstract fractal-like imagery and interactive mindfulness interventions in virtual reality. *Virtual Reality (Waltham Cross)*, *28*(1), 53. Advance online publication. DOI: 10.1007/s10055-023-00916-7

Basu-Ray, I., Metri, K., Khanra, D., Revankar, R., Chinnaiyan, K. M., Raghuram, N., Mishra, M. C., Patwardhan, B., Sharma, M., Basavaraddi, I. V., Anand, A., Reddy, S., Deepak, K. K., Levy, M., Theus, S., Levine, G. N., Cramer, H., Fricchione, G. L., & Hongasandra, N. R. (2022). A narrative review on yoga: A potential intervention for augmenting immunomodulation and mental health in COVID-19. *BMC Complementary Medicine and Therapies*, *22*(1), 191. DOI: 10.1186/s12906-022-03666-2 PMID: 35850685

Battur, R.; Kunchur, P.; Bangarashetti, S.; Managuli, M.; Kulkarni, G.L. (2023). Artificial Intelligence and Machine Learning Techniques for Analysis of Yoga Pose. *Lecture Notes in Electrical Engineering*, 1007 LNEE, 457–466.

Bawistale, K., and S. R, (2025). "Machine Learning based Yoga Guidance Approach for The Third-Trimester Pregnant Womens Originated with Lloyd's k-Means Algorithm," *2025 Third International Conference on Augmented Intelligence and Sustainable Systems (ICAISS)*, Trichy, India, pp. 1378-1385, .DOI: 10.1109/ICAISS61471.2025.11041857

Biswas, I., Kaur, J., Pearce, F., Lewis, S., & Chattopadhyay, K. (2025). E076 Key features of effective yoga interventions for treating rheumatoid arthritis: A systematic review and meta-analysis. *Rheumatology (Oxford, England)*, *64*(3, Supplement_3), keaf142.311. Advance online publication. DOI: 10.1093/rheumatology/keaf142.311

Bodempudi, S., Nikhitha, K. D., Niharika, T., Snehith, N., Shameem, S., & Namgiri, J. V. (2023). "Mudras and Yoga Positions Detection and Recognition using YOLOv7 and Faster R-CNN," *2023 7th International Conference on Electronics, Communication and Aerospace Technology (ICECA)*, Coimbatore, India, pp. 1254-1259, DOI: 10.1109/ICECA58529.2023.10395497

Bolpagni, M., Pardini, S., & Gabrielli, S. (2024). Human centered design of AI-powered Digital Therapeutics for stress prevention: Perspectives from multi-stakeholders' workshops about the SHIVA solution. *Internet Interventions : The Application of Information Technology in Mental and Behavioural Health*, *38*, 100775. Advance online publication. DOI: 10.1016/j.invent.2024.100775 PMID: 39314669

Borthakur, D., Paul, A., Kapil, D., & Saikia, M. J. (2023). Yoga pose estimation using angle-based feature extraction. *Health Care*, *11*(24), 3133. DOI: 10.3390/healthcare11243133 PMID: 38132023

Bostrom, N., & Yudkowsky, E. (2014). The ethics of artificial intelligence. In K. Frankish & W. Ramsey (Eds.), The Cambridge handbook of artificial intelligence (pp. 316–334). Cambridge University Press. DOI: 10.1017/CBO9781139046855.020

Brewer, J. A., Worhunsky, P. D., Gray, J. R., Tang, Y. Y., Weber, J., & Kober, H. (2011). Meditation experience is associated with differences in default mode network activity and connectivity. *Proceedings of the National Academy of Sciences of the United States of America*, *108*(50), 20254–20259. DOI: 10.1073/pnas.1112029108 PMID: 22114193

Bryant, E. F. (2009). *The Yoga Sutras of Patanjali: A new edition, translation, and commentary*. North Point Press.

Bryant, E. F. (2009). *The Yoga Sutras of Patañjali: A new edition, translation, and commentary*. North Point Press.

Büssing, A., Ostermann, T., Lüdtke, R., & Michalsen, A. (2012). Effects of yoga interventions on pain and pain-associated disability: A meta-analysis. *The Journal of Pain*, *13*(1), 1–9. DOI: 10.1016/j.jpain.2011.10.001 PMID: 22178433

C, H. B., & Kumari, S. (2022). Yoga Ai Trainer Using Tensorflow. Js Posenet. Www .Irjmets.Com @*International Research Journal of Modernization in Engineering, 503*(02).

Cao, Z., Simon, T., Wei, S. E., & Sheikh, Y. (2017). Realtime multi-person 2D pose estimation using part affinity fields. In *Proceedings of the IEEE Conference on Computer Vision and Pattern Recognition (CVPR)* (pp. 7291–7299). https://doi .org/DOI: 10.1109/CVPR.2017.143

Chahar, K., Sharma, Y., Kumar, M., Kumari, L., Mishra, L., Patel, P., & Kurmi, B. D. (2023). A recapitulation of the polycystic ovarian disorder in adult women and the risk of disease associated with the polycystic ovarian disorder. *Health Sciences Review (Oxford, England)*, *8*, 100110. DOI: 10.1016/j.hsr.2023.100110

Chakrabarty, J., Vidyasagar, M., Fernandes, D., Joisa, G., Varghese, P., & Mayya, S. (2015). Effectiveness of pranayama on cancer-related fatigue in breast cancer patients undergoing radiation therapy: A randomized controlled trial. *International Journal of Yoga*, *8*(1), 47–53. DOI: 10.4103/0973-6131.146062 PMID: 25558133

Chatterjee, A., & Prinz, A. (2022). Personalized Recommendations for Physical Activity e-Coaching (OntoRecoModel): Ontological Modeling. *JMIR Medical Informatics*, *10*(6), e33847. Advance online publication. DOI: 10.2196/33847 PMID: 35737439

Chatterjee, S., & Bose, R. (2022). AI-based predictive healthcare monitoring using wearable devices. *International Journal of Medical Informatics*, *164*, 104812. DOI: 10.1016/j.ijmedinf.2022.104812

Chauhan, S., Chetwani, P. S., & Mahajan, S. (2024). Yoga Pose Recognition through Fine-Tuned ResNet50V2 Model with Projection Head. In: *IC3TES* (Conference paper). DOI: 10.1109/IC3TES62412.2024.10877545

Chen, R. J., Wang, J. J., Williamson, D. F. K., Chen, T. Y., Lipkova, J., Lu, M. Y., Saber, S., & Mahmood, F. (2024). Algorithmic fairness in artificial intelligence for medicine and healthcare. *Nature Biomedical Engineering*, *7*(6), 719–742. DOI: 10.1038/s41551-023-01056-8 PMID: 37380750

Chi Lee, A. (2018). Acceptance and Commitment Therapy: A Mindfulness and Acceptance-Based, Value-Driven Approach to Human Flourishing With Christian Spirituality Considerations. *Acceptance & Commitment Therapy: A Mindfulness & Acceptance-Based, Value-Driven Approach to Human Flourishing With Christian Spirituality Considerations.*

Chithra, S., Sriram, S., Rajalakshmi, P., & Brindha, P. (2024). Yoga theraphy in the management of polycystic ovarian disease –. *RE:view, 9*(4).

Creswell, J. D., & Goldberg, S. B. (2025). Mindfulness apps and health: Perspectives and prospects. *Annual Review of Psychology, 76*. Advance online publication. DOI: 10.1146/annurev-psych-011624-025753

De Michelis, E. (2004). A history of modern yoga: Patanjali and Western esotericism. *Continuum.*

Demir, E., Uğurlu, B. N., Uğurlu, G. A., & Aydoğdu, G. (2025). Artificial intelligence in otorhinolaryngology: Current trends and application areas. *European Archives of Oto-Rhino-Laryngology : Official Journal of the European Federation of Oto-Rhino-Laryngological Societies (EUFOS) : Affiliated with the German Society for Oto-Rhino-Laryngology - Head and Neck Surgery, 282*(5), 2697–2707. DOI: 10.1007/s00405-025-09272-5 PMID: 40019544

Desai, M., & Mewada, H. (2023). A novel approach for yoga pose estimation based on in-depth analysis of human body joint detection accuracy. *PeerJ. Computer Science, 9*, e1607. DOI: 10.7717/peerj-cs.1152 PMID: 37346636

Devi, C. R., & Rani, N. J. (2022). Exploring on the Comparative Merit of Allopathy Medicine and Yoga Therapy for PCOD Condition. *International Journal of Health Sciences (Qassim), III*, 308–324. DOI: 10.53730/ijhs.v6nS3.5187

Dhakate, H., Anasane, S., Shah, S., Thakare, R., & Rawat, S. G. (2024). "Enhancing Yoga Practice: Real-time Pose Analysis and Personalized Feedback," *2024 International Conference on Emerging Systems and Intelligent Computing (ESIC)*, Bhubaneswar, India, pp. 35-40, DOI: 10.1109/ESIC60604.2024.10481659

Dhanasekar, S., & Sindhu, S. (2025). "Asana AI – Yoga Pose Detection Using Pose Estimation and Real-Time Feedback System," *2025 International Conference on Computational Robotics, Testing and Engineering Evaluation (ICCRTEE)*, Virudhunagar, India, pp. 1-6, DOI: 10.1109/ICCRTEE64519.2025.11052949

Dhanyal, S. S., & Nandyal, S. S. (2023). Yoga pose annotation and classification by using time-distributed convolutional neural network. *Indonesian Journal of Electrical Engineering and Computer Science, 32*(3), 1639–1647. DOI: 10.11591/ijeecs.v32.i3.pp1639-1647

Dilip, D. K. A., & Prashant, D. D. (2023). *IMPORTANCE OFAAHAR VIHAR IN PCOD. 12*(13).

Divino, F. (2024). From meditation to techno-mindfulness: On the medicalization of contemplative practices and future prospects. *Histories, 4*(1), 125–143. DOI: 10.3390/histories4010008

Doshi, M., ... (2025). "Enhancing FMCG sales prediction using recurrent neural networks and economic indicators," *Parul University International Conference on Engineering and Technology 2025 (PiCET 2025)*, Hybrid Conference, Vadodara, India, pp. 1223-1230, DOI: 10.1049/icp.2025.1574

Drigas, A. S., & Karyotaki, M. (2019). A layered model of human consciousness. *International Journal of Recent Contributions from Engineering. Science & IT, 7*(3), 41–50. DOI: 10.3991/ijes.v7i3.11117

Duggal, A., Kumar, S., & Tripathi, P. (2025). Exploring AI Techniques for Yoga Image Classification: A Focus on Machine Learning and Deep Learning. In: *ICISCN* (Conference paper). DOI: 10.1109/ICISCN64258.2025.10934197

Duppala, V. R.. (2024). "Aatma Yoga: Automation of Yoga Pose Recognition and Recommendation using Deep Learning," *2024 International Conference on Inventive Computation Technologies (ICICT)*, Lalitpur, Nepal, pp. 1315-1322, DOI: 10.1109/ICICT60155.2024.10544761

Easwaran, E. (2007). *The Bhagavad Gita* (2nd ed.). Nilgiri Press.

Elavarasi, S. A., Ankit Kumar, P., & Jayanthi, J. "Development of Ai-Based Posture Monitoring System to Assist Yoga Training," *2023 International Conference on Research Methodologies in Knowledge Management, Artificial Intelligence and Telecommunication Engineering (RMKMATE)*, Chennai, India, 2023, pp. 1-4, DOI: 10.1109/RMKMATE59243.2023.10368735

Elavsky, S., & McAuley, E. (2007). Physical activity and mental health outcomes during menopause: A randomized controlled trial. *Annals of Behavioral Medicine : A Publication of the Society of Behavioral Medicine, 33*(2), 132–142. DOI: 10.1007/BF02879894 PMID: 17447865

Esteva, A., Robicquet, A., Ramsundar, B., Kuleshov, V., DePristo, M., Chou, K., Cui, C., Corrado, G., Thrun, S., & Dean, J. (2019). A guide to deep learning in healthcare. *Nature Medicine*, *25*(1), 24–29. DOI: 10.1038/s41591-018-0316-z PMID: 30617335

Ezer, T. S., Giron, J., Erel, H., & Zuckerman, O. (2024). Somaesthetic meditation wearable: Exploring the effect of targeted warmth technology on meditators' experiences. DOI: 10.1145/3613904.3642557

Farb, N. A. S., Segal, Z. V., Mayberg, H., Bean, J., McKeon, D., Fatima, Z., & Anderson, A. K. (2007). Attending to the present: Mindfulness meditation reveals distinct neural modes of self-reference. *Social Cognitive and Affective Neuroscience*, *2*(4), 313–322. DOI: 10.1093/scan/nsm030 PMID: 18985137

Feuerstein, G. (1998). *The Yoga tradition: Its history, literature, philosophy and practice*. Hohm Press.

Feuerstein, G. (2003). *The deeper dimension of yoga: Theory and practice*. Shambhala Publications.

Field, T. (2016). Yoga research review. *Complementary Therapies in Clinical Practice*, *24*, 145–161. DOI: 10.1016/j.ctcp.2016.06.005 PMID: 27502816

Floridi, L., Cowls, J., Beltrametti, M., Chatila, R., Chazerand, P., Dignum, V., Luetge, C., Madelin, R., Pagallo, U., Rossi, F., Schafer, B., Valcke, P., & Vayena, E. (2018). AI4People—An ethical framework for a good AI society. *Minds and Machines*, *28*(4), 689–707. DOI: 10.1007/s11023-018-9482-5 PMID: 30930541

Fonseca, A. A., Espinosa-Parra, I. M., Dávalos, M. B. M., & Montoya, C. D. C. R. (2025). Exploring experiences: A qualitative study on ai-enhanced mindfulness for neurodivergent individuals. *Journal-health education and welfare*. https://doi.org/ DOI: 10.35429/JHEW.2025.9.16.4.1.7

Gadhvi, R., & Desai, P. Siddharth (2026). PosePilot: An Edge-AI Solution for Posture Correction in Physical Exercises. *Lecture Notes in Computer Science*, 15938 LNCS, 208–219.

Gal, E., Irme, S., & Kube, T. (2024). Mechanisms of change in app-based mindfulness interventions: A systematic review. *Mindfulness*, *15*, 2105–2131. DOI: 10.1007/s12671-024-02426-w

Ganesh, K. and Ramudhin (2025), A. Leveraging AI to Mitigate Risks in Yoga Practice: A Real-Time Posture Correction Application. In Proceedings of the 12th International Conference on Sport Sciences Research and Technology Support (icSPORTS 2024), pages 241-250 ISBN: 978-989-758-719-1; ISSN: 2184-3201 DOI: DOI: 10.5220/0013063300003828

Garg, A. (2025). AI-Powered Yoga Pose Detection and Feedback System. *International Journal for Research in Applied Science and Engineering Technology*, *13*(5), 6224–6230. Advance online publication. DOI: 10.22214/ijraset.2025.70581

Garg, S., Saxena, A., & Gupta, R. (2023). Yoga pose classification: A CNN and MediaPipe inspired deep learning approach for real-world application. *Journal of Ambient Intelligence and Humanized Computing*, *14*(12), 16551–16562. Advance online publication. DOI: 10.1007/s12652-022-03910-0

Gayakwad, M. (2024). Web Service Implementation "AI Yoga Trainer Using Human Pose Estimation" for Web Discovery. *Journal of Electrical Systems*, *20*(2), 2167–2176. Advance online publication. DOI: 10.52783/jes.1985

Ghosh, S., Chanda, D., & Mukhopadhyay, C. (2025). Efficacy of wearable AI driven mindfulness practices in the management of stress. *Advances in computational intelligence and robotics book series*, 85-120. DOI: 10.4018/979-8-3373-0467-0.ch004

Gonem, S., Sherif, M., Taylor, J., Lord, W., & Bafadhel, M. (2020). Applications of artificial intelligence and machine learning in respiratory medicine. *Thorax*, *75*(8), 695–701. DOI: 10.1136/thoraxjnl-2020-214556 PMID: 32409611

Gosalia, M., Dedhia, R., Doshi, S., Sharma, R., & Mangla, M. (2024). "Individualized Guidance in Yoga Practice: A Comparative Analysis of Technology Solutions," *2024 International Conference on Electrical Electronics and Computing Technologies (ICEECT)*, Greater Noida, India, pp. 1-6, DOI: 10.1109/ICEECT61758.2024.10739307

Gowrish, G., Vineeth, Y. S., & Thenmozhi, M. (2024). "AI Powered gym tracker using AI Pose estimation," *2024 2nd International Conference on Networking and Communications (ICNWC)*, Chennai, India, pp. 1-6, DOI: 10.1109/ICNWC60771.2024.10537312

Goyal, M., Singh, S., Sibinga, E. M., Gould, N. F., Rowland-Seymour, A., Sharma, R., Berger, Z., Sleicher, D., Maron, D. D., Shihab, H. M., Ranasinghe, P. D., Linn, S., Saha, S., Bass, E. B., & Haythornthwaite, J. A. (2014). Meditation programs for psychological stress and well-being: A systematic review and meta-analysis. *JAMA Internal Medicine*, *174*(3), 357–368. DOI: 10.1001/jamainternmed.2013.13018 PMID: 24395196

Gupta, H., Arora, P., & Malhotra, S. (2021). Privacy and security challenges in AI-driven healthcare monitoring systems. *Journal of Information Security and Applications*, *58*, 102765. DOI: 10.1016/j.jisa.2021.102765

Hasan, M. K., Azad, M. K., & Hossain, M. S. (2025). 'Dharana' as the Gateway: Meditative Wit(H)Nessing and the transformation of trauma in Han Kang's The White Book. *INTERNATIONAL JOURNAL OF MULTIDISCIPLINARY RESEARCH AND ANALYSIS, 8*(4). Advance online publication. DOI: 10.47191/ijmra/v8-i04-30

Hirapara, J.. (2025). "Precision Agriculture: Forecasting Crop Prices Through Advanced Data Mining and Machine Learning Models," *2025 International Conference on Networks & Advances in Computational Technologies (NetACT)*, Trivandrum, India, pp. 1-6, DOI: 10.1109/NetACT65906.2025.11188961

Hirpara, J., Doshi, M., Patel, A., & Choudhury, K. (2025). A Study on Machine Learning Algorithms: Forecasting Crop Prices. In Rajagopal, S., Popat, K., Meva, D., Bajeja, S., & Mudholkar, P. (Eds.), *Artificial Intelligence Based Smart and Secured Applications. ASCIS 2024. Communications in Computer and Information Science* (Vol. 2427). Springer., DOI: 10.1007/978-3-031-86299-1_4

Hochreiter, S., & Schmidhuber, J. (1997). Long short-term memory. *Neural Computation, 9*(8), 1735–1780. DOI: 10.1162/neco.1997.9.8.1735 PMID: 9377276

Ihde, D. (1990). *Technology and the lifeworld: From garden to earth.* Indiana University Press. DOI: 10.2979/3108.0

Irfan, M., Ali, A., & Rehman, A. U. (2025). Integrating artificial intelligence with naturopathy and yoga for chronic disease management: A systematic review. *Journal of Integrative and Complementary Medicine, 31*(2), 115–134.

Irfan, N., Zafar, S., Shakil, K. A., Wani, M. A., Kumar, S. N., Jaiganesh, A., & Abubeker, K. M. (2025, July 4). Integrating AI predictive analytics with naturopathic and yoga-based interventions in a data-driven preventive model to improve maternal mental health and pregnancy outcomes. *Scientific Reports, 15*(1), 23878. DOI: 10.1038/s41598-025-07885-8 PMID: 40615420

Jain, I., Srivastava, R., Srivastava, V., Sinha, V., & Juneja, A. (2025). Ethical Decision-Making in Yoga Posture Detection through AI: Fostering Responsible Technology Integration. Ethical Decision-Making Using Artificial Intelligence: Challenges, Solutions and Applications, 99-123.

Jerath, R., Edry, J. W., Barnes, V. A., & Jerath, V. (2015). Physiology of long pranayamic breathing. *Medical Hypotheses, 85*(5), 486–496. DOI: 10.1016/j.mehy.2015.07.004 PMID: 16624497

Jo, B. J., & Kim, S. K. (2022). Comparative Analysis of OpenPose, PoseNet, and MoveNet Models for Pose Estimation in Mobile Devices. *TS. Traitement du Signal, 39*(1), 119–124. Advance online publication. DOI: 10.18280/ts.390111

Jorge, M. P., Santaella, D. F., Pontes, I. M. O., Shiramizu, V. K. M., Nascimento, E. B., Cabral, A., Lemos, T. M. A. M., Silva, R. H., & Ribeiro, A. M. (2016). Hatha Yoga practice decreases menopause symptoms and improves quality of life: A randomized controlled trial. *Complementary Therapies in Medicine*, *26*, 128–135. DOI: 10.1016/j.ctim.2016.03.014 PMID: 27261993

Joshi, A., Kiran, R., Raj, R., & Agarwal, R. (2020). Stress management of engineering students through deep breathing yoga. *International Journal of Work Organisation and Emotion*, *11*(2), 140. Advance online publication. DOI: 10.1504/IJWOE.2020.110625

Kabat-Zinn, J. (2003). Mindfulness-based interventions in context: Past, present, and future. *Clinical Psychology : a Publication of the Division of Clinical Psychology of the American Psychological Association*, *10*(2), 144–156. DOI: 10.1093/clipsy.bpg016

Kaplan, J. (2016). *Artificial intelligence: What everyone needs to know*. Oxford University Press. DOI: 10.1093/wentk/9780190602383.001.0001

Kaprekar, H., Thakurta, A. G., & Shirsekar, S. S. (2024). Virtual reality makes mindfulness accessible. https://doi.org/DOI: 10.58532/V3BDSO24P1CH1

Keesara, S., Jonas, A., & Schulman, K. (2020). Covid-19 and health care's digital revolution. *The New England Journal of Medicine*, *382*(23), e82. DOI: 10.1056/NEJMp2005835 PMID: 32240581

Keny, V. (2025). Can artificial intelligence experience spirituality?. *Journal of advances in science and technology, 22* (2). DOI: 10.29070/3t5w4a12

Khan, M. N. H., Creswell, D., & Albert, J. O'CONNELL, P., Fallon, S., Polowitz, M., Xu, X., &Islam, B. (2025). Mindfulness meditation and respiration: Accelerometer-based respiration rate and mindfulness progress estimation to enhance app engagement and mindfulness skills. *Proceedings of the ACM on interactive, mobile, wearable and ubiquitous technologies, 9*, 95:1-95:32. https://doi.org//arxiv.2507.17688DOI: 10.48550

Kim, D.-K., Rhee, J.-H., & Kang, S. W. (2014). *Reorganization of the brain and heart rhythm during autogenic meditation*. https://www.frontiersin.org/journals/integrative-neuroscience/articles/10.3389/fnint.2013.00109/full

Kim, H., Zala, A., Burri, G., & Bansal, M. (2021).. . *FIXMYPOSE: Pose Correctional Captioning and Retrieval. AAAI, 14B*, 13161–13170.

Kirk, M. A., Taha, B., Dang, K., McCague, H. P., Hatzinakos, D., Katz, J., & Ritvo, P. (2022). A Web-Based Cognitive Behavioral Therapy, Mindfulness Meditation, and Yoga Intervention for Posttraumatic Stress Disorder: Single-Arm Experimental Clinical Trial. *JMIR Mental Health*, *9*(2), e26479. Advance online publication. DOI: 10.2196/26479 PMID: 34499613

Kishore, D. M., Bindu, S., & Manjunath, N. K. (2022). Smart yoga instructor for guiding and correcting yoga postures in real time. *International Journal of Yoga*, *15*(3), 254–261. DOI: 10.4103/ijoy.ijoy_137_22 PMID: 36949838

Kumar Mishra, A., & Mishra, K. (2024). YogaSiddhi: AI-Powered Pose Analysis using MoveNet for Yoga Refinement. *Article in International Journal of Computer Applications, 186*(8).

Kumar, A., Sankhyan, S., Tripathi, K., Rao, A. K., Bhavsar, A., & Dutt, V. (2024). Vrzm: Exploring the psycho-physiological benefits of zen meditation in immersive environments. DOI: 10.1109/ISMAR-Adjunct64951.2024.00063

Kumar, A., Sankhyan, S., Tripathi, K., Thakur, S., Bhavsar, A., & Dutt, V. (2024). Vrzm: Exploring the effect of zen meditation on eeg patterns in immersive environments. DOI: 10.1109/SMC54092.2024.10831479

Kumar, D., Verma, C., & Illés, Z. (2025). Federated learning with explainable AI for liver disease prediction: A privacy-preserving approach, Intelligence-Based Medicine,Volume 12, 2025, 100285, ISSN 2666-5212, DOI: 10.1016/j.ibmed.2025.100285

Kumar, N., & Singhal, D. (2024). Empowering mental well-being: Ai-guided self-recognition and support. *International research journal of computer science, 11* (05),465-470. DOI: 10.26562/irjcs.2024.v1105.06

Kumar, D.. (2025). *Federated learning with explainable AI for disease prediction.* ScienceDirect.

Kumar, R., & Srivastava, S. (2023). Wearable sensor data for stress and affective state monitoring: Challenges and opportunities. *Sensors (Basel)*, *23*(4), 2215. PMID: 36850813

Kumar, S., Mehta, A., & Joshi, V. (2021). Wearable sensor-based health monitoring systems using Internet of Things and Artificial Intelligence. *Journal of Healthcare Engineering*, *2021*, 1–12. DOI: 10.1155/2021/9983652

Labde, S. (2025). Real Time Yoga Posture Recognition and Correction. *International Journal for Research in Applied Science and Engineering Technology*, *13*(5), 4922–4927. Advance online publication. DOI: 10.22214/ijraset.2025.71355

LeCun, Y., Bengio, Y., & Hinton, G. (2015). Deep learning. *Nature, 521*(7553), 436–444. DOI: 10.1038/nature14539 PMID: 26017442

Liu, J., & Zhou, Z. (2024). "A Real-Time Yoga Instruction Method Based on Lightweight Human Pose Estimation," *2024 4th International Conference on Computer Science, Electronic Information Engineering and Intelligent Control Technology (CEI)*, Guangzhou, China, pp. 122-125, DOI: 10.1109/CEI63587.2024.10871775

Long, C., Jo, E., & Nam, Y. (2022). Development of a yoga posture coaching system using an interactive display based on transfer learning. *The Journal of Supercomputing*, *78*(4), 5269–5284. DOI: 10.1007/s11227-021-04076-w PMID: 34566258

Loughnane, C., Laiti, J., O'Donovan, R., & Dunne, P. J. (2025). Systematic review exploring human, AI, and hybrid health coaching in digital health interventions: trends, engagement, and lifestyle outcomes. In *Frontiers in Digital Health* (Vol. 7). DOI: 10.3389/fdgth.2025.1536416

Lu, H. B., Ma, R. C., Yin, Y. Y., Song, C. Y., Yang, T. T., & Xie, J. (2024). Clinical Indicators of Effects of Yoga Breathing Exercises on Patients with Lung Cancer after Surgical Resection: A Randomized Controlled Trial. *Cancer Nursing*, *47*(3), E151–E158. Advance online publication. DOI: 10.1097/NCC.0000000000001208 PMID: 36716034

Lukoff, K., Yu, C., Kientz, J., & Hiniker, A. (2018). What makes smartphone use meaningful or meaningless? *Proceedings of the ACM on Interactive, Mobile, Wearable and Ubiquitous Technologies*, *2*(1), 1–26. DOI: 10.1145/3191754

Luo, Y. (2025). How AI transforms mental wellness: From applications to essential questions. https://doi.org/DOI: 10.59350/mn6az-tfm26

Luo, C., Chu, X., & Yuille, A. (2018). Orinet: A fully convolutional network for 3D human pose estimation. *British Machine Vision Conference 2018, BMVC 2018.*

Lupton, D. (2016). *The quantified self: A sociology of self-tracking*. Polity Press.

Madhu, S., Kumar, P., & Chandra, S. (2025). Ensemble Learning based EEG Classification – Investigating the Effects of Combined Yoga and Rajyog Meditation. *Journal of Scientific and Industrial Research, 84*(1), 36–47.

Mallinson, J., & Singleton, M. (2017). *Roots of yoga*. Penguin Classics.

Manikumar, T., Kankanala, J., Kishore, K., & Sriram, L. (2024). "Real Time Yoga Posture Location and Assessment Utilizing Deep Learning," *2024 International Conference on Sustainable Communication Networks and Application (ICSCNA)*, Theni, India, pp. 751-756, DOI: 10.1109/ICSCNA63714.2024.10863926

Manisha, G., Meenakshi, N. A., Srinithi, S., Murugesan, R., & Sheikh Mastan, S. A. R. (2025, June). VR-based yoga posture detection, classification and correction. *ICTACT Journal on Data Science and Machine Learning*, *6*(3), 829–834. DOI: 10.21917/ijdsml.2025.0166

Manoni, A., Loreti, F., Radicioni, V., Pellegrino, D., Della Torre, L., Gumiero, A., Halicki, D., Palange, P., & Lukowicz, P. (2020). A machine learning approach for monitoring respiratory events during sleep. *MDPI Sensors*, *20*(20), 5785. DOI: 10.3390/s20205785

Marade, A., Suvarna, K., Chaudhari, P., & Bhandiwad, P. V. (2025). Spiritual.ai: An ai-driven platform for enhancing mental, emotional, and spiritual well-being. *International Journal for Research in Applied Science and Engineering Technology*, *13*(4), 4211–4216. DOI: 10.22214/ijraset.2025.64703

Mathur, D. A. (2023). *Endowing to good Health: A Case Study on Managing PCOD through Yoga. 10*(6).

McCarren, L., & Kuoppamäki, S. (2024). The use of a voice-based digital mindfulness app to facilitate self-perceived bodily and emotional well-being among older adults: A mixed method study. DOI: 10.2196/preprints.67533

Meghana, J. H., Chethan, H. K., Santhosh Kumar, K. S., & Shiva Prakash, S. P. S. (2025). Comprehensive Analysis of Pose Estimation and Machine Learning Classifiers for Precise Yoga Pose Detection and Classification. *Procedia Computer Science*, *258*, 3345–3356. DOI: 10.1016/j.procs.2025.04.592

Meng, X., & Liu, Z. (2025, May 27). Yoga pose recognition using dual structure convolutional neural network. *PeerJ. Computer Science*, *11*, e2907. https://www.cloudthat.com/resources/blog/the-ethics-of-ai-addressing-bias-privacy-and-accountability-in-machine-learning. DOI: 10.7717/peerj-cs.2907 PMID: 40567706

Mitsea, E., Drigas, A., & Skianis, C. (2023). Digitally Assisted Mindfulness in Training Self-Regulation Skills for Sustainable Mental Health: A Systematic Review. In *Behavioral Sciences* (Vol. 13, Issue 12). DOI: 10.3390/bs13121008

Mitsea, E., Drigas, A., & Skianis, C. (2024). Artificial intelligence, immersive technologies, and neuro-technologies in breathing interventions for mental and emotional health: A systematic review. *Electronics (Basel)*, *13*(12), 2253–2253. DOI: 10.3390/electronics13122253

Mittal, A., Krishna, N. R., Singh, D., & Kavuri, V. (2025). Study Protocol for a Yoga-Based Lifestyle Modification Program for Leucorrhea Disorders. *Cureus*. Advance online publication. DOI: 10.7759/cureus.78294 PMID: 40027048

Mohan, V., Srivastava, S., & Kiran, M. (2022). Deep learning-based yoga posture recognition system. *International Journal of Engineering Research & Technology (Ahmedabad)*, *11*(5), 134–140.

Mohseni, M., Eghbali, M., Bahrami, H., Dastaran, F., & Amini, L. (2021). Yoga Effects on Anthropometric Indices and Polycystic Ovary Syndrome Symptoms in Women Undergoing Infertility Treatment: A Randomized Controlled Clinical Trial. *Evidence-Based Complementary and Alternative Medicine : eCAM*, *5564824*, 1–9. Advance online publication. DOI: 10.1155/2021/5564824 PMID: 34221076

Muktibodhananda, S. (2006). *Hatha yoga pradipika* (4th ed.). Bihar School of Yoga.

Nalbant, G., Hassanein, Z. M., Lewis, S., & Chattopadhyay, K. (2022). Content, Structure, and delivery Characteristics of Yoga Interventions for Managing Hypertension: A Systematic Review and Meta-Analysis of Randomized Controlled Trials. *Frontiers in Public Health*, *10*, 846231. Advance online publication. DOI: 10.3389/fpubh.2022.846231 PMID: 35419342

Narayanan, M. M. (2025). Yoga AI - Integrating artificial intelligence with yoga and therapy for personalized healthcare. *Annals of Geriatric Education and Medical Sciences*, *11*(2), 68–70. Advance online publication. DOI: 10.18231/j.agems.2024.015

Narimani, M., & Naeim, M. (2025). Artificial intelligence in mental health: Integrating opportunities and challenges of multimodal deep learning for mental disorder prevention and treatment. *Annals of Medicine and Surgery (London)*, *87*(9), 5757–5761. Advance online publication. DOI: 10.1097/MS9.0000000000003624 PMID: 40901142

National Center for Complementary and Integrative Health. (2024). *Yoga: What the science says*. National Institutes of Health. https://www.nccih.nih.gov/health/yoga-what-the-science-says

Nesin, J., & Sathyamoorthy, G. (2025). Psychoneuroimmunology of yoga and meditation: Mechanisms and clinical applications. In Sharma, S., & Gupta, R. (Eds.), *Indian Knowledge Systems in Modern Healthcare* (pp. 112–145). IGI Global.

Nidhi, R., Padmalatha, V., Nagarathna, R., & Amritanshu, R. (2012). Effect of holistic yoga program on anxiety symptoms in adolescent girls with polycystic ovarian syndrome: A randomized control trial. *International Journal of Yoga*, *5*(2), 112–117. DOI: 10.4103/0973-6131.98223 PMID: 22869994

Nidhi, R., Padmalatha, V., Nagarathna, R., & Ram, A. (2012). Effect of a yoga program on glucose metabolism and blood lipid levels in adolescent girls with polycystic ovary syndrome. *International Journal of Gynaecology and Obstetrics : The Official Organ of the International Federation of Gynaecology and Obstetrics, 118*(1), 37–41. DOI: 10.1016/j.ijgo.2012.01.027 PMID: 22507264

Olivelle, P. (1996). *Upanishads*. Oxford University Press.

Omotoyosi Adeyemi, J. (2024). Enhancing Elderly Wellness through AI-Powered Yoga and Exercise Support Systems. *Biomedical Journal of Scientific & Technical Research, 54*(4). Advance online publication. DOI: 10.26717/BJSTR.2024.54.008579

Özsezer, G., & Mermer, G. (2025). Real-Time Prediction of Correct Yoga Asanas in Healthy Individuals With Artificial Intelligence Techniques: A Systematic Review for Nursing. *Nursing Open, 12*(8), e70278. DOI: 10.1002/nop2.70278 PMID: 40768382

Özsezer, G., & Mermer, G. (2025). Real-time prediction of correct yoga asanas using artificial intelligence. *Nursing Open*. PMID: 40768382

Pal, R., Adhikari, D., Heyat, M. B. B., Ullah, I., & You, Z. (2023, April 9). Yoga Meets Intelligent Internet of Things: Recent Challenges and Future Directions. *Bioengineering (Basel, Switzerland), 10*(4), 459. DOI: 10.3390/bioengineering10040459 PMID: 37106646

Pandey, P. K., Gupta, P., Chaudhary, S., Miyapuram, K. P., & Lomas, D. (2022). Real-time sensing and neurofeedback for practicing meditation using simultaneous eeg and eye tracking. https://doi.org/DOI: 10.1109/TENSYMP54529.2022.9864414

Parab, N. P., Rampurawala, A. A., Khade, S. S., & Mahato, M. (2023). Personalised AI Based Yoga-Pose Recommendation System Using Game Theory. In: *ICACTA* (Conference paper). DOI: 10.1109/ICACTA58201.2023.10393658

Parashar, D., Mishra, O., Sharma, K., & Kukker, A. (2023). Improved yoga pose detection using MediaPipe and MoveNet in a deep learning model. *Revue d'Intelligence Artificielle, 37*(5), 1197–1202. DOI: 10.18280/ria.370511

Park, C., Youn, I., & Han, S. (2022). Single-lead ECG based autonomic nervous system assessment for meditation monitoring. https://www.nature.com/articles/s41598-022-27121-x

Patel, R., & Sharma, P. (2022). Artificial intelligence techniques for yoga posture detection and correction. *International Journal of Advanced Computer Science and Applications, 13*(4), 210–218.

Patel, S., Park, H., Bonato, P., Chan, L., & Rodgers, M. (2012). A review of wearable sensors and systems with application in rehabilitation. *Journal of Neuroengineering and Rehabilitation*, *9*(1), 21. DOI: 10.1186/1743-0003-9-21 PMID: 22520559

Pawar, M. P. U., & Kulkarni, M. H. H. (2025). Real Time Yoga Pose Detection Using AI. *International Journal of Latest Technology in Engineering Management & Applied Science*, *14*(10), 151–155. DOI: 10.51583/IJLTEMAS.2025.1410000020

Peake, J. M., Kerr, G., & Sullivan, J. P. (2018). A critical review of consumer wearables, mobile applications, and equipment for providing biofeedback, monitoring stress, and sleep in physically active populations. *Frontiers in Physiology*, *9*, 743. DOI: 10.3389/fphys.2018.00743 PMID: 30002629

Purser, R. (2019). *McMindfulness: How mindfulness became the new capitalist spirituality*. Repeater Books.

Radhakrishnan, S. (1948). *The Bhagavadgita*. George Allen & Unwin.

Raj, gokul, Ramakrishnan, R., Parasuraman, T., Ganesh, R., & Natesamurthy, V. (2025). *Pose Estimation in Yoga: A Bibliometric Exploration of Technological Advancements in Sports Sciences | Journal of Neonatal Surgery*. https://www.jneonatalsurg.com/index.php/jns/article/view/1689?utm_source=chatgpt.com

Rajendran, A. K., & Sethuraman, S. C. (2025). YogAngleNet: Body angle-based yogic posture classification approach using MediaPipe from single-person images. *Turkish Journal of Electrical Engineering and Computer Sciences*, *33*(5), 613–630. DOI: 10.55730/1300-0632.4147

Rajgure, E. G., & Patidar, R. (2025). The Scientific Analysis on Effective Yoga Posture Recognition Techniques. *Lecture Notes in Electrical Engineering, 1211 LNEE*. DOI: 10.1007/978-981-97-4359-9_13

Rajput, G. S., Khan, M. A., Jain, T., Khandelwal, T., & Sharma, U. (2024). Exploring Chakra Balancing Practices in Software Applications. In: *ACROSET* (Conference paper). DOI: 10.1109/ACROSET62108.2024.10743620

Rao, S., & Nishmitha, B. A. Dinamani, C. T, D. D. N and Rakshitha. (2024). "TechAsanaAdvancer Technical Mastery of Yoga Poses with AI," *2024 Second International Conference on Advances in Information Technology (ICAIT)*, Chikkamagaluru, Karnataka, India, pp. 1-7, DOI: 10.1109/ICAIT61638.2024.10690406

Rao, K., Prakash, M., & Iyer, S. (2020). Real-time human pose estimation and yoga monitoring using computer vision techniques. *Procedia Computer Science*, *171*, 1450–1459. DOI: 10.1016/j.procs.2020.04.155

Reyes, A. P., Jefferson Gabutan, M., Villacarlos, A. P., Lyn Sta Romana, C., & Aliac, C. J. (2023). "Motion: A Mobile Application for Yoga Pose Accuracy and Consistency," *2023 3rd International Conference on Electrical, Computer, Communications and Mechatronics Engineering (ICECCME)*, Tenerife, Canary Islands, Spain, pp. 1-6, DOI: 10.1109/ICECCME57830.2023.10252614

Reyes, A. P., Gabutan, M. J., Villacarlos, A. P., Romana, C. L. S., & Bacallan, N. "A Yoga Pose Evaluation System for Enhanced Yoga Education," *2023 International Conference on Computer Applications Technology (CCAT)*, Guiyang, China, 2023, pp. 80-85, DOI: 10.1109/CCAT59108.2023.00022

Rieke, N., Hancox, J., & Li, W.. (2020). The future of digital health with federated learning. npj. *Digital Medicine*, *3*(1), 119. PMID: 33015372

Rony, M. K. K., Parvin, M. R., & Ferdousi, S. (2023). Advancing nursing practice with artificial intelligence: Enhancing preparedness for the future. *Nursing Open*, *11*(1), nop2.2070. Advance online publication. DOI: 10.1002/nop2.2070 PMID: 38268252

Rosario, C. D. P. D., Fernández, L., Agustin, V. A., Centeno, C. J., Mangrobang, M. B., &Cortez, D. M. A. (2024). Ai-powered intelligent mindfulness-based cognitive therapy companion for emotion recognition and context-aware therapy. DOI: 10.1109/ISAS64331.2024.10845635

S Bhat, G., IL, S., Hariharan, H., & Swamy, H. (2023). Yoga AI Assistant with ReactJS. *INTERANTIONAL JOURNAL OF SCIENTIFIC RESEARCH IN ENGINEERING AND MANAGEMENT, 07*(04). DOI: 10.55041/IJSREM18878

Sabry, F., Eltaras, T., Labda, W., Alzoubi, K., & Malluhi, Q. (2022). Machine learning for healthcare wearable devices: The big picture. *Journal of Healthcare Engineering*, *4653923*, 1–25. Advance online publication. DOI: 10.1155/2022/4653923 PMID: 35480146

Saeidnia, H. R., Firuzpour, F., Kozak, M., & Majd, H. S. (2025). Advancing cancer diagnosis and treatment: Integrating image analysis and AI algorithms for enhanced clinical practice. *Artificial Intelligence Review*, *58*(4), 105. Advance online publication. DOI: 10.1007/s10462-025-11117-w

Sahu, V. S. (2026). The changing scenario of yoga education with artificial intelligence. *Research Hub.*, *07*(1), 230–233. DOI: 10.63665/rh.v7i2.39

Saini, N. (2024). Exploring The Synergy Of Ai And Yogic Practices: A Future-Oriented Approach For Holistic Wellbeing. *Educational Administration: Theory and Practice*, *30*(5), 15412–15420. DOI: 10.53555/kuey.v30i5.9101

Sak, J., & Suchodolska, M. (2021). Artificial Intelligence in Nutrients Science Research: A review. *Nutrients*, *13*(2), 322. DOI: 10.3390/nu13020322 PMID: 33499405

Sapci, A. H., & Sapci, H. A. (2020). Artificial Intelligence Education and Tools for Medical and Health Informatics Students: Systematic review. *JMIR Medical Education*, *6*(1), e19285. Advance online publication. DOI: 10.2196/19285 PMID: 32602844

Sapna, D. (2025). Yoga and Artificial Intelligence: A Review of The Potential Applications of AI in Yoga Research and Practice for Neurological Disorders. *Indian Journal of Ayurveda & Alternative Medicines*, *2*(1), 8–14.

Saravanapandian, M. J. B, K. B, V. S, J. R. J. Shiney and S. S. S. (2025). "Smart Yoga Mat: An AI-Integrated Affordable Yoga Mat for Personalized Guidance and Progress Tracking," *2025 7th International Conference on Signal Processing, Computing and Control (ISPCC)*, SOLAN, India, pp. 858-862, DOI: 10.1109/ISPCC66872.2025.11039326

Saxena, P., Sharma, V., Yadav, A., Singh, R. P., & Laiphrakpam, L. D. (2025). An Algorithmic and Machine Learning Approach for Yoga Asanas Feedback. In: *ISACC* (Conference paper), 7–12. DOI: 10.1109/ISACC65211.2025.10969307

Selvaraj, V., Vanitha, J., Dhanaraj, F. M., Sekar, P., & Babu, A. R. (2020). Impact of yoga and exercises on polycystic ovarian syndrome risk among adolescent schoolgirls in South India. *Health Science Reports*, *3*(4), e212. DOI: 10.1002/hsr2.212 PMID: 33305014

Selye, H. (1956). *The stress of life*. McGraw-Hill.

Sengar, S. S., Hasan, A. B., Kumar, S., & Carroll, F. (2024). Generative artificial intelligence: A systematic review and applications. *Multimedia Tools and Applications*, *84*(21), 23661–23700. DOI: 10.1007/s11042-024-20016-1

Seoni, S., Jahmunah, V., Salvi, M., Barua, P. D., Molinari, F., & Acharya, U. R. (2023). Application of uncertainty quantification to artificial intelligence in healthcare: A review of last decade (2013–2023). *Computers in Biology and Medicine*, *165*, 107441. Advance online publication. DOI: 10.1016/j.compbiomed.2023.107441 PMID: 37683529

Shajari, S.. (2023). The emergence of AI-based wearable sensors for digital healthcare applications. *Sensors (Basel)*, *23*(23), 9498. DOI: 10.3390/s23239498 PMID: 38067871

Shamekhi, A., & Bickmore, T. (2015). Breathe with me: A virtual meditation coach. DOI: 10.1007/978-3-319-21996-7_29

Shankar, R., Devi, F., & Xu, Q. (2025). Mindfulness-based interventions using artificial intelligence: A systematic review protocol. DOI: 10.1101/2025.06.20.25329981

Sharma, H. K., Choudhury, T., Mahapatra, S., Satish Kumar, G. A. E. S., & Maganti, S. B. (2024). Deep Learning based approach for Prediction of Yoga Posture using Yoga Asana Images. *AIP Conference Proceedings*, *2942*(1), 20006. DOI: 10.1063/5.0197215

Sharma, P., & Yadav, R. (2024). Artificial intelligence in yoga therapy: A transformative approach to holistic health management. In *Advances in computational intelligence for healthcare* (pp. 215–234). Springer., DOI: 10.1007/978-3-031-60542-7_11

Shih, C.-L., Liu, J.-Y., Anggraini, I. T., Xiao, Y., Funabiki, N., & Fan, C.-P. (2024). *"Difficulty Evaluation of Yoga Poses by Angular Velocity and Body Area Calculation for GPU-Based Yoga Self-Practice System," 2024 IEEE Gaming, Entertainment, and Media Conference*. GEM., DOI: 10.1109/GEM61861.2024.10585480

Shourie, P., Anand, V., Upadhyay, D., Devliyal, S., & Gupta, S. (2024) "YogaPoseVision: MobileNetV3-Powered CNN for Yoga Pose Identification," *2024 7th International Conference on Circuit Power and Computing Technologies (ICCPCT)*, Kollam, India, pp. 659-663, DOI: 10.1109/ICCPCT61902.2024.10673072

Singh, B., & Kaunert, C. (2024). Augmented reality and virtual reality modules for mindfulness. *Advances in medical technologies and clinical practice book series*,111-128. https://doi.org/DOI: 10.4018/979-8-3693-1123-3.ch007

Singh, S., Pandey, P. K., Chaudhary, S., Miyapuram, K. P., & Lomas, J. D. (2022). Towards the development of personalized and generalized interfaces for brain signals across different styles of meditation. DOI: 10.1145/3571600.3571656

Singh, D., & Verma, N. (2023). Machine learning approaches for personalized yoga recommendation systems. *International Journal of Intelligent Systems and Applications*, *15*(2), 45–56.

Singleton, M. (2010). *Yoga body: The origins of modern posture practice*. Oxford University Press. DOI: 10.1093/acprof:oso/9780195395358.001.0001

Sinha, N., & Sinha, R. K. (2024, September-December). Harnessing the Potential of Artificial Intelligence in Yoga Therapy. *International Journal of Yoga*, *17*(3), 242–245. DOI: 10.4103/ijoy.ijoy_124_24 PMID: 39959510

Sinpichetkorn, T., Chaunchaiyakul, R., Yang, A. L., Lin, Y. Y., & Masodsai, K. (2022). Effects of Vinyasa Yoga on Stress and Health Benefits in Office Workers. *Journal of Exercise Physiology Online*, *25*(4).

Skelly, A. C., Chou, R., Dettori, J. R., Turner, J. A., Friedly, J. L., Rundell, S. D., Fu, R., Brodt, E. D., Wasson, N., Winter, C., & Ferguson, A. J. R. (2018). *Noninvasive nonpharmacological treatment for chronic pain: A systematic review* (Comparative Effectiveness Review No. 209). Agency for Healthcare Research and Quality. DOI: 10.23970/AHRQEPCCER209

Soni, R., & Muniyandi, M. (2019). Breath Rate Variability: A Novel Measure to Study the Meditation Effects. *International Journal of Yoga, 12*(1), 45–54. DOI: 10.4103/ijoy.IJOY_27_17 PMID: 30692783

Suryawanshi, Y., Gunjal, N., Kanorewala, B., & Patil, K. (2023). Yoga dataset: A resource for computer vision-based analysis of Yoga asanas. *Data in Brief, 48*, 109257. DOI: 10.1016/j.dib.2023.109257 PMID: 37383745

Swain, D., Satapathy, S., Acharya, B., Shukla, M., Gerogiannis, V. C., Kanavos, A., & Giakovis, D. (2022). Deep Learning Models for Yoga Pose Monitoring. *Algorithms, 15*(11), 403. Advance online publication. DOI: 10.3390/a15110403

Talaat, A. S. (2023). Novel deep learning models for yoga pose estimator. *SN Applied Sciences, 5*(12), 341. Advance online publication. DOI: 10.1007/s42452-023-05581-8

Telles, S., Raghavendra, B. R., Naveen, K. V., Manjunath, N. K., Kumar, S., & Subramanya, P. (2012). Changes in autonomic variables following two meditative states described in yoga texts. *Journal of Alternative and Complementary Medicine (New York, N.Y.), 19*(1), 35–42. DOI: 10.1089/acm.2011.0282 PMID: 22946453

Telles, S., Singh, N., Gupta, R. K., & Balkrishna, A. (2016). A selective review of dharana and dhyana in healthy participants. *Journal of Ayurveda and Integrative Medicine, 7*(4), 255–260. DOI: 10.1016/j.jaim.2016.09.004 PMID: 27889426

Thakur, K. (2025). INDIAN KNOWLEDGE TRADITIONS: INTEGRATING MIND, BODY & SPIRIT FOR HOLISTIC WELLNESS. *International Journal of Research and Analytical Reviews, 12*(2). Advance online publication. DOI: 10.56975/ijrar.v12i2.312734

Tripathi, A., Tyagi, A., Dubey, A., Vijh, S., & Verma, P. (2025). Enhancing Virtual Yoga Training: Real-time Pose Assessment with Voice-guided Accuracy Feedback. In: *ICETM* (Conference paper).

Tripathi, R. L. (2025). AI meets mindfulness: Redefining spirituality and meditation in the digital age. https://doi.org/DOI: 10.53032/tvcr/2025.v7n1.03

Tripathi, S. M. (2021). Yogic theory of consciousness and its neuroscientific correlates: Chitta, vritti, and the default mode network. *Journal of Consciousness Studies, 28*(5–6), 112–145.

Tripathi, S. M. (2021). Yogic theory of consciousness and its neuroscientific correlates: Chitta, Vritti, and the default mode network. *Journal of Consciousness Studies, 28*(5–6), 112–145.

Tripathi, V., & Bharadwaj, P. (2021). Neuroscience of the yogic theory of consciousness. *Neuroscience of Consciousness, 2021*(2), niab030. Advance online publication. DOI: 10.1093/nc/niab030 PMID: 34925910

Tunduny, T., & Shibwabo, B. (2026). Explainable AI Approaches in Federated Learning: Systematic Review. *JMIR AI, 5*, e69985. https://ai.jmir.org/2026/1/e69985. DOI: 10.2196/69985 PMID: 41632959

Uma, G. (2024). *An Analytical Study about Awareness and Knowledge on PCOD among Coimbatore People. 1043.*

Upadhyay, A., Basha, N. K., & Ananthakrishnan, B. (2023). Deep learning-based yoga posture recognition using the Y_PN-MSSD model for yoga practitioners. *Health Care, 11*(4), 609. DOI: 10.3390/healthcare11040609 PMID: 36833142

Vasu, R. B. S. (2003). *The Shiva Samhita.* Munshiram Manoharlal. (Original work published 1914)

Vats, S., & Mehta, S. (2024). “Advances in Yoga Training Tools: A CNN-RF Based Pose Identification System,” *2024 15th International Conference on Computing Communication and Networking Technologies (ICCCNT)*, Kamand, India, pp. 1-6, DOI: 10.1109/ICCCNT61001.2024.10725347

Vivekanandha, S., Bhargavi, N., Srinivas, I., Harika, K., & Raju, K. (2025). Enhancing Yoga with AI: Accurate Pose Detection Using Machine Learning. *International Journal of Computer Techniques, 12.*

Walia, A. (2024). Integrating classical yoga and modern psychology: Insights from neuroimaging and AI on mind transformation. *International Journal for Multidisciplinary Research, 6*(5), 27627. Advance online publication. DOI: 10.36948/ijfmr.2024.v06i05.27627

Walsh, K. M., Saab, B. J., & Farb, N. A. S. (2019). Effects of a mindfulness meditation app on subjective well-being: Active randomized controlled trial and experience sampling study. *JMIR Mental Health, 6*(1), e10844. DOI: 10.2196/10844 PMID: 30622094

Wang, H. (2021). Neural Network-Oriented Big Data Model for Yoga Movement Recognition. *Computational Intelligence and Neuroscience, 2021*(1), 4334024. DOI: 10.1155/2021/4334024 PMID: 34751226

Wang, L., Guo, X., Zhang, Z., & Lee, C. (2025). Metaverse-Enabled Yoga Coach Avatar Using AI-Enhanced Multimodal Insole Sensing System. *Advanced Functional Materials.*

Wang, S., Zhou, G., Ma, Y., Hu, L., Chen, Z., Chen, Y., & Zhao, H. (2011). Wearable respiratory biofeedback system based on body sensor network. *Procedia Engineering, 15*, 3296–3300. DOI: 10.1016/j.proeng.2011.08.618

Wieczorek, A., Pintz, F., & Wagner, M. (2025). Physiological and psychological health effects of a mobile vr-based mindfulness breathing meditation with integrated biofeedback: A replication study. *Virtual Reality (Waltham Cross), 29*(4), 152. Advance online publication. DOI: 10.1007/s10055-025-01235-9

Woodyard, C. (2011). Exploring the therapeutic effects of yoga and its ability to increase quality of life. *International Journal of Yoga, 4*(2), 49–54. DOI: 10.4103/0973-6131.85485 PMID: 22022122

Yadav, M., Sharma, A., & Sharma, I. (2025). The impact of Pragya Yoga and Savita Dhyana on stress levels and sleep quality of women. *Dev Sanskriti Interdisciplinary International Journal, 26*, 01–06. https://doi.org/DOI: 10.36018/dsiij.26.376

Yadav, R., Chaudhary, R., Istwal, S., Kumar, S., Bohra, M., & Kumar, I. (2023). Development of an AI Enabled Yoga Posture (Aasans) Prediction System Using Deep Neural Network Model. *2023 International Conference on Sustainable Emerging Innovations in Engineering and Technology, ICSEIET 2023*. DOI: 10.1109/ICSEIET58677.2023.10303586

Yadav, S. K., Singh, A., Gupta, A., & Raheja, J. L. (2019). Real-time Yoga recognition using deep learning. *Neural Computing & Applications, 31*(12), 9349–9361. Advance online publication. DOI: 10.1007/s00521-019-04232-7

Yenishettil, S., Karajkhede, G., & Panat, L. (2024). Virtual Yoga Teacher with AI Model for Yoga Posture Correction for Good Health. *2024 ITU Kaleidoscope. Innovation and Digital Transformation for a Sustainable World, ITU K, 2024*, 1–8. Advance online publication. DOI: 10.23919/ITUK62727.2024.10772930

Yom-Tov, E., Feraru, G., Kozdoba, M., Mannor, S., Tennenholtz, M., & Hochberg, I. (2021). Encouraging physical activity in patients with diabetes: Intervention using a reinforcement learning system. *Journal of Medical Internet Research, 19*(10), e338. DOI: 10.2196/jmir.7994 PMID: 29017988

Yu, A., Lee, G., Liu, Y., Zhang, M., Jung, S. E., Park, J., Rhee, J., & Cho, K. (2025). Development and evaluation of an immersive metaverse-based meditation system for psychological well-being using llm-driven scenario generation. *Systems*, *13*(9), 798–798. DOI: 10.3390/systems13090798

Zakaria, T. M., Langi, A. Z. R., Nazaruddin, M. S., & Anshori, I. (2025). Artificial Intelligence (AI) in Neurofeedback Therapy Using Electroencephalography (EEG), Heart Rate Variability (HRV), and Galvanic Skin Response (GSR): A Review. *IEEE Access : Practical Innovations, Open Solutions*, *13*, 133078–133112. DOI: 10.1109/ACCESS.2025.3582805

Zhang, J., Li, W., Ogunbona, P., Wang, P., & Tang, C. (2020). RGB-D-based action recognition datasets: A survey. *Pattern Recognition*, *60*, 86–105. DOI: 10.1016/j.patcog.2016.05.019

Zhu, X., Li, X., & Liu, S. (2024). Predicting mental health from physiological signals: A review of machine learning approaches using wearable data. *PLOS Digital Health*, *3*(1), e0000312.

About the Contributors

Ayoub Khan (Senior member IEEE) received his Ph. D (Electrical Engg.) from Jamia Millia Islamia, New Delhi, India, and Master of Technology (Computer Science and Engineering) from Guru Gobind Singh Indraprastha, New Delhi, India. Presently, he is working as Deputy Director, Smart Cyber-Physical System (CPS) Research Centre, University of Bisha, Saudi Arabia with interests in Internet of Things, RFID, Wireless Sensors Networks, Ad Hoc Network, Smart Cities, Industrial IoT, and signal processing, NFC, Routing in Network-on-Chip, Real Time and Embedded Systems. He is a certified Chief Information Security Officer (CISO) and Certified Information Security Manager (CISM). He has more than 14 years of experience in his research and consultancy area.

Raghav Mehra is a Professor and Program Leader of AIML at Chandigarh University with over 21 years of academic and research experience. He has served as HOD, Dean of Academics, and Assistant Director in reputed AICTE and UGC-approved institutions, leading them to achieve ISO, NBA, and NAAC accreditations. He holds an MCA, M.Tech., Ph.D. in Computer Science (Genetics & AI), and an M.A. in Yog. His expertise spans AI, ML, IoT, Cloud Computing, Networking, and Software Engineering. Dr. Mehra has guided 17 Ph.D. scholars, published 50+ research papers, authored books, and filed 20+ patents in AI and wellness technologies. He has received multiple AICTE grants, delivered lectures internationally, and developed advanced labs and academic programs. A member of IEEE, ISTE, CSI, and IAENG, Dr. Mehra continues to contribute to education, research, and innovation at the intersection of technology and human well-being.

Kanaga Suba Raja is a Professor and Associate Dean at the School of Computing, SRM Institute of Science and Technology, Tiruchirappalli, with over 20 years of teaching and research experience in Computer Science and Engineering. He has supervised 13 Ph.D. scholars, published more than 120 international journal papers, including 23 in SCI/WoS-indexed journals, and authored 9 book chapters.

His research spans Artificial Intelligence, Data Science, Cloud Computing, Wireless Networks, and Healthcare Informatics. He has secured funded projects, including a 17 lakh grant for an AI-based smart parking system, and holds 2 granted and 5 published patents. A dedicated academic leader, Dr. Suba Raja has served as Head of Department at Easwari Engineering College and SRM IST, contributed to curriculum design, and organized numerous international conferences and faculty development programs. He is a member of IEEE, ACM, ISTE, IAENG, and other professional bodies. With over 1200 citations and an H-index of 18, Dr. Suba Raja continues to advance impactful research while mentoring future scholars and fostering global academic collaborations.

Pushkar Praveen ran Assistant Professor in the Department of Electronics and Communication Engineering at G.B. Pant Institute of Engineering and Technology, Pauri Garhwal, Uttarakhand, India. He received his Ph.D. in Electronics and Communication Engineering from Uttarakhand Technical University and M.Tech. in VLSI Design from CDAC Noida. He has over 13 years of academic and industry experience. His research interests include electronic device and circuit design, VLSI systems, embedded systems, Internet of Things (IoT). Dr. Praveen has published several research articles in reputed SCI/SCIE and Scopus- indexed journals and conferences. He has also contributed to multiple edited books and book chapters. He is actively involved in organizing faculty development programs, conferences, and research projects funded by national and international agencies. Dr. Praveen is a member of professional organizations including IEEE, IAENG, and ISTE.

Rijwan Khan is currently working as Professor and Dean Faculty of Computer Applications at Marwadi University, Rajkot, Gujrat. He also served as Dean Emerging Technologies and Training at ABES Institute of Technology, Ghaziabad. He completed his PhD in 2017 from Jamia Millia Islamia University, New Delhi, India. He has more than 20 years' experience of teaching. He served as Head of Department-CSE in ABESIT and also Dean Research in ABESIT. He is editor in chief of Journal of Engineering, Science and Mathematics (JESM). He is guest editor of more than 15 journals. He edited 10 books in Elsevier, IGI Global, CRC and Bentham Science. He published 12 SCI Indexed Journal Papers, 22 Scopus Indexed Journal Papers and 22 Conference papers and 20 book chapters. He was keynote speaker in an international conference in Muscat, Oman conducted by Ministry of Agriculture, Oman. He has H index 24 and I index 40 and number of citations are more than 2400. He is member of ACM, ISTE, IETE

***

Hannan Akhtar is a final-year undergraduate student in Electronics & Communication Engineering at G B Pant Institute of Engineering & Technology, Pauri, Uttarakhand, India. His areas of interest include embedded systems, digital electronics, microprocessors, microcontrollers and iot. He has worked on academic projects related to embedded systems and is keen to further explore research and innovation in this domain.

Garima Anand received her B.Tech degree in Information Technology from GGSCMT, PTU, Jalandhar in 2009, her Master of Engineering degree in Computer Science & Engineering from BBSBEC, Fatehgarh Sahib, PTU, Jalandhar in 2015 and is pursuing her Ph.D from Christ University, Bengaluru, India. She has an experience in academia & teaching for more than 15 years. She is currently employed with Christ University, Bengaluru as Assistant Professor. Her research interest is in Artificial Intelligence and Deep Learning

Anushka Banerjee is studying B.Tech. in Artificial Intelligence and Data Science at Ajeenkya DY Patil University. She had started solidifying her programming skills by completing certification courses on Data Structures in C, Tableau functions and Operating Systems along with doing few projects using Python, C, C++ and Web Page using HTML, CSS and Java Script. She had also attended an Arduino-Based Automation course at Dolphin Labs to enhance my software knowledge. There, she learned how to work with sensors, microcontrollers, and circuit design. She has also written multiple review papers on topics such as Geographic Information Systems, Swiss Bank vs. European Central Bank: Data Analysis. She is also researching and learning many topics such as AI in the Digital Era, Bibliometric Analysis, etc. Because of her interest in latest technologies, she participated in Global Hyperloop Competition hosted by IIT Madras representing the college as team Vac-Vectoor where she learnt many subtopics from the mentors.

Susanta Das is a seasoned educator with a proven record of teaching and mentoring diverse students, working at multiple institutions, and providing service to the various initiatives of organizations. He received his Ph.D. and M.A. degrees from Western Michigan University (WMU), USA, and M.Sc. degree from Banaras Hindu University (BHU), India all in Physics. He continued his research as a Marie-Curie post-doctoral fellow at Stockholm University, Stockholm, Sweden on beam diagnostics for the DESIREE (Double ElectroStatic Ion Ring ExpEriment) in the project DITANET (Diagnostic Techniques for particle Accelerators – a Marie-Curie initial training NETwork), at the Indian Institute of Science Education and Research-Kolkata, India on high-pressure physics as a Project Scientist-B, and at the University of Electro-Communications, Tokyo, Japan on ion-surface interactions as a

Post-doctoral fellow. Throughout his career, Dr. Das worked and collaborated with many researchers, Ph.D., master, and visiting students from different countries. He further visited many countries to discuss research and an international conference participant (UK, Italy, Germany, Greece, Belgium, Bulgaria, Romania, Brazil etc.). He worked at several institutions before assuming his current role at Ajeenkya D Y Patil University. He received the Marie-Curie post-doctoral fellowship in Sweden, Science Academies' Summer Research Fellowship in India, Gowen Frostic Doctoral Fellowship, Department Graduate Research and Creative Scholar Award by WMU, and Leo R. Parpart Doctoral Fellowship by Dept. of Physics, WMU, among many others, throughout his academic journey. He co-authored several research articles in WoS/Scopus indexed international journals, conference proceedings, and scholarly book chapters and co-edited several books published by renowned international publishing houses (IGI-Global, Springer Nature, Nova Science Publishers, Wiley, Scrivener-Wiley, Notion Press). At present, Dr. Das continues to delve into cutting-edge fields, with a keen interest in nanotechnology, UN SDGs, and data science. His multifaceted contributions, spanning teaching, research, and administrative leadership, showcase a dedicated professional who is instrumental in advancing the vision and mission of the institutions he serves.

Siddharth Gaur is a researcher and technology practitioner with interests in artificial intelligence, nutrition informatics, and digital wellbeing. His work explores the integration of AI-driven food analysis, mindful eating frameworks, and holistic health principles. He is currently engaged in the development of MERN-based systems and applied machine-learning solutions for public health and user-centered wellness applications.

Awesh Khati is a committed Ph.D. scholar in Physical Education Pedagogy at the prestigious Lakshmibai National Institute of Physical Education (LNIPE), Gwalior. With a strong academic background and a deep passion for advancing the field of physical education, he has authored several research papers and book chapters, including publications in Scopus-indexed journals. He is also the author of a published book on football, reflecting his blend of academic rigor and practical insight. Alongside his scholarly work, Mr. Khati is an accomplished football player, bringing valuable on-field experience to his research. His contributions demonstrate a dedication to promoting holistic physical development and enriching sports education, positioning him as a promising voice in the realm of physical education and sports science.

Kunj Bihari Meena is a faculty member and researcher in Computer Science and Engineering at Jaypee University and Engineering Technology Guna. Dr. Meena has published multiple papers in reputed international journals and conferences, including SCI and Scopus-indexed publications. He has received Best Paper Awards for his research contributions and serves as a reviewer for prestigious SCI/Scopus journals and conferences. His areas of research include image processing, digital image forensics, deep learning, and blockchain.

Richa Kapoor Mehra is working as an Associate Professor of Philosophy and Area chair of Social Sciences and Humanities (SSH) at O.P Jindal Global University, India, she has earned her PhD in Philosophy from Jawaharlal Nehru University, Delhi. While pursuing PhD, she was recipient of Junior Research Fellowship from prestigious Indian Council of Philosophical Research (ICPR). She has completed Masters and bachelor's in philosophy from Miranda House, University of Delhi. She was awarded with Miranda House award and Delhi University rankers prize for scoring highest marks in bachelor's program. She has also worked at Miranda House, University of Delhi, Amity University, Noida, B.M.L Munjal University and IIIT Kalyani. Recently she has designed a course on Critical Thinking and Analysis for undergraduate business students at O.P Jindal Business School. Dr. Mehra has launched the department of philosophy at Amity University, Noida and hence designed various philosophy course for undergraduate students. She has been awarded with the Excellent Academician Award, in an International Conference organized by University of Sri Jayewardenepura, Sri Lanka. She has presented several research

Rajesh Prasad is currently working as Professor in the Department of Computer Science and Engineering at Ajay Kumar Garg Engineering College, Ghaziabad, India. He received the M.Tech. degree in Software Engineering and the PhD degree in Computer Science and Engineering from the Motilal Nehru National Institute of Technology, Allahabad, India. He has more than 23 years of teaching experience in various universities and higher Institutions. He has published more than 70 research papers in various journals and conferences. He is a reviewer of various reputed journals. His research interests include data mining, artificial intelligence, data compression, algorithms, and bioinformatics

Shree Ram is a dedicated Computer Science engineering student with a strong focus on software development and intelligent systems. He has hands-on experience in building scalable applications using Java, Spring Boot, React, PostgreSQL, and modern cloud technologies. His academic interests include microservices architecture, AI-driven automation, and system optimization. Known for his analytical mindset and project leadership, he consistently applies practical problem-solving to real-world technical challenges. He aims to contribute meaningful innovations in large-scale software engineering.

Sandeep Kumar Singh is a faculty in the area of Information Systems and Analytics at Jindal Global Business School, O.P. Jindal Global University, Sonipat. Prior to joining Jindal Global Business School, he worked as an Assistant Professor at JKLU Jaipur for two years. He has earned his Ph.D. in computational physics from Antwerpen University, Belgium. His PhD work focused on mathematical modeling and simulation of two-dimensional materials. Post to his PhD, he worked as a research scientist in Sweden for four years in energy storage systems, bioelectronics. He also did MTech in industrial mathematics and scientific computing from IIT Madras, Chennai. His current research interests are to apply complex mathematical modeling in the business and financial world.

Somya Singh is a B. Tech. student in the Department of CSE, Ajay Kumar Garg Engineering College, Ghaziabad, India. Her research interest includes: Machine learning and Game design.

Mehak Srivastava is a B. Tech. student in the Department of CSE, Ajay Kumar Garg Engineering College, Ghaziabad, India. Her research interest includes: Algorithms and block chain.

Nithya T is working as Assistant Professor in Velalar College of Engineering and Technology

Vipin Tyagi is a distinguished academician, researcher and author, currently serving as Dean (Academic and Research) at Jaypee University of Engineering and Technology in Guna, Madhya Pradesh. With a rich background in Computer Science, his expertise spans across Image Processing, Cyber Forensics, and Speech Recognition. Prof. Tyagi has a prolific publication record, contributing significantly to his fields of interest. His scholarly work includes numerous journal articles, conference papers, and books. Some of his notable publications are in the areas of image forgery detection, image denoising, and content-based image retrieval. He has authored and edited several books and papers in the field of computing and data sciences, such as "Digital Image Forgery Detection: Techniques, Challenges and Applications", "Predictive Computing and Information Security" and "Content-Based Image Retrieval: Ideas, Influences, and Current Trends" published by Springer Singapore. His book "Understanding Digital Image Processing" using MATLAB, published by Taylor and Francis is highlighted by Mathworks at: https://in.mathworks.com/academia/books/understanding-digital-image-processing-tyagi

.html His scholarly work has earned him a respectable h-index and numerous citations in the academic community.

Agya Ram Verma is a dedicated academician, researcher, and educator in the field of Electronics and Communication Engineering. Currently serving as an Assistant Professor (Regular) in the Department of Electronics and Communication Engineering at Govind Ballabh Pant Engineering College, Pauri Garhwal, Uttarakhand, he has made significant contributions to teaching, research, and academic development. Dr. Verma completed his Ph.D. in January 2019 from GB Pant Engineering College, with a research focus on "Filter Design Using Evolutionary Technique for Biomedical Signal Application." His academic journey includes an M.Tech in Electronics and Communication Engineering from IIIT Jabalpur, where he secured 78% marks, and a B.Tech in Electronics and Instrumentation Engineering from Rohilkhand University with a CGPA of 7.66. He also achieved an All India Rank of 2191 in GATE 2010. With over a decade of teaching experience, Dr. Verma began his career as an Assistant Professor at Rajasthan Institute of Engineering and Technology, Jaipur, in 2013. He then joined Govind Ballabh Pant Engineering College as a contractual faculty member and was later appointed as a regular faculty member in 2019. Throughout his career, he has taught a wide range of subjects including Machine Learning, Analog Communication, VHDL, Python Programming, Signal Compression, Optimization Techniques, and Internet of Things (IoT). Dr. Verma's research interests lie in multirate signal processing, filter and filter bank design, biomedical signal processing, ECG signal analysis, and communication systems. He has published numerous research papers in reputed international journals such as Springer, Elsevier, and IEEE conferences. His work focuses on advanced signal processing techniques, optimization algorithms, and machine learning applications in healthcare systems. He has successfully completed and led several sponsored research projects funded by organizations like MHRD, AICTE, and MeitY. His ongoing projects include research in IoT with Artificial Intelligence and sustainable water resource management for Himalayan communities. Dr. Verma is also an innovator with two granted international patents in the field of biomedical signal processing and neuromuscular disorder detection. In addition to research, he has contributed to academia through authorship of multiple books on machine learning, Python programming, and smart infrastructure systems, published by reputed international publishers. An active academic contributor, Dr. Verma serves as a reviewer for several SCI and Scopus-indexed journals and has been recognized with awards such as the Best Paper Award at an international conference (CCSN 2023). He has also received fellowships like the MHRD scholarship during his M.Tech and the Summer Faculty Research Fellowship from IIT Delhi. Beyond research and teaching, Dr. Verma has guided numerous M.Tech and B.Tech students in their dissertations and projects, particularly in areas like ECG signal processing, image enhancement, and machine learning applications. He has also organized and coordinated multiple workshops, faculty development programs, and international conferences. Dr. Verma actively contributes to institutional development through various administrative roles, including M.Tech Coordinator, Lab In-charge, Hostel Warden, and Deputy Proctor. His commitment to education, research, and innovation continues to inspire students and contribute to advancements in engineering and technology.

Muskan Wahi is a B. Tech. student in the Department of CSE, Ajay Kumar Garg Engineering College, Ghaziabad, India. Her research interest includes: Machine learning and AI.

Index

N

P

R

S

T

W

Y

www.ingramcontent.com/pod-product-compliance
Lightning Source LLC
LaVergne TN
LVHW081525300926
849161LV00006B/1305